THE COMPUTERIZATION OF BEHAVIORAL HEALTHCARE

The Jossey-Bass Managed Behavioral Healthcare Library
Michael A. Freeman, General Editor

NOW AVAILABLE

Marketing for Therapists: A Handbook for Success in Managed Care
Jeri Davis, Editor

The Computerization of Behavioral Healthcare:
How to Enhance Clinical Practice, Management, and Communications
Tom Trabin, Editor

Behavioral Risk Management: How to Avoid
Preventable Losses from People Problems at Work
Rudy M. Yandrick

The Complete Capitation Handbook
Gayle L. Zieman, Editor

Inside Outcomes: The National Review of Behavioral Healthcare Outcomes
Tom Trabin, Michael A. Freeman, and Michael Pallak

Managed Behavioral Healthcare: History, Models,
Strategic Challenges, and Future Course
Tom Trabin and Michael A. Freeman

Behavioral Group Practice Performance Characteristics:
The Council of Group Practices Benchmarking Study
Allen Daniels, Teresa Kramer, and Nalini Mahesh

How to Respond to Managed Behavioral Healthcare:
A Workbook Guide for Your Organization
Barbara Mauer, Dale Jarvis, Richard Mockler, and Tom Trabin

FORTHCOMING

Forming and Managing a Group Practice
Stuart J. Ghertner and Ronald B. Hersch, Editors

Legal and Ethical Challenges in Managed Behavioral Healthcare
John Petrila, Editor

THE COMPUTERIZATION OF BEHAVIORAL HEALTHCARE

How to Enhance Clinical Practice, Management, and Communications

A VOLUME IN THE JOSSEY-BASS
MANAGED BEHAVIORAL HEALTHCARE LIBRARY

Tom Trabin, EDITOR

Foreword by Michael A. Freeman,
GENERAL EDITOR

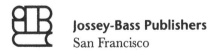

Jossey-Bass Publishers
San Francisco

A volume in the Jossey-Bass Managed Behavioral Healthcare Library.

Copyright © 1996 by Jossey-Bass Inc., Publishers, and CentraLink, 1110 Mar West, Suite E, Tiburon, CA 94920 (415/435-9821), in cooperation with the Institute for Behavioral Healthcare, 4370 Alpine Road, Suite 108, Portola Valley, CA 94028 (415/851-8411).

Substantial discounts on bulk quantities of Jossey-Bass books are available to corporations, professional associations, and other organizations. For details and discount information, contact the special sales department at Jossey-Bass Inc., Publishers (415) 433–1740; Fax (800) 605–2665.

For sales outside the United States, please contact your local Simon & Schuster International office.

Library of Congress Cataloging-in-Publication Data

The computerization of behavioral healthcare: how to enhance clinical
  practice, management, and communications/Tom Trabin, editor;
  foreword by Michael A. Freeman.
      p.   cm.—(A volume in the Jossey-Bass managed behavioral
  healthcare library)
    Includes bibliographical references and index.
    ISBN 0-7879-0221-7 (alk. paper)
    1. Psychiatry—Data processing.   2. Mental health services—Data
  processing.   I. Trabin, Tom.   II. Freeman, Michael A.   III. Series:
  Jossey-Bass managed behavioral healthcare library.
  RC455.2.D38C67   1996
  616.89'00285—dc20

95-26784
CIP

FIRST EDITION
PB Printing 10 9 8 7 6 5 4 3 2 1

CONTENTS

Foreword   ix

Michael A. Freeman

Introduction   xiii

Tom Trabin

PART ONE: CLINICAL PRACTICE

1   How Information Technologies Are
    Transforming Behavioral Healthcare   3

Marion J. Ball, Judith V. Douglas

2   Clinical Decision Support Systems   11

Wallace J. Gingerich, Anthony Broskowski

3   The Use of Computers in Therapy   39

Roger L. Gould

4   Clinical Assessment and Outcomes Measurement   63

Murray P. Naditch, Kevin L. Moreland

PART TWO: MANAGEMENT

5   Easing the Transition from Paper
    to Computer-Based Systems 87

    Larry D. Rosen, Michelle M. Weil

6   Computerization in Group Practices 108

    Peter S. Currie

7   Computerization in County and
    Community Mental Health Centers 124

    Tuan D. Nguyen, Gary Olsen

8   Computerization in Hospital-Based Delivery Systems 151

    Warner V. Slack, Charles Safran, Howard L. Bleich

9   Computerization in Managed
    Behavioral Healthcare Companies 172

    William R. Maloney, Eugene D. Hill III

PART THREE: COMMUNICATIONS

10 The Need to Know Versus the Right to Privacy 191

    Robert Gellman, Kathleen A. Frawley

11 The Rapid Growth of Electronic Communication 213

    Michael W. Hurst, William A. Roiter

12 How to Use the Internet and Electronic Bulletin Boards 228

    Dick Schoech, Katherine Kelley Smith

13 The Past, Present, and Future of Data Standards 254

    Ronald W. Manderscheid, Marilyn J. Henderson

Epilogue 270

    Tom Trabin

About the Authors 272

Index 282

FOREWORD

Behavioral healthcare has changed. The old and familiar professional landscape now seems disorienting and altered. The familiar landmarks that were well known to mental health administrators, clinicians, insurance executives, EAP directors, and academic researchers are fading off the map. Vanishing or gone are the employers who didn't pay attention to healthcare costs, the insurance plans that would reimburse on a fee-for-service basis, the hospitals with beds filled by patients with coverage encouraging long lengths of stay, the solo clinicians with full practices of affluent patients seeking long-term insight-oriented therapy, and the community mental health centers that worked in a system of their own.

The scenery of today is different. Health maintenance organizations and managed behavioral health plans have replaced the insurance companies. Employers and purchasing cooperatives are bypassing even these new organizations and purchasing directly from providers. Clinicians are forming group practices. Groups are affiliating with facilities. Facilities are forming integrated delivery systems. Integrated delivery systems are building organized systems of care that include HMOs, care management, and sophisticated management information systems. These information systems are linking payers, managers, and providers into coordinated and comprehensive systems with new levels of accountability. The boundaries of the public sector are eroding, and the distinction between public and private has become more difficult to perceive.

Methods

How can we operationalize the new paradigms, the new models and systems of care needed to make the promise of managed care come true? New methods of benefit administration and health services delivery will be required to implement this vision within realistic financial limits.

At the broadest level, these methods include the core technologies used to manage benefits, care, and the health status of individuals and defined populations. At the level of frontline operations, these methods include continuous quality improvement, process reengineering, outcomes management, public-private integration, computerization, and delivery system reconfiguration in the context of capitation financing. These are the skill sets that the Managed Behavioral Healthcare Library helps you build through an ongoing series of pragmatic professional publications.

New methods of direct clinical care are also required. Instead of treating episodes of illness, disease-state management methods will allow clinicians in future managed and integrated behavioral healthcare systems to reduce morbidity and mortality for individuals and for groups. The Managed Behavioral Healthcare Library also provides frontline clinicians and delivery system managers with the skills that enable our healthcare systems to truly provide scientifically validated bio-psycho-social treatments of choice in behavioral healthcare.

Adjusting to this "brave new world" is challenging enough, and many mental health professionals are tempted to give up and opt out now. But for most of us the challenge is worth facing. While this period is fraught with difficulty and risk, there are a number of opportunities. Whenever a paradigm shifts, those having a stake in the previous paradigm risk losing their place in the one that emerges. In a nutshell, the Managed Behavioral Healthcare Library will help you identify and confront the challenges you will face as the prevailing healthcare paradigms change. Moreover, the volumes in this series will provide you with pragmatic strategies and solutions you can call upon to sustain your importance in the healthcare systems of the future.

In spite of the upheavals transforming the behavioral healthcare enterprise, many basic goals remain the same. In fact, managed behavioral healthcare has come about largely because our previous way of doing things failed to solve fundamental problems related to the cost, quality, access, and outcomes of care. The promise of "managed behavioral healthcare"—whatever this concept may eventually come to mean—holds out the hope of affordable, appropriate, and effective mental health and addiction treatment services for all. The various initiatives and efforts that are under way to reach this new plateau will result in a vast array of professional opportunities for the behavioral healthcare specialists whose talents are required to make this promise come true.

By reading the books and reports in the Managed Behavioral Healthcare Library, you will learn how to respond to the perils and possibilities presented by the shift to managed behavioral healthcare. The authors of this book and other volumes in this series recognize the need for direct and pragmatic solutions to the challenges posed by the new landscape that is becoming the home for our efforts.

To help readers obtain the resources and solutions required, each chapter of each publication is written by an outstanding expert who can communicate in a pragmatic style to help you make a difference. In this way, the Managed Behavioral Healthcare Library provides resources to help readers meet each of the key challenges posed by the new landscape in behavioral healthcare. This volume and the others planned for the series help you improve your effectiveness at pricing, financing, and delivering high-quality, cost-effective care. Future volumes will provide straightforward solutions to the ethical challenges of managed behavioral healthcare and offer advice about practice management and marketing during a period of industry consolidation.

You can look forward to still other books and reports about developing and managing a group practice, creating workplace-based behavioral healthcare programs, measuring outcomes, computerizing delivery systems, and other ways of "benchmarking" and comparing your own organization or practice with others that face similar challenges.

Since the landscape of behavioral healthcare is in flux, professionals in the field need to be aware of alternative future scenarios that might emerge and develop the skill sets for success within each one. For behavioral healthcare leaders, it is critical to have the vision to select the best options that accord with shared values and the skills to put these possibilities into practice. For this reason, the themes of vision, action, and results are incorporated into the volumes you read in the Managed Behavioral Healthcare Library.

Vision

In the context of the current debate and upheavals in healthcare, we have seen broad agreement regarding the importance of behavioral health security for all Americans, at an affordable price. The Managed Behavioral Healthcare Library offers publications that show how universal coverage for affordable, appropriate, accessible, and effective mental health and addiction treatment benefits and services can be achieved.

Action and Results

Knowing that we are in a period of change, and even having the desire to make the changes that are needed, makes little difference without actions based on methods that can produce results. Since you and the readers of this library take action and produce results through day-in, day-out application of your professional expertise, the Managed Behavioral Healthcare Library is action-oriented to provide the greatest possible benefit to you and your colleagues.

◆ ◆ ◆

Cost-effective use of computers and networked, interactive information technologies is a new concern for most behavioral healthcare professionals. As the revolutionary impact of the information age continues to be felt, many behavioral healthcare specialists will suffer from the same "computer phobia" or aversion that has been experienced by midcareer professionals in other sectors of the economy. Resistance to computerization must be overcome if behavioral healthcare providers, health plan managers, EAPs, and others are to sustain and improve their effectiveness within the next three to five years. Given the rapid computerization of the entire healthcare industry, simply staying in business will be contingent on effective use of clinical and management information systems and networked, interactive information technologies. *The Computerization of Behavioral Healthcare* will help you meet this objective and more, through friendly and accessible—but also sophisticated—explanations of computer applications across the breadth of the behavioral healthcare enterprise.

An outstanding group of authors has pooled its expertise to inform you about the ways in which computerization and networked, interactive information technologies are being used for clinical practice enhancement, operations management, and communications in the behavioral healthcare field. Furthermore, critical, related issues—such as making the transition from paper to electronic files, the need to know versus the right to privacy, and emerging data standards—are addressed within this volume.

We hope this book, along with the other volumes in the Managed Behavioral Healthcare Library, provides the information and inspiration essential for all professionals who want to understand the challenges and opportunities available today.

January 1996

Michael A. Freeman, M.D.
Tiburon, California

INTRODUCTION

Tom Trabin

We live in the midst of a technological revolution that is having an impact on every aspect of our lives. Computers and networked, interactive information services and systems are at the center of this revolution, transforming every major industry. Behavioral healthcare lags behind but has not escaped this trend, despite the resistance of many providers. The entire field, including service providers, delivery system managers, and health plan executives, faces a rising tide of choices on hardware, software, and integrated information services and systems. No longer are these decisions in the distant province of information system executives or computer consultants to large organizations. Instead, clinicians in solo practice and the clinical and administrative staff of even the smallest group practices now select and use computers and computer software.

The pace of work and many other aspects of our lives have accelerated, for better and for worse. Technologies that transformed how we travel and how we transmit information have made the world seem smaller. We become accustomed to continuing developments in these directions and adjust our expectations accordingly. Behavioral healthcare is not immune to these expectations. We expect technology to make data entry easier, data processing faster, and the communication of complex and voluminous information much more feasible and effective.

The Emerging Context

A man in a cartoon states that he doesn't mind "smart" houses, but he is becoming irritated with his toaster calling him an idiot.

This cartoon reflects a changing reality that touches the behavioral healthcare field. A virtual world is emerging through computers that is truly amazing. In some group practices, patients can schedule appointments through the Internet. Clinicians are beginning to enter and transmit data electronically without completing paper forms. Electronic bulletin boards provide disorder-specific support groups online. Consumers of healthcare services can use self-help software to address some problems, thus obviating even the need for an office visit. Virtual reality programs are in use to treat fear of heights. Tremendously exciting possibilities are opening up for the use of technology to enhance patient care.

We are, as an industry, under intense pressure to contain costs and to measure and improve clinical outcomes. These pressures, in combination with competitive market forces, are the main drivers of adoption of new technology. In particular, the substantial cost savings that can be achieved through simplifying administrative processes requires computerized, highly efficient information systems. This is the most fundamental computerization project for most if not all behavioral healthcare organizations.

Increasingly, payers are beginning to value providers who can use outcome data to demonstrate the quality of their services. To respond adequately to this relatively new payer trend, providers must computerize their clinical assessments to facilitate rapid data entry, analysis, and reporting. Similarly, as payers begin to require consistent provider adherence to practice guidelines, providers will need easy access to decision support software and online clinical information services. In addition, market pressures demanding much faster communication between providers, payers, and purchasers have stimulated the application of many methods of electronic data interchange developed relatively recently for some other industries.

Decision makers in behavioral healthcare organizations of any size, from small group practices to large managed care companies, face some of their most daunting and expensive decisions in the purchase and development of their organization's information systems. The stakes are high. The basic system they select and the additional software and hardware they install have profound impacts on the efficiency and effectiveness of their organization's operations, on their staff morale and job satisfaction, on their organization's image in the marketplace, and on the patients and providers with whom they interact. Yet technological innovations in the computer industry and changing information requirements in the marketplace are occurring at such a dizzying pace that costly mistakes in buying antiquated "legacy" systems and inadequately designed data base systems are all too easy to make. It is critical for behavioral healthcare professionals to obtain up-to-date information on implementing these new technologies in our industry.

The decision to buy a new computer or computer information system is only the beginning of a series of challenges. Any organization that shifts from paper- to computer-based information systems experiences fundamental changes in their entire work flow process. These changes affect how tasks are prioritized and carried out, and which details in the work flow process get the most attention. Computerization is also likely to impact how staff relate to each other and to their customers, including patients. Many human issues are raised regarding data privacy and other ethical concerns, morale and job satisfaction, communication, the quality of patient care, and the like.

Structure of the Book: An Overview

This book addresses how the rapid restructuring of the behavioral healthcare industry is reflected in and made possible by dramatic innovations in computerized information services and systems throughout every segment of the field. The authors describe advances in different types of software and online services, and they examine the profound impact that these new technologies have upon patients, clinicians, and behavioral healthcare organizations. They also describe what organizations are doing to accommodate these changes, examine what will be required of these organizations in the near future, and give practical advice on how to get there.

The book is designed to address a broad range of the major challenges facing the behavioral healthcare industry. As the book's subtitle implies, the book is divided into sections according to the three major functions that computers in behavioral healthcare are designed to support: clinical practice, management, and communications. Part One, the clinical section, examines developments in the computerization of patient records and clinical decision support. The management section, Part Two, describes how to manage the transition from paper to computers and how computerization is impacting specific types of organizations and industry segments. As for communications, Part Three introduces policy guidelines for protecting the privacy of patient data and new methods and services available for electronic communication of information; this part also looks at how emerging standardization initiatives will influence the kind of information we choose or are required to communicate to others.

These chapters combine practical explanations and suggestions with discussions of policy implications. Most chapters begin with historical developments pertaining to the chapter topic, provide an overview of current developments and trends with specific examples, examine the major challenges, and suggest future directions. No matter what the topic, each chapter includes an examination of implications for patients, clinicians, and/or various types of organizations within the behavioral healthcare industry.

Clinical Practice

Part One of this book focuses on the direct impact of computerization on clinical practice and will be of great interest to a wide range of readers. It begins with a visionary chapter by Marion Ball, past president of the International Medical Informatics Association, on how fully computerized, networked, and interactive information systems will likely impact the management and delivery of care within the behavioral healthcare industry. She writes with a highly informed perspective on current developments in informatics throughout the world, as well as from professional experience as the chief information officer of a large organization.

Chapter Two provides an excellent introduction to various types of computer-assisted decision support, with particular focus on aspects of treatment planning. Wally Gingerich and Tony Broskowski, both widely published experts with many years of experience, begin with a historical overview of clinical decision support tools and then provide a framework for the reader to distinguish between different types of tools. They offer examples of current tools in use for triage, treatment planning, and case management, followed by their vision of how these and future tools are likely to transform different segments of the behavioral healthcare industry.

The next two chapters in Part One examine other ways in which computers are used to assist clinical decision making. Roger Gould gives an overview of computer-assisted therapy programs: how they work, what advantages they offer, what limitations they contain, and why attitudinal resistance to their adoption prevails within the professional community. The author is a clinician and also the inventor of a computer-assisted therapy program. In the last chapter of this part, Murray Naditch and Kevin Moreland examine the history of assessment and outcome measurement efforts, especially with the aid of computerization, and provide examples from among the most current efforts to computerize these processes. Both authors have been eminent pioneers in this area for many years, and they present readers with a compelling vision of how new technologies can open up tremendous advances in decision support for enhanced quality of patient care.

Management

In Part Two, we begin with Chapter Five, which addresses a vital challenge: how can staff with widely differing attitudes toward computers be trained effectively and efficiently to use a new system? All readers, including those not technically oriented, will easily understand and appreciate this chapter. Its authors, Michelle Weil and Larry Rosen, provide an excellent analysis of various human obstacles to computerization within behavioral healthcare organizations, and how customized training programs can be set up to assist people with different types of computer fears. Weil and Rosen have conducted extensive research for over ten years and across fourteen countries, the findings from which have been disseminated via many publications, radio, and television.

The next four chapters in Part Two address computerization issues as they pertain to specific types of behavioral healthcare organizations. Peter Currie, a group practice administrator who has developed a computerized patient record, writes about the computer needs and challenges for group practices at different stages of development. Tuan Nguyen and Gary Olsen, both information systems (IS) executives for county and community mental health centers, describe the main financial, management, and clinical issues facing their types of organizations throughout the country, and how these issues impact computer information system requirements. Warner Slack, a world-renowned expert in many areas of medical informatics, and his colleagues Charles Safran and Howard Bleich describe the lengthy, complex, but highly successful process of computerization within a hospital system, and what the essential ingredients are for success. William Maloney and Eugene Hill, both experienced executives in treatment delivery and managed care organizations, provide an excellent historical summary of computer information system developments within the insurance and hospital industries; they review how those systems' elements are gradually being combined within evolving managed care and integrated delivery system organizations.

Communications

To begin Part Three, Chapter Ten examines the most controversial issues in computerization: the individual right to privacy versus the public need to know. Robert Gellman and Kathleen Frawley examine recent policy initiatives that attempt to set protection standards for patient confidentiality and data privacy within computerized information systems. The authors have contributed substantially to recent initiatives in Congress, the American Health Information Management Association, and other healthcare organizations.

Chapters Eleven and Twelve focus on very recent developments in our industry which will have profound implications for the future. The first chapter, on the rapid growth of electronic communication, reviews industrywide developments intended to replace telephonic and postal communications with direct computer-assisted electronic interchange of data. The authors, Michael Hurst and William Roiter, are former clinical and managed care executives who helped invent new methods for electronic data interchange; they draw upon their industry knowledge to describe how electronic approaches are revolutionizing how professionals communicate with each other across organizations. Chapter Twelve, on the Internet and electronic bulletin boards, describes how behavioral health professionals and consumers can access services of interest to them; the chapter lists many of these services and gives examples of how they are being used. The authors, Dick Schoech and Katherine Kelley Smith, are both experts with extensive experience in this area; Schoech began the first electronic bulletin board service for human service professionals many years ago.

The last chapter examines the history of efforts in standardization development, what the major ongoing efforts are, and how they can be expected to impact the entire industry and field. The authors, Ron Manderscheid and Marilyn Henderson, are widely respected, Manderscheid notably for his leadership role in supporting and helping to coordinate many of these initiatives in both the public and the private sectors through his work with the U.S. Department of Health and Human Service's Center for Mental Health Services.

Begin Your Adventure

As you may note from an overview of the chapters, this book provides you with a great adventure. It chronicles an important historical juncture in the field of behavioral healthcare. Computerization is changing how we work, how we communicate, how we build accountability for containing costs and improving quality effectively, and how we achieve our mission of improving the welfare and well-being of our patients.

You will find that the authors give an excellent portrayal of the incredibly wide range of developments in behavioral healthcare computing. They are eminent in their respective fields and acutely aware of the leading developments and trends. For this reason, and despite the speed with which computer innovations keep arriving, the book you are about to read will provide you with information that will be extremely useful for many years to come. Enjoy your adventure.

Acknowledgments

Several friends and colleagues provided encouragement and inspiration. I am especially grateful to Michael Freeman, Gerry Piaget, and Joan Piaget, without whom this book would not have been possible. They envisioned the importance of computerization for the behavioral healthcare industry years ago and provided me with the resources and inspiration to undertake many rewarding projects that led eventually to this book. I also would like to thank Malcolm Harriman, Gene Hill, and Saul Feldman, each of whom encouraged me to undertake this book at its inception. Once I was under way, Alan Rinzler from Jossey-Bass was a wonderful editor with whom I worked; his enthusiastic support and skillful collaboration added considerably to the quality of the book and to my experience in putting it together.

The chapter authors are extremely bright and dedicated individuals who are eminent experts in their respective fields. As such, they are also busy professionals. I am grateful to them for giving me the honor of working with them and for taking time to share their knowledge with others through the medium of this unique book. I hope you, the reader, find their writing as captivating and informative as I did.

The role of editor provides at least as many administrative challenges as literary ones. Thankfully, I had some assistance with those matters. I appreciate the help provided to me by Majella Uzon and Adam Richmond, with whom I work closely at CentraLink, and Katie Levine at Jossey-Bass.

Last and most especially, I would like to acknowledge my wife, Nancy, for her patient understanding throughout the editorial process. The book was designed, organized, and edited by taking time away from our weekends and evenings. I thank her for her loving support throughout the process.

To my wife, Nancy,
doctor of oriental medicine,
who builds bridges between traditional Eastern and
Western medicine, and uses practice management
software to computerize her clinical practice

PART ONE

CLINICAL PRACTICE

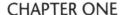

HOW INFORMATION TECHNOLOGIES ARE TRANSFORMING BEHAVIORAL HEALTHCARE

Marion J. Ball and Judith V. Douglas

Information technology holds great promise for behavioral healthcare. Still largely unautomated, behavioral healthcare can benefit from the kinds of technological advances that have been made in medical and surgical care, where computer applications have been further developed, and also from recent work with health information networks (HINs). Behavioral healthcare is in the enviable position of having had much of its groundwork done by other areas within healthcare, from whose successes it can benefit while avoiding their failures.

The New Information Technology Environment

The entire field of healthcare is now being transformed by information technology. The Institute of Medicine within the National Academy of Sciences set the stage for change by forming its Committee to Improve the Patient Record in 1990. It has drawn upon the work of many, including pioneers such as Larry Weed, who saw the need more than twenty years ago to use computers to manage information and extend the capabilities of the human mind.

The Computer-Based Patient Record

The Committee to Improve the Patient Record envisioned the computer-based patient record (CPR) as both an artifact and an agent of change. This vision of the CPR remains valid today. The CPR Institute was formed soon after in response to the committee's report. Using available technologies, it and other organizations are striving to implement the vision by supporting creation of a new and improved CPR which can replace traditional paper-based patient records.

Since 1990 the environment nurturing the CPR concept has changed remarkably. With the director of the National Library of Medicine serving as the first director of the Office for High Performance Computing and Communications (HPCC), healthcare became an active player within the high-stakes world of advanced technology. The Internet has mushroomed in size and spread into all sectors of American life. In healthcare, picture archiving and communications systems (PACS) and computerized imaging have underscored the need for high-speed data networks. Specialized research data bases have grown in number, scope, and complexity, as have remote access to the biomedical literature. The early 1990s saw the beginnings of tremendous developments in electronic communication of clinical applications, and electronic billing became an increasingly routine function.

Today, the CPR is viewed as one element within this rich and complex information environment. Organizations and working groups are addressing issues critical to the CPR. Among these are standards and security, both essential to the networks that comprise the health information infrastructure, or "infostructure." These issues are also being addressed as they apply to the health professional's workstation, which serves as an "enabler" for the CPR, giving users necessary capabilities. In August 1994, an international working conference on hospital information systems (HIS) extended its view beyond hospital boundaries and placed the CPR within the context of health information systems broadly.

As it comes to embody the longitudinal concept of "womb to tomb," the CPR will play a critical role in wellness and preventive care, providing clinicians with readily accessible records and better real-time decision support, and assisting patients in the search for individualized care. Within managed care settings, the CPR will streamline the delivery of care, as patients move among providers to obtain the levels and types of services they need. For healthcare managers, policy makers, and researchers, the CPR will offer better data bases. For the increasingly mobile patient population, it will create the transferable records that are essential to continuing good care.

Creating a Healthcare Network

Chief information officers and other healthcare managers and planners are working to take strategic advantage of this new information technology environment. But the creation of a healthcare information infrastructure is no trivial task. *The challenge is to make getting on the network worthwhile for healthcare practitioners.* Once the linkages are up and working, features and capabilities can be added. For the network to succeed, the linkages have to be designed with full attention to standards and with future developments planned for in the aggregate. Advances in this area can be concurrent with development of the CPR.

To create truly multidisciplinary, community-based healthcare, information networks must link all healthcare providers, wherever they may practice and deliver their services. Linking so many groups presents very real technical problems, which must have technical solutions. More importantly, it involves political and organizational issues, and they will be infinitely more troublesome. We have to go beyond the model set by the propriety networks maintained by an insurer or hospital. Ultimately, all health professionals need to be linked, including physical therapists, labs, nurse-run clinics, dental offices . . . in short, the full array of healthcare providers.

Because managed care involves different providers who in turn may be linked contractually with multiple managed care entities, networking on a community or regional level is essential to the health infostructure. The extent and pervasiveness of networking we are now beginning to see will ultimately support advances in telemedicine, among them electronic house calls and teleconsults using visual transmissions along with clinical data. Specialty areas have tested teleconsults, using nurse practitioners, visiting nurses, and home health aides with physicians on call. Corporations and health centers have piloted programs providing healthcare consumers with health information upon request via fax and/or computer. We will definitely see more telehealth applications supporting primary care through access to medical specialties and to secondary- and tertiary-level care.

Other Initiatives

The benefits of informatics do not come cheaply. They require considerable investment in planning, infrastructure, equipment, applications, and organizational development. Fortunately, behavioral healthcare can piggyback on work being done elsewhere.

Although information technologies are being used to address the problems of data security, the protection of patient confidentiality remains a more complex policy issue. Long of concern to physicians, the success of the computer-based patient record will ultimately depend upon resolution of this issue. Patient confidentiality is an exponentially more sensitive issue within behavioral healthcare, given cultural attitudes and concerns regarding employers having access to records. To further complicate matters, questions have recently arisen regarding emerging data repositories for the health insurance industry. We need to bring this issue into the larger context of privacy in the information age. We may also need to consider nationwide standards through federal legislation.

The eventual realization of CPRs and an effective health infostructure depends on the willingness of providers to enter complete and accurate data. This will require user-friendly interfaces, which at this point are still too complicated and too technically oriented. Information handling in healthcare presents a profound and multidimensional challenge which is not purely technical in nature. The cognitive sciences, which have not been highly involved in technology, are becoming increasingly active in the development of truly user-friendly interfaces. Once we understand information-seeking behaviors, we can make the computer "know" the user—rather than make the user "learn" the computer. Workstation development is dependent upon easy-to-use, "intuitive" interfaces, which will improve health professionals' access to the network and use of its resources as well as the workstation's capabilities. Together, the workstation and the network constitute the enabling technologies which must underlie the computer-based patient record.

Standards are critical to the information infrastructure. Technical complexities are being addressed by a host of organizations. In healthcare, arriving at standards is phenomenally complex. Even if we had the technologies for a computer-based patient record today, the existence of diverse, even conflicting, terminologies for diagnosis, treatment, and outcomes would make the record meaningless. This is much more difficult to address than technical standards.

As networks develop, the CPR will provide the data required for monitoring and managing care. Eventually we will have data repositories which we can use to evaluate practice patterns and care delivery. Access to large datasets will eliminate some of the uncertainties associated with limited data. Yet the reliability and validity of our analyses will be determined by our successes (or failures) in developing standard nomenclature and understanding the representation of knowledge in healthcare. We cannot measure "outcomes" without knowing "inputs," and inputs vary widely now. This problem will be even greater in the behavioral healthcare field than in biomedicine, since behavioral healthcare involves practitioners from quite different professional backgrounds.

Over the past several years, amid talk of "reengineering" and "reforming" healthcare, the emphasis has been on the financial bottom line—not on the mission and content of healthcare itself. The failure of large-scale federal reform has led us to look at the whole picture, at healthcare across the community, as provided by different practitioners and in different settings. Healthcare, and especially behavioral healthcare, should look beyond the mechanistic reengineering model to the more organic and humanistic organizational development model. We need to examine the premises behind the delivery system we have now. We need to determine if indeed we can avert some of the costs associated with illness care by providing behavioral healthcare services. We may well find direction from our European counterparts, who, unlike us, have long focused on primary care and whose family doctors know their patients as individuals.

Finally, we need to involve individuals in their own healthcare. With the growth of the Internet, we are seeing more and more networking opportunities for individuals concerned about their own health. Multimedia are being used to help patients make informed choices about treatment options as well as to guide them through their personal health histories.

Information Technology in Managed Behavioral Healthcare

Developed in the 1980s as a separate "carve-out" from regular healthcare insurance, managed behavioral healthcare has special needs for information technology. These needs are significant: today over one hundred million Americans receive their coverage for mental health and substance abuse through a managed behavioral healthcare vendor. Like the rest of the managed care sector, the behavioral carve-out industry has realized both the cost savings and the cost shifting made possible by benefit plan design and has made significant headway in controlling long-term costs through the management of care.

Methods for managing care are extensive, ranging from standardized pretreatment assessment and treatment planning to practice pattern analysis and provider profiling. These methods and others not mentioned here are all information-dependent. While this alone would make information technology critical to the industry, it is compounded by the provider network model prevalent in behavioral healthcare. The contracted network of independent providers most common today requires the linkages which communications technologies can provide. Certain product lines offered by the managed behavioral carve-out industry, such as telephonic utilization review and provider referral, further involve information technology. This applies to organizations of all sizes and levels of complexity, from large managed care companies to relatively small group practices without walls.

While other areas of healthcare are focusing on health information networking—to support multiple hospital systems, link satellite clinics and physician offices with hospitals, and create community health information networks—managed behavioral healthcare is targeting provider network management. This well-defined purpose increases the probability of success; yet provider network management includes a wide range of functions and potential applications specific to behavioral healthcare. Additional opportunities exist, but most likely they will be explored in a second informatics initiative, after provider network management efforts have achieved their goals.

Provider Network Management: Functions and Applications

Although practice guidelines are now being developed in managed healthcare, the behavioral carve-out industry has not given them a high priority and tends to regard them as somewhat controversial. It is most definitely easier to document removal of an appendix than removal of anxiety, and also easier to evaluate the outcome of the procedure. But given the need for accountability, no matter how demanding it is, guideline development will become increasingly important in behavioral healthcare. Here, as in general healthcare, outcomes research requires substantive definition, proven methodologies, and a robust data base for analysis before it can deliver upon its promise. Technical networking provides the infrastructure that makes the data repository possible. It is up to provider network management to utilize those capabilities and to leverage them into a strategic advantage. Within provider network management, case managers play a critical role; the more support provided to them on the screen, the more effective they can be in a number of areas.

Fortunately, health informatics is beginning to draw upon the cognitive sciences for determining optimal design of the human/machine interface required by the computer-based patient record and its enabling technology, the professional workstation. Computerizing existing paper forms offers limited benefits; the development of new screens based upon an understanding of how individuals seek, process, and use information offers far greater utility and the capability to transform how work is done. This understanding should determine how much information is presented on the screen and how it is arranged and displayed. These design characteristics are as critical to the success of any application as its own internal logic and validity.

A key application for case managers in behavioral healthcare is decision support for level-of-care treatment planning. Decisions as to whether inpatient, day patient, or outpatient placement is most appropriate have both therapeutic and financial implications; such decisions clearly merit a high level of support. Expert systems to support clinical decision making can be of assistance here, using severity, chronicity, and work functioning to determine level of care and to raise red flags. The experience of hospital-based acute medical/surgical care in developing, validating, and using such systems should be studied for possible insights.

A second application area is provider listing for referral purposes. Increasingly, the industry is relying on provider profiles and ratings which allow the case manager to vouch for the quality of providers and to determine the best patient-provider match. Such systems enable the case manager to determine which providers are geographically accessible to a patient and to identify the professional credentials (M.D., Ph.D., M.S.W., etc.) and other characteristics (gender, age) of those providers. Effective management of care requires that the match be made appropriately. Referring a patient to a psychiatrist when a social worker is qualified to handle a particular problem does not make therapeutic or business sense; yet a limited number of encounters with a psychologist may be less costly and more effective than ongoing meetings with a counselor. And the professional who treats depression successfully may be less effective with patients presenting with agoraphobia.

In short, evaluating performance and developing provider profiles can be invaluable to provider network management. The inevitable sensitivities of the provider community can to some extent be offset if the process is not a "black box" but rather an acknowledged and open methodology, itself subject to evaluation and review. Such a methodology may be unnecessary in a staff model; within a network model, it is essential if quality is to be maintained. Within the latter model, network management provides the standards to its far-flung, part-time contractual providers that person-to-person supervision provides in the staff model. Under the network model, provider network management is not a technical function. It is much more. Provider network management, not human resources management, establishes the corporate identity, ethos, and standards.

Thus the psychological consulting field of organizational development (OD) assumes new significance, especially the new subspeciality that addresses the organizational impact of health informatics. The fact is that, with the exception of claims processing, the industry is not highly automated at this time, and this intensifies the need for OD as informatics technologies are introduced.

Case managers are often the first contact for those providing and those seeking and receiving services. Over the course of treatment, queries are frequently directed to claims managers as well. Especially within the provider network model, the case manager's queries are often the only points of contact between managed care staff and the treatment delivery system. Their roles are critical to the provision of quality services. As informatics technologies are introduced, both case and claims managers will require training to acculturate them to new ways of doing business. As more and more functions are automated, the conversations that case managers hold with providers and patients will be shaped by the fields displayed on the screens of their workstations. Again, these conversations identify the level of service needed and make provider-patient matches. In essence, one role these case managers perform is telephonic triage—not unlike the role of paramedics who deliver telemedicine—and they need on-the-job training. As the carve-out industry evolves to absorb both the impact of informatics and the advances in behavioral healthcare, continued training will be required. This is the essence of highly pragmatic OD.

Automation can support basic managed care functions, such as entering and forwarding care authorizations, tracking records, and verifying that they include clinical rationale. Automation can also provide expert system support for higher-level functions, such as the level-of-care triage decisions mentioned earlier. This latter application manifests relatively low-level complexity and high-level business need. Level of placement directly affects costs, as do onsite staff requirements.

Expert systems can help to contain both, by ensuring appropriate placement as well as limiting the need for large numbers of highly educated case managers.

Looking to the Future

There is no doubt that information technology will play a major role in managed behavioral healthcare. It is critical to remember, however, that the role will be that of an "enabler" only. Patient care must remain the focal point for management, which must take upon itself the responsibility for using the new enabling technologies to improve care, support professional practice, and address critical issues. Technology cannot be either the driver or the scapegoat. Human aspects of care cannot and must not be subjugated to what is just conveniently accomplished by the technology.

If we use these powerful new enablers to help us reengineer and redesign the healthcare system—or the sector of it which we are charged to manage—we can create a kinder and more caring system that puts the patient first.

Notes

P. 3, *pioneers such as Larry Weed:* Weed, L. L. (1991). *Knowledge coupling: New premises and new tools for medical care and education.* New York: Springer-Verlag.

P. 3, *as both an artifact and an agent of change:* Dick, R., & Steen, E. (1991). *The computer-based patient record.* Washington, DC: National Academy Press; Ball, M. J., & Collen, M. F. (1992). *Aspects of the computer-based patient record.* New York: Springer-Verlag.

P. 4, *an "enabler" for the CPR, giving users necessary capabilities:* Ball, M. J., Silva, J. S., Douglas, J. V., Degoulet, P., & Kaihara, S. (1994). The health professional workstation. *International Journal of Bio-Medical Computing, 34*(1–4).

P. 4, *the context of health information systems:* Hammond, W. E., Bakker, A. B., & Ball, M. J. (1995). Information systems with fading boundaries. *International Journal of Bio-Medical Computing, 39*(1).

P. 5, *via fax and/or computer:* Anderson, E. L. (1995). Technology for consumers and information needs in health care. In Ball, M. J., Simborg, D. W., Albright, J. W., & Douglas, J. V. (Eds.). *Healthcare information management systems: A practical guide* (2nd ed., pp. 3–16). New York: Springer-Verlag.

P. 6, *organic and humanistic organizational development model:* Lorenzi, N. M., Riley, R. T., Ball, M. J., & Douglas, J. V. (1995). *Transforming health care through information: Case studies.* New York: Springer-Verlag.

P. 7, *guide them through their personal health histories:* Anderson, E. L. (1995). Technology for consumers and information needs in health care. In Ball, M. J., Simborg, D. W., Albright, J. W., & Douglas, J. V. (Eds.). *Healthcare information management systems: A practical guide* (2nd ed., pp. 3–16). New York: Springer-Verlag.

P. 7, *coverage for mental health and substance abuse through a managed behavioral healthcare vendor:* Trabin, T., & Freeman, M. (1995). *Managed behavioral healthcare: History, models, strategic challenges and future course.* Tiburon, CA: CentraLink.

CHAPTER TWO

CLINICAL DECISION SUPPORT SYSTEMS

Wallace J. Gingerich and Anthony Broskowski

Computers are just beginning to move out of the business offices of behavioral healthcare companies and into the hands of practicing clinicians. This trend is due to a number of factors, but the primary force for change is the development of decision support systems, computer applications that can help providers deliver higher-quality behavioral health services more efficiently and more reliably.

This chapter begins by looking briefly at how decision support systems (DSSs) developed, and why they are just now beginning to be used in behavioral healthcare. Then we will take a closer look at what DSSs are and the main technologies employed in decision support systems today. We then look at clinical decision making in behavioral health, to see how and where DSSs might be helpful to clinicians. Then we look at some of the current DSSs available today to give you an idea of what you can expect such a system to do for you. We also consider some of the factors you should consider when selecting a DSS. Finally, we offer some speculations about the future of DSSs in behavioral healthcare.

Brief History of Decision Support Systems

DSSs as we know them today evolved over time, as computing technology became more powerful and users demanded more helpful outputs.

Transaction Processing Systems

Computers moved out of the laboratory and into the workplace in 1951 when UNIVAC, the first commercial electronic computer, was installed at the U.S. Bureau of the Census. UNIVAC became a household word one year later when CBS television used it to project Dwight Eisenhower as the winner of the 1952 presidential election on the basis of only 3 percent of the vote. While this forecast was arguably a decision support application of early computing technology, most decision support applications in the 1950s were more accurately considered *transaction processing systems*, processing huge data bases for universities, government, and large financial institutions. In those early days of commercial computing, computers were large and expensive and required skilled personnel to operate them.

Information Reporting Systems

In the 1960s managers and researchers began to demand that the data contained in the huge data banks be processed and output in such a way that it would be more accessible and useful for decision making. These *information reporting systems,* as they were called, produced standardized reports and printouts that managers could use to get detailed information on their organizations. Although managers now had access to information, the detailed reports they received were often not responsive to their immediate decision-making needs. Furthermore, these systems ran on large mainframe computers operable only by data processing professionals. It often took weeks or months to reprogram these large computers to perform new analyses and reports.

By the end of the 1960s distributed computer systems came to be used in some industries such as banking, allowing managers to have terminals on their desks and giving them direct access to the data. (Distributed systems have only recently come to be used in behavioral health.) This new capability in computerized information systems raised the demands of managers still more: they wanted to be able to do ad hoc queries and analyses of their data that addressed specific decision-making needs, and they wanted an immediate response.

Decision Support Systems

Independently from the data-oriented computer information systems described above, operations researchers had over the years learned how to develop mathematical models and simulations that could be used to solve a wide variety of complex problems, such as planning military strategies and managing plant production and inventory. In the early 1970s, these two developments came together, combining the model-oriented capabilities of operations research with the data-oriented information processing systems, and decision support systems were born.

The term *decision support system* was first used by Gorry and Scott Morton in 1971 to refer to interactive computer systems which could help managers solve relatively unstructured problems. These systems combined data-based information with a model or simulation of the decision-making process in order to support the decision-making task of the user. Some of the first applications of these decision support systems were designed to help users manage factory production or process loan applications. The single best known decision support application developed during this time was the electronic spreadsheet, known originally as Visi-Calc. This program quickly became indispensable to accountants and financial planners because of its capability to help them do ad hoc "what-if" analyses.

With the advent of personal computing in the late 1960s and the continuing development of decision support technology, DSSs have proliferated in business and industry. DSSs have been adopted slowly in behavioral health practice, however. But before we examine the reasons why, let us take a closer look at just what a DSS is and at some of the DSS technologies that are available today.

What Are Decision Support Systems?

Generally speaking, decision support systems (DSSs) are interactive computer-based systems that help decision makers utilize data and models to solve unstructured problems. The key idea here is that the computer system helps the user make decisions in situations where it would be difficult to do so without this assistance and where the information processing needs outstrip human capacities. Operationally, DSSs usually include one or more of the following functions: ad hoc data retrieval, graphical presentation of complex information in order to see patterns, the capacity to explore different scenarios through what-if analyses, statistical analysis and model fitting, or some form of expertise or artificial intelligence applied to the data. According to Vogel, the essential characteristics of DSSs include the following:

- DSSs are intended to *support* decision makers, not replace them.
- DSSs are aimed at *less well structured* problems that tend to lack complete specification.
- DSSs seek to *combine* the use of *models* and analytic techniques with customary *data* access and retrieval functions.
- DSSs are *interactive and friendly* to the decision maker, including users who are not technically sophisticated.

- DSSs are intentionally *flexible* in order to adapt to changes in the environment and the user's needs.
- DSSs are often used to draw conclusions from *large data bases* which are difficult to analyze without sophisticated tools.

Structural Definition

DSSs include three basic components. A DSS always includes a *data base management* system, or knowledge system. The data may be included within the DSS in the form of rules, it may reside in existing data bases in the user's environment, or it may be input by the user while using the system. The second component is a *model base management* system, or problem processing system, which provides for analysis and interpretation of the data. The model base component may be a mathematical model, a logical deductive system, or an inferencing system, and it may contain "intelligence." Finally, a DSS always contains a *dialogue management system,* or user interface. This component gets input from the user, manages the interaction between the user and the data base and model base components, and responds to the user's request.

In practice, DSS denotes a heterogeneous grouping of systems. They are defined more by function than structure, and in all cases they must provide *support* to the user in a *decision-making* task. In concept, however, all DSSs contain the aforementioned three components: data, a model, and an interactive interface. It is particularly important to know and understand what goes into the data base and model base components, because they become the basis for the decision support the system will provide. The user of a DSS is responsible to use it appropriately.

Types of Decision Support Systems

A variety of approaches have been employed to give DSSs the capability to support the user in decision making. While not all of the approaches have been implemented in commercially available behavioral health applications, most of them have been tried in research and experimental settings. A brief discussion of these main types of DSSs and examples of each will give you an idea of the kinds of systems we might expect in the not-too-distant future.

Structured Computerized Clinical Records

Perhaps the simplest type of DSS is one in which information in the clinical record is structured and computerized in such a way that it can be easily reviewed, summarized, and analyzed. Structured records make possible decision aids such as ticklers of upcoming tasks, trend analysis, and graphical display of client change. There are many challenges in structuring clinical information, which by nature is largely unstructured, and many attempts have been made over the last several decades to accomplish it.

A 166-bed psychiatric hospital in Israel recently computerized patient records to assist in clinical decision making and help with treatment planning. The system allows the clinician to review case notes, and it can compile a discharge summary based on information in the record. It also produces routine reports and reminders, and it assists the clinician in writing goals. Similar systems have been implemented in the United States and elsewhere, in several public and private hospitals. The value of this type of DSS is dependent upon the extent to which the system represents the relevant information about the client effectively and enables the clinician to analyze it for treatment and case management decisions.

Algorithmic Models

Another type of DSS applies mathematical or algorithmic models to datasets in order to see patterns or predict future behavior. For example, statistical models have been used to predict heart disease and asthma relapse. These two models were predicated on analyses of large patient populations in which various patient indicators were shown to correlate with illness outcomes. These statistical models, built from the larger data base, can then be applied to similar patients in order to predict their outcomes. A critical issue with such systems is the validity of the model used to make the prediction, and whether the model applies to the particular patient being considered. When these conditions are satisfied, however, these DSSs can provide information to the clinician that is simply beyond the information processing capacity of the unassisted human.

Decision-Tree Systems

Another common type of DSS is the decision-tree system. For example, DTREE is a DSS that uses an expanded version of the DSM-III-R decision trees to guide the clinician through the process of making a psychiatric diagnosis. The DSS asks a series of yes-no questions to elicit symptom behaviors of the patient being considered. As in many such systems, DTREE decides which areas need detailed exploration based on the clinician's answers to basic screening questions. In addition to providing the DSM-III-R diagnosis, the system can provide the clinician with an explanation of its diagnostic reasoning. The validity of a decision-tree DSS is based on the soundness of the knowledge and the reasoning process embedded in the decision tree itself. Decision-tree DSSs can serve a very useful reminder function for clinicians and can increase the consistency with which clinical decisions are made throughout an organization.

Expert Systems

The field of artificial intelligence must be credited for the development of a relatively new and potentially useful type of DSS, that of expert systems. Artificial intelligence (AI) is the branch of computer science that attempts to create computer programs to perform tasks that would be considered intelligent if done by a human. To accomplish this objective, AI has traditionally used symbolic (rather than numeric) and nonalgorithmic methods which can be applied to ill-defined and unstructured problems.

Expert systems are programs that are designed to function like human consultants, providing expert advice to the user in a specified problem area. Expert systems typically contain a set of if-then rules to represent specialized knowledge about the problem area. For example, one of the rules in MYCIN, the famous expert system for diagnosing infectious diseases, states "IF the site of the culture is throat, and IF the identity of the organism is streptococcus, THEN there is strongly suggestive evidence (.8) that the subtype of the organism is not group-D." Rules are organized hierarchically so that one rule can be used to determine the presence (or absence) of the IF condition in another rule, as shown in the preceding example. Further, rules may lead to conclusions with some uncertainty, as the .8 probability in the example illustrates.

The complete set of rules in an expert system is known as the rule-base or knowledge-base; it can be thought of as the data base management component of the DSS. The model base management component of an expert system is the *inference engine,* which controls the order in which rules are tested or "fired," how uncertainty is handled, and other aspects of the reasoning process. A standard capability of expert systems is the ability to explain to the user why a certain question is being asked, and provide the logical and factual basis for the conclusion it reaches. This capacity for feedback is possible because the rules are usually expressed within the system in ordinary language, such as English. Thus, expert systems can be used to educate users. They also allow the user to query the system to evaluate the quality of its advice, much as a clinician would ask a human consultant for an explanation.

Expert systems technology is well enough developed by now that expert system shells (the inferencing system and user interface) can be purchased and the user can add his or her own rules. PATHware, reviewed later on, is an example of an expert system shell. Expert system shells are analogous to data base systems, where the information processing capability is provided and the user has only to add the information—rules in this case—to make the system functional. Although it is possible to create a functioning expert system quite easily with one of these shells, the development and validation of a rule base that provides competent advice is well beyond the scope of this brief discussion.

Neural Networks

A second type of DSS to come out of the field of artificial intelligence is neural networks. Neural networks represent a revolutionary new direction in computing technology, one in which the design of computing machines is inspired by the structure of biological systems. Ordinary digital computers have a microprocessor, which acts on instructions from the software program stored in its memory and executes operations. Fundamentally, digital computers add, move, and compare numbers in a serial, step-by-step fashion. Consequently, they have been good at structured tasks involving mathematical manipulation and accessing large amounts of data from memory. Ordinary computers are not well suited to pattern-matching tasks such as understanding speech, recognizing a face, or reaching a conclusion based on incomplete information. These are the kinds of tasks that neural network computers perform well, a capability that holds considerable promise for the use of computing technology in behavioral health.

A neural network comprises many small processing elements, called nodes or neurons. The neurons are organized into layers, with each neuron in a layer connected to every neuron in the adjoining layer by a pattern of variable weights. Rather than being programmed like a traditional digital computer, a neural network is trained by being presented with many cases or instances until it "learns" a pattern of interconnected weights that maximizes the association between the inputs of the cases and the outputs. Then, when presented with a new case, one that it has never seen before, the network can assign it to the correct outcome group.

Neural networks blur the traditional boundaries between the data base management and model base management components of a DSS. In a fully trained neural network, these two components are essentially merged. The validity of the processing model depends, of course, on how representative the cases are that were used to train the system, and the quality of the case data that were fed into the network.

For example, one neural network was developed to predict admission decisions to a psychiatric emergency room. The developers found that the system, based on training from 658 previous admission cases, was able to predict the actual decisions made by experienced clinicians. Similarly, another neural network was trained to predict the length of stay of patients in a state psychiatric hospital. Again, the developers found that the neural net DSS performed at least as well as a team of clinicians.

It is important to note that, unlike expert systems rule bases, neural networks make no a priori assumptions about how decisions should be made. Rather, during the training period they simply evolve a series of weighted connections that successfully relate the clinical outcomes to the client characteristics that have been inputs. Because of this, the decision-making knowledge contained in neural networks is difficult to interpret.

Clinical Decision Making

Before we look at some current examples of behavioral DSSs, it would be well to consider the nature of decision making, and those elements of the process that lend themselves to computerized decision support systems.

Decision Making Defined

Decision making is best thought of as a process that occurs over time, a process through which decisions are made, rather than a single event at a specific point in time. It is a complex information-seeking and problem-solving activity with four phases: (1) *intelligence,* or finding occasions for making a decision; (2) *design,* or finding possible courses of action; (3) *choice,* or choosing among the alternatives; and (4) *review,* or evaluating past choices. Decision making is an interactive and cyclic process in which information at each phase affects the process, and feedback from previous decisions may serve as information for future decisions.

Some common needs for improved decision making are better detection of problems that require attention, fuller exploration of alternative courses of action, enhanced coping when faced with unclear objectives, reduction of systematic cognitive biases, and clearer structuring of the decision-making process itself.

Common Behavioral Health Decisions

Many behavioral health clinical decisions come to mind for which a DSS might be a helpful support to the clinician. While the distinctions or boundaries between these various types of decisions is never exact, the potential user of decision support systems needs to be clear about the types of decisions the system claims to support and whether or not those are the decisions that the user needs to make.

Data Collection and Assessment. Some systems are nothing more than a computer-assisted tool to support the collection of data from the patient or others and then to make its storage, tabulation, or communication more reliable, consistent, and efficient. While not a decision support system in the sense of using the computer program's inferential or numerical processing powers, such a system can support decision making through its ability to standardize the data and its presentation to the decision makers. This is a significant and necessary precondition to the more advanced types of computerized decision support systems that rely on a structured and formalized process for entering information, although the sequence of data capture and entry may be dynamic. The PsychAccess system reviewed in this chapter is an example of such an application, as are emerging automated medical record applications.

Screening and Diagnosis. Some systems, such as the Problem Knowledge Coupler reviewed later, are designed to help the provider make a better assessment or diagnosis of the patient's condition, along with the other decisions they are designed to support. Logic may be embedded in such systems to prompt specific questions based on the answers to earlier questions, or the logic can "screen in" or "screen out" alternative diagnoses, or "screen for" the patient's appropriateness or likelihood to benefit from alternative forms of intervention.

For example, the system may help decide whether a patient with a disease at a given stage of progression and severity is a good candidate for a new form of drug treatment or surgery. Such systems are likely to have high payoff when a differential diagnosis or assessment implies specific forms of treatment known to be effective. Because of the low reliability in making psychiatric diagnoses, and the lack of systematic research linking specific diagnoses to specific treatments and specific outcomes, this application of decision support in behavioral healthcare lags behind its comparable development in other areas of general medicine.

Level of Treatment. Some of the earliest behavioral health DSSs concerned themselves with decisions regarding the necessity to admit a person with a behavioral health problem to a hospital and, once admitted, the necessity of continuing the stay versus referring the patient to other "levels" of treatment, such as residential alternatives, partial hospitalization, outpatient, or home-based care. While only a very gross distinction, these triage or level-of-treatment decisions—particularly the decision whether or not to hospitalize—were critical to most payers and most hospital providers. Hospitalization was clearly associated with the most common high-cost (from the payer's perspective) or high-revenue (from the provider's perspective) interventions available, which were routinely covered by insurance plans.

Secondary to costs and revenue concerns were questions about the effectiveness of hospitalization and whether or not more was better than less. When the supply of hospital beds increased, so did their utilization, raising doubts about whether hospitalization was being driven by clinical needs or by supplier-induced demand. Hospital length-of-stay and readmission rates appeared to be more related to insurance benefit design than clinical conditions.

Whether computerized or not, most formalized managed care decision support tools in the behavioral health industry started from the seeds of making decisions about levels of treatment. Many of the current systems continue to focus on this early and very important decision.

Treatment Planning. Once a level-of-treatment decision is made, there remain additional questions. What set of interventions, therapies, or drugs is most appropriate for this patient? What combinations? How much? And how intensive must these interventions be? The questions imply that there are distinctive alternative methods or intensities of treatment within any given level of treatment, and that there are well-known relationships between characteristics of the patients and their problems and the types of treatment that will be most effective. The Psych-Pro system, for example, offers one of five treatment "categories" nested within the recommendation for an outpatient level of treatment.

Some research and much debate centers around assumptions of specific treatment assignment as they apply to the behavioral health industry. Over time there has been increasing differentiation among the specific types of treatments available within any given level: more therapeutic drugs with specific indications for use, more specific methods of psychotherapy or behavior and cognitive change, more specific methods of family and marital interventions. Although there are notable exceptions, the optimal match between type of patient, type of problem, and type of treatment has yet to be demonstrated empirically for many disorders. Nevertheless, since treatment planning decisions must be made, formalized rule-based or empirically validated DSSs may prove to be useful to decision makers.

Also embedded in this general category of decisions is the issue of "matching" the patient to a specific therapist once the decision is made to treat the person at the outpatient level. This issue is widely discussed now that outpatient therapy has become a more prevalent method of treatment. There are a variety of therapists and modalities available, ranging from those doing long-term psychoanalysis to those doing planned brief-term, problem-focused therapy. Recognizing that many therapists are likely to provide only one form of therapy regardless of who the referred patient is, many managed care companies consider it important to identify for each patient the therapist most likely to be a cost-effective provider for their specific problems.

At least one of the systems reviewed in this chapter (as well as in Chapter Four, on outcome assessment), COMPASS, is based on the premises that therapy is effective (up to a point), proportional to the number of sessions; that it progresses in a specific sequence of stages; and that a critical factor in the effectiveness of the therapy is the nature of the alliance or bond between the therapist and the patient. Clearly such a theory of therapy suggests that some therapists might be more effective than others for specific patients, and that data collected over time across various therapist-patient combinations will support more effective patient-therapist assignment decisions in the future.

Practice Guidelines. The early 1990s have witnessed the development of disease-specific treatment guidelines in general healthcare, due largely to widespread variation in physician practice patterns even when strong research evidence was available to indicate the greater effectiveness of a specific procedure for a given disease.

There is no single template used to present practice guidelines. To the extent that they reflect either findings from the research literature or the consensus opinions of acknowledged experts, practice guidelines vary in their details and the degree of prescriptive directions they provide. As the term *guideline* suggests, they are intended to provide recommendations as to what the provider should try, what general outcomes to expect within a given time period following the intervention, and what to try next if the first interventions do not work as expected.

This chapter cannot address all the issues inherent in the various methods for developing such guidelines and the factors that affect their use and validation. However, practice guidelines in behavioral healthcare have arrived and their use will continue to spread. Decision support systems are being developed, such as the QualityFIRST system reviewed in this chapter, that attempt to identify and recommend for use the most appropriate guideline for a given patient.

Critical Clinical Pathways. Well beyond practice guidelines in their specificity, critical pathways are statements about the exact sequence and duration of activities that should take place in the treatment of a given condition. Critical pathways are most often used in hospital settings for specific acute diseases and medical or surgical procedures.

As an example, for a coronary artery bypass graft the pathway will specify which test should be conducted before hospitalization, and what should happen during the first day in the hospital and before, during, and after the day of surgery, with the expectation that if all goes according to "normal" expectations the patient will be discharged after the fourth day. Currently, we know of no decision support system that is providing this type of specificity for the treatment of behavioral healthcare conditions.

Disease Management Protocols. Building on the concept of practice guidelines and pathways, disease management protocols are becoming popular as mechanisms to provide the proper level of integration and continuity of care required by diseases that demand multiple and diverse resources being applied over time and distance, especially for chronic conditions.

For example, persons with such diseases as diabetes, asthma, and schizophrenia require a multidisciplinary team of providers offering a range of different services centered on that patient; these services must be provided over time and across settings. Systems such as the Problem Knowledge Coupler provide disease management protocols online to the providers having case management responsibilities for the patient.

Examples of Current Behavioral Health DSSs

Having looked at decision support systems in general, and the kinds of behavioral health decisions that lend themselves to computerized decision support systems, we take a look at some of the DSSs we mentioned above. All of these systems are currently available to providers. Some of the systems we review have been in use for several years or more; others are just coming to the marketplace.

Information on the DSSs we review was obtained from marketing materials provided by each vendor and interviews with their development or marketing staff. The reader is advised to directly contact the company developing a particular system for more detailed and up-to-date information.

The systems reviewed here illustrate the types of DSSs described above. Most systems contain elements of more than one type; for example, a DSS that we classify as a structured clinical record may also contain algorithms to guide the user in the sequence and branching of questions asked of the patient.

We do not review all of the DSSs in existence, but we have attempted to cover the best known and most available ones. Contact information is included at the end of the chapter. Because we can expect to see many more behavioral health DSSs introduced in the next several years, this is in a sense a preview of the kinds of systems one can expect to see in the near future.

COMPASS

Although the COMPASS system is reviewed in Chapter Four with regard to its use as an outcomes assessment system, we review it here as an example of a DSS based on a structured clinical record. COMPASS uses patient and therapist ratings on a number of scales intended to reflect the severity of the patient's condition at the start of outpatient psychotherapy, and to monitor the progress and effectiveness of treatment.

COMPASS is based on the extensive "dose-effect" research of Ken Howard. It assumes that successful therapy progresses in three stages: remoralization, remediation, and rehabilitation. The patient completes scales assessing his or her level of well-being, symptoms, and "life functioning." The therapist also assesses the patient's level of functioning. Upon scoring, COMPASS provides an overall rating of the patient's status, called the Mental Health Index, as well as intermittent progress reports and ratings on the various symptom and functioning scales.

COMPASS is used primarily to measure progress and outcomes of adult outpatient psychotherapy. However, to the extent that COMPASS tracks and identifies trends in treatment progress over sessions, it can also be used in clinical supervision or case management to support decisions to alter or terminate a given outpatient treatment modality when there are no demonstrated improvements which would otherwise be expected at that point in treatment. The system claims it is able to detect early in the process if the therapy is ineffective, as well as how much improvement may be possible with additional treatment. The system would serve to support decisions about the type of therapy being provided as well as decisions to be made by a third-party review organization regarding the need for additional treatment.

Furthermore, with an accumulation of a data base on multiple therapists using COMPASS over a large number of their patients, it would be feasible to construct provider profiles on each therapist and the cost-effectiveness of their respective treatments for different categories of patients. Such a data base could presumably support decisions for assigning patients to therapists using rules or algorithms based on a "best fit," given the characteristics and problems of the patient. Such a data base could also support decisions about the relative effectiveness of different networks of therapists.

While these potentials exist, and COMPASS does report its use in managed care systems covering over four million lives and multiple networks, there is currently no demonstration known to these authors that any COMPASS users have, in fact, built a sufficiently large data base over a sufficient number of patients, therapists, and networks to support using COMPASS for treatment assignment and network evaluations.

The developers of the COMPASS system claim that in at least one application it has reduced overall treatment costs by 47 percent and lowered outpatient costs by 62 percent while it "significantly raised the quality of care." However, from the information provided it is not possible to isolate the effects of COMPASS independently from other interventions and changes that may have been implemented concurrently within this group of employees, as from case management, benefit plan changes, changes in preferred providers, etc.

It should be noted that COMPASS applications are currently limited to outpatient treatment, although inpatient applications were in development at the time of this writing. The measures included in COMPASS appear suited mainly to a population of adults, and possibly adolescents, but provide little decision support for treating children.

The cost of using the COMPASS system depends on the volume of instruments required as well as the number and frequency of reports requested. Currently COMPASS operates as a service, receiving forms and providing reports. Connectivity is available via networks or modems for data transfer. A software version that can run on a workstation will be available in the future.

PsychPro

According to the developers, there are two distinct tools within the PsychPro system. The first is an Acute Precertification Tool, to be used by the provider or an external review organization for making recommendations regarding the necessity of inpatient or residential care for patients in an acute crisis. The second tool is an Outpatient Decision Support tool, for recommending treatment and monitoring progress. The former was designed primarily to support the external review done by third-party review organizations; the latter is designed for use by organized managed care service delivery organizations that wish to make appropriate treatment assignments and review progress independently of external review organizations. Like COMPASS, the assumption is that with enough data on enough therapists and patients, the data base can be used to inform decisions regarding the relative effectiveness of different therapists with different types of patients.

The Acute Precertification tool uses clinician's ratings on eight subscales, embedded within a "smart questioning algorithm" that asks subsequent questions based on answers to previous questions. Using this algorithm, the system produces a recommendation regarding which of seven levels of treatment is most appropriate for the patient, ranging from inpatient to routine outpatient. If the recommendation is for routine outpatient treatment, the system recommends which of five categories of treatment would be most appropriate: brief EAP intervention, psychotherapy, substance-abuse counseling, psychiatric assessment and medication, or group therapy. Clinician ratings are focused on case-mix factors (patient diagnostic and historical factors) and behavioral impairments, while the patient's ratings are on symptoms and opinions regarding the therapeutic alliance and their satisfaction with treatment.

The Outpatient Decision Support tool tracks scores on three symptom and satisfaction scales based on the patient's ratings and three behavioral impairment scales based on the clinician's ratings. Further, the system claims to track outcomes throughout treatment by comparing the "clinical trajectory of change for a particular patient profile . . . with the actual trajectory of change." When the actual is outside the range of the expected, the system will flag the case, suggest an alternative course of treatment, and identify the reason for the suggested alternative. The system uses guidelines developed for hypothetical average patients and applies them to a particular patient at a particular time. There is no information on how these guidelines were developed, although in the PsychPro materials we received there is reference to depression guidelines from the Agency for Health Care Policy and Research (AHCPR) that call for a moderately depressed client to respond partially or fully by the sixth session. PsychPro embodies that guideline in its decision support tool.

PsychPro claims to use patient risk factors to adjust their expected scale scores. There are two risk-adjustment scores, one based on diagnostic categories and the other based on historical factors in the patient's life (for example, previous treatments and types of treatment, history of physical or sexual abuse, etc.). Our review did not encompass the specific methodology being used by PsychPro to do the risk adjustment and calculate the "expected trajectory" of progress.

The systems offered by PsychPro run on Windows-based stand-alone PCs or LAN-based workstations. The data base created by PsychPro can interface with a number of data base management systems. Users of PsychPro can have paper forms mailed, faxed, or sent by modem to a central source, where they are downloaded, scored, and analyzed; or they can enter the rating directly on their own PCs or LAN workstations. The system provides monthly, quarterly, and annual reports. The developers claim the system can also produce individual provider, group, and facility profiles and report cards.

PsychPro is being used by Aetna and Human Affairs International, the Oxford Health Plan, and Community Health Plan of Albany, New York. Licenses are priced according to the membership of the enrolled population on which it will be applied or on the number of workstations or PCs on which the system is installed.

QualityFIRST Behavioral Health Guidelines

QualityFIRST Behavioral Health Guidelines, as its name indicates, provides decision support for treatment planning through practice guidelines. It utilizes a decision-tree procedure to determine the diagnosis, select the level of care and the treatment and resources needed, and support the ongoing management of specific behavioral health problems. The levels of care addressed by the system include inpatient psychiatric care, inpatient detoxification or rehabilitation, partial hospitalization, intensive and routine outpatient treatment, aftercare, medication management, and self-help group support. The guidelines in the system can be used for retrospective, concurrent, or prospective review. They are described as "boundary guidelines" inasmuch as they provide only the framework for thinking about what to consider and not specifying exactly what to do. The boundary guideline sets up each case for prospective care management and subsequent outcomes measurement.

Based on DSM-IV diagnoses and severity of symptoms, patient characteristics, and other clinician inputs, QualityFIRST recommends treatment options but allows the practitioner to vary from the recommendation. It captures the clinician's departures from the recommended guidelines and the reasons for them in subsequent analyses.

Guidelines are developed by a multidisciplinary panel of experts who are asked to interpret peer-reviewed clinical and research literature, including publications by federal government agencies such as AHCPR and those developed by medical specialty societies. On the basis of this review, a treatment algorithm or practice guideline is produced and refined over time. Each guideline is supported by a fully referenced position paper that provides an overview of the diagnostic and treatment considerations for the specific condition. Currently, Version 3.7 provides guidelines for fifteen specific psychiatric disorders, of which three are specific to children and adolescents, and four guidelines for substance-abuse disorders, one of which includes adolescents. Four more guidelines are under development at the time of this review. Once released, each guideline and supporting position paper is reviewed annually and updated on the basis of literature and client feedback.

Because the behavioral health guidelines are only a subset of a larger number of medical and surgical care guidelines, the developers addressed the issue of integrating behavioral and medical care. The guidelines note common medical syndromes that should be ruled out in the diagnosis of a behavioral disorder. Disability, return-to-work parameters, and case management considerations are also included in each guideline, making them applicable to managing care for workers' compensation programs and short-term disability management.

The software runs under Windows with a point-and-click decision-tree logic that takes the user through a short sequence of pass-fail or multiple-choice questions to arrive at treatment recommendations. The relevant position papers and extensive help notes are also online. The system can run on a notebook, a desktop PC, a LAN, or a mainframe computer. The system is available for a licensing and monthly subscription fee based on the number of guidelines and the number of workstations using the software. Users receive quarterly releases with new guidelines and annual revisions of existing guidelines.

The developer of QualityFIRST claims the system's software architecture allows it to interface with an organization's existing treatment pathways and guidelines, clinical and patient satisfaction and outcomes data, and existing continuous quality improvement (CQI) processes. There were no examples of the system's reports or recommendations available for this review. However, the developer offers prospective buyers the ability to experience a remote demonstration of the system if they have a modem on their local computer.

QualityFIRST is a fairly new product. Its installed base is limited to some HMOs, two disability companies who use them as part of an integrated medical/surgical and disability package, and the parent company (Health Risk Management), which uses it for their contracted review services.

Internal research is being planned to determine if reviewers' use of the guidelines affects utilization parameters in comparison to settings where the guidelines are not used.

PsychAccess

Unlike most other systems in this review, PsychAccess is not a decision support system that uses computer processes to make diagnoses, assign patients to levels of care, or recommend any specific treatment. Rather, PsychAccess is a computerized method of standardizing, recording, and communicating information needed by various decision makers along the provider-reviewer-payer continuum. As such, we consider PsychAccess an example of a structured clinical record DSS.

PsychAccess is designed primarily to ease the task of recording and sharing clinical information between providers and other parties responsible for authorizing or paying for care. PsychAccess does this by standardizing the documentation methodologies already endorsed by several major managed care organizations (MCOs), allowing reports generated by the system to be used by these particular MCOs, and allowing clinical data from these reports to be used by the provider to document the quality of care to still other providers. Two versions and several enhancements are available.

The first version is a set of forms compatible with standard fax equipment, allowing practitioners to fax completed treatment-related documents to an authorized service center where they are converted to customized paper reports or electronic records and then transmitted to the appropriate payer or MCO. The receiving organization can purchase PsychAccess software to build a data base from these forms if they so desire.

The other version is a Windows-based application used by the clinician. There is a Care Management module for MCOs, which performs case management or utilization review activities, allowing the reviewers to view clinical reports from providers, record assessments of risk, and issue and send treatment authorizations electronically. A second module, Case Supervision and Reporting, is designed for supervisors who manage the caseload of staff and profile network providers.

The various forms embedded in either version reflect the usual paperwork flow that unfolds during treatment, starting with intake, assessment/diagnosis, initial and revised treatment plans, concurrent review and progress notes, claims, claims inquiries, and appeals, as well as closing and discharge plans. In addition to these forms, the software version allows the clinician to maintain progress notes, display trends in the patient's condition, track outstanding authorizations, and send and receive documents directly from their computer.

In addition to recording patient history, mental status, and all DSM IV axes, the provider selects from a "collection of 63 behaviorally descriptive terms, called impairments" to further describe the patient and justify the necessary treatment. Each impairment can be further rated on a four-point severity scale to describe the effects of the impairment on the patient's functioning. It is hoped that this increased specificity "will result in more informed resource allocation and utilization management." The terminology *impairments* is said to be independent of discipline or theoretical orientation and easy to learn how to use with "little or no training." While citing the literature on the source and the popularity of impairments as a descriptive language, the developer acknowledges that the necessary reliability, validity, and temporal stability research studies are not yet completed, although the preliminary results are described as "promising."

The software can be run on stand-alone PCs or on client-server based platforms. At the time of this writing the system was not yet available and was scheduled for release in late 1995. The developer indicates that MEDCO Behavioral Health Care, Inc., intends to use PsychAccess for interactions with its eighteen thousand contracted providers. No information was available on the method of pricing the various versions and add-on modules.

PATHware

PATHware uses smart algorithms and a rule base to trigger treatment recommendations. It is an example of an expert system DSS.

PATHware is a DSS shell that gives the user's application development team (ADT) an "artificial intelligence protocol configuration tool" to design a DSS suited to its needs, using fixed data elements embedded in the system's menus or various check boxes.

Up to sixteen "issues" can be defined, each with up to sixteen factors. Each factor can have as many as five response options or answers. The entire set of issues, factors, and response options is called a "protocol." Up to six protocols form a "configuration." Protocols can use any words, phrases, or languages that are readily understood by the individuals using the system: providers, patients, or family members. Questions can be written so as to allow branching as well as embedded "help" and warning texts contingent on responses.

The ADT can assign weights to each possible response or question. These weights can be summed into various scales considered to be important in the decision-making process. The team can also specify that the answer to a specific question contributes different weights to different scales.

The ADT specifies certain decisions or "treatments." "Rules" are the conditions for which a recommendation for a specific treatment is triggered. Treatment rules can be based on (1) the scores of various scales, (2) a specific response to a single question, (3) an interaction between two scales, or (4) an interaction between a scale score and any range of response options to a single factor. The software uses an "inferential engine" that allows the decision rules to be triggered independently of the sequence in which the data is collected and entered. While entering data, the user can move from one item to another in whatever sequence the respondent offers the information. However, the ADT can design the protocol to make some data elements mandatory or prerequisite to others.

Once the protocol and configuration is created, a run-time, Windows-based version of the DSS can be created and multiple copies distributed to as many end users as necessary. PATHware's rules and the data entered by the user are stored in a Microsoft Access relational data base, which can be accessed through a wide range of other software products designed to query or manipulate data bases, including SQL and various report writers.

The system provides a variety of standard reports: all the assessment data collected, numerical indicators reflecting severity, three sets of bar graphs containing up to ten risk severity scales each, five "risk mitigation" scales, a single "roll-up" graph, and a listing of recommended treatments. Presumably, with repeated application of a protocol with a patient at different time periods, one could access the data base to produce before-and-after comparisons or trendlines.

PATHware runs on a stand-alone PC or a client-server platform. The PC must have at least an Intel 486 CPU running at 33 Mhz, a minimum of 8 megabytes of RAM, and 2 megabytes of free space on the hard drive.

In essence, everything in PATHware is customizable, an advantage to users who need more than what most off-the-shelf DSSs offer. For example, users may need DSS protocols for specific populations which do not readily fit into other systems (children, serious and persistently mentally ill patients, medical patients with psychiatric co-morbidities, etc.). The disadvantage is the work required to define all the questions, issues, weights, and related logic to trigger the decisions. While users should understand all the logic and rules in any predesigned, off-the-shelf DSS, not every organization can invest the time and effort required to create and make explicit all the decisions they currently make implicitly.

PATHware leaves unanswered the issues of reliability and validity. Having created scales, scores, and treatment rules, will the allure of automation tempt the ADT into believing these issues do not need to be addressed? Fortunately, PATHware does allow for refinements or modifications to the protocol. If reliability and validity studies suggest modifications, the ADT can make them without waiting for a software vendor to make changes. While easy customization makes for easy updates, consistency in the data base could suffer.

Pricing is based on client-specific needs. In some cases PATHware staff will initially consult with and train the user organization on how to use the software to develop various protocols or will design one for them. This cost is added to the software costs. Ongoing training and support is priced at approximately 20 percent of the software purchase price.

Problem Knowledge Couplers

An entirely different approach to clinical decision support is exemplified by the Problem Knowledge Coupler (PKC). Problem Knowledge Couplers are computer-based tools that can be used by the provider at the point of patient service to better identify the patient's problems and risk factors, record clinical findings, and develop refined diagnostic and patient care management strategies.

The primary designer behind PKC is Dr. Larry Weed, pioneer developer of the problem-oriented medical record. The PKC system is an effort to abstract the most current knowledge for diagnosing and treating diseases into a useable "knowledge network" or "knowledge base" and couple that base to an interactive tool to be used by the provider at the point of service to the patient. Couplers come in three varieties: (1) as screening tools to identify problems and risk factors, (2) for recording presenting problems that could have different diagnostic and care management implications, and (3) for recording problems of patients with known diagnoses which require management.

Using point-and-click screens, the clinician selects from a high-level list of major complaints (for example, "Depression, Fatigue, Apathy," "Headaches," Chest Pain," etc.), called the Coupler Index. The next screen offers options to record the specific "finding," such as type of onset and associated symptoms. Findings can be recorded as positive, negative, or uncertain. This information is then used by a "medical knowledge base" which is coupled to the system to produce a summary of the findings, an index of possible causes or relevant management options, and detailed displays of information for each specific cause and management option. The Findings Summary screen includes all positive and negative findings organized into broad groups specific to each Coupler.

Comments are provided that relate each finding to one or more of the possible causes, provide information for managing and monitoring the patient's status, or suggest further investigations that need to be carried out to better define and diagnose the problem. Comments include literature citations. The Cause Index screen lists the possible causes for the patient's clinical findings and, for each cause, the number of findings associated with the patient that are associated with a given disease/diagnosis. Further details can then be obtained to rule in or rule out different diagnoses based on findings inconsistent with those reported by the patient.

The thinking behind the PKC method is not artificial intelligence, but rather a pure combinatorial approach of relating all findings with all possible causes and letting the human provider use this information to make better decisions. To the extent that there are well-known causes that lead to a diagnosis that lead directly to a known treatment, such a parsing of knowledge at the point of the intervention is likely to have a large payoff. When specific treatments to "cure" the disease are not known, the system can certainly deliver to the provider the best knowledge of how to manage the care of the patient over time.

There are presently sixty-two Couplers available, with a set of nine in the behavioral health area: history and comprehensive screening; anxiety, panic, and phobias; psychotic behavior; depressed feelings, fatigue, and apathy; depression management; personality problems; suicidal thinking and behavior; male erectile dysfunction; and obsessive-compulsive disorders. Each Coupler is based on an extensive literature review and is updated as new research knowledge grows. At the time of this review there was no information available specific to the extent of use or effectiveness of these behavioral health Couplers.

Information is stored in a dBase-compatible file using FoxPro indexing. Each record contains patient and provider identification, date/time stamps, and space for optional free-text comments. Any patient information can be retrieved to add or delete findings, and old information can be stored without being overwritten. The output can be on hard copy that is then incorporated in the paper medical record, or the system can be integrated within a computer-based medical record. Information can also be exported into other PC applications such as Word, WordPerfect, Excel, and any OLE-compliant applications. The system can run on a laptop or desktop (386 CPU or better) machine and requires at least 20 megabytes of available hard disk space. The system can also be operated on a LAN or WAN network, allowing rapid communication among staff who may be involved in the patient's care.

The price structure in the first year is based on covered lives or number of providers who use the system. Pricing includes installation, training, and support. In subsequent years users pay a subscription fee to continue to receive updates and new Couplers.

Criteria for Selecting a DSS

Now that we have examined decision making in behavioral healthcare, and reviewed some of the DSSs currently available, it is time to think about how one decides whether to purchase a DSS and, if so, which one. Many considerations come into play in such a decision, some of them economic, but we will consider here some of the more substantive issues you should take into account.

What Decision Will the DSS Help You With?

Is the DSS designed to help with diagnosing, treatment planning, determining level of care, or following practice guidelines? Is it intended to support the clinician in terms of making his or her work better or easier, is it intended to help the provider organization achieve more consistency or efficiency in services it provides, or will it do both? If the system is designed to benefit the organization, will the clinician users view this as important and will they use it? It is important to bring clinicians into the decision to use a DSS, at least to the extent that they understand why it is being implemented and how it will ultimately benefit the organization and its consumers.

What Is the Basis (Validity) for the Decision Support?

Many DSSs include a model base component, as described earlier. This might be an expert system rule base, a decision tree to help with diagnoses, or a set of practice standards against which the clinician's work is being compared.

It is important to understand the basis for the decision advice. Is it based on normative data, empirical studies, or expert opinion? Or is the model base that is embedded in the DSS mandated by organizational policy, such as standards for care or critical clinical pathways? Whatever the philosophical or empirical basis for the DSS, one must consider whether it is compatible with and acceptable to the providers who will be using it, and whether it meets accepted standards of professional practice.

Is the DSS Compatible with Your Existing Data Base?

To be effective, a behavioral health DSS must be compatible with existing clinical data required to arrive at the needed decision-making advice. Some DSSs are stand-alone systems that ask the user to input the necessary information. Others may have the capacity to access existing clinical information so long as it is stored in a compatible data base. Thus it is important to know whether the DSS can access existing records, end up duplicating already existing record-keeping systems, or actually require the organization to convert to a different record-keeping system altogether. One should think not only about how the DSS will interface with the organization's current information system but also whether it will be adaptable to future needs.

How Will the DSS Work in Day-to-Day Practice?

This is a more practical (and subjective) concern. How will clinicians or patients use the DSS? Will it fit in naturally and unobtrusively with their practice and office environment, or does it impose too much user burden? Will clinicians find that the benefits of using the DSS justify any inconveniences or time costs in using it? When it comes right down to it, will they use it?

Historically, clinicians have been slow to adopt computerization aids in the delivery of human services. A DSS may have value, but only if it will be used. For this reason, it is often important to involve clinicians in deciding whether to use a DSS, and if so, which one.

Will the Benefits of the DSS Outweigh Its Costs?

Using a DSS will most certainly entail some costs along with the presumed benefits. It is important to anticipate realistically what the costs of using a DSS will be. Of course, costs include purchase of the DSS software itself and the equipment to run it, and any ongoing software support costs as well as equipment maintenance. What is often overlooked, however, is the time needed initially to train staff as well as the time needed for ongoing training and support. Also, it is vital to determine if use of the DSS will require clinicians or other staff to devote additional time to their cases and related responsibilities.

On the plus side, what tangible benefits can the organization expect from using the DSS? Will it result in improved care for clients in terms of more immediate or longer lasting results, or improved consumer satisfaction? Will the DSS help the organization avoid costly mistakes and legal costs? Will it reduce the length of care? Will it maximize matching the treatment to the client?

It is useful to attach actual dollar values to the anticipated costs and benefits for implementing a DSS, so you can see clearly if the system will be worthwhile overall to your organization.

Future Directions for DSS in Behavioral Health

Up to this point, we have focused on the current state of the art in DSSs for behavioral health practitioners. Decision support is a rapidly developing area, however, so we want to consider some directions we can expect to see in the not-too-distant future.

DSS Technology Will Become More Powerful

Decision support technology, as well as computer technology in general, will develop rapidly during the next decades. Much of this development will come in the form of refinements and extensions of the types of DSSs we see today. Expert systems technology is certain to become more powerful. For example, we can expect to see new methods and tools for "mining and refining" practice expertise and representing it in rule bases that expert systems can use.

As alluded to above, neural-network computing technology will likely have a major impact on behavioral health practice. Compared with conventional digital computers, neural network computers are in their infancy. And compared with the sophistication of biologically based neural structures, neural networks are extremely limited and primitive. However, if neural computers are able to perform complex (and humanlike) information processing activities such as understanding human speech, reaching reliable conclusions in the face of incomplete information, and recognizing patterns in unstructured data, they can have an enormous impact on behavioral health practice. Computers will be able to respond to spoken commands from the user rather than requiring keyboard input, which will make them easier and less obtrusive to use. They will be able to advise on diagnosis and treatment even though information may not be complete. Perhaps most importantly, neural computers will be able to help us detect patterns in large client data bases that will enable us to make more accurate and reliable assessments and develop more specific treatments for selected conditions.

Behavioral Health Practice Will Become More Standardized

A major impediment to the use of DSSs in behavioral health has been the lack of standardization in clinical data. Compared with the financial and retailing industries, which have become heavily automated in recent years, behavioral health has a very limited nomenclature with which to describe diagnoses, treatments, or clinical outcomes. Continuing research is likely to lead to a better understanding of various mental health problems and the treatments that are effective for each, and this knowledge will lead to more standardization in clinical assessment and treatment planning. As our diagnostic and treatment protocols become more proceduralized, clinical decision making will lend itself more and more to DSSs.

The Types and Applications of DSSs Will Proliferate

As DSSs improve, and as they demonstrate their value in behavioral health practice, we can expect to see their numbers and applications increase. Users will be able to select from a number of competing DSSs to aid in DSM-IV diagnoses, for example. Some DSSs will be small, inexpensive, stand-alone systems that run on ordinary microcomputers, whereas others will be large, custom-designed systems tailored specifically to the needs of large networks or companies. As their use increases, and the competition among DSS developers becomes keener, we will see more powerful DSSs that are easier to use.

DSSs Will Be Used to Encode and Disseminate Best Practices

As behavioral health practice becomes more standardized, and DSS technology improves, we will see DSSs used increasingly to encode best practices, such as diagnostic protocols and treatment guidelines. This will be particularly advantageous for large organizations and networks that wish to standardize their practice and keep current with the latest treatment knowledge. For example, as new treatments for depression become available, developers of the treatment-planning DSS can distribute updated versions of the software that incorporate the new treatment in recommendations, and provide explanations to the practicing clinician. Had such a system been available for advising on diagnoses, it no doubt would have eased and quickened the transition from DSM-III-R to DSM-IV.

Managed Behavioral Healthcare Will Increasingly Rely on DSSs

As DSSs become more capable and demonstrate their value in providing high quality healthcare, providers will increasingly be expected to use them. For example, managed care companies, particularly the large and highly integrated companies who hire their own clinical staff, will probably use expert systems to handle routine authorizations for treatment. Only exceptional cases would be reviewed by a case manager. If a DSS has been shown to improve reliability and consistency in diagnosing, providers may be required to use it to justify authorization for treatment. Similarly, as practice standards become established for various diagnostic groupings, providers will be expected to demonstrate that they meet those standards.

Use Issues for DSSs Will Continue

As DSSs demonstrate their usefulness in behavioral health decision making, there will be a growing tendency to use them to do more than *support* the decision maker.

They may come to *replace* the decision maker instead. As was noted above, DSSs were originally designed to support the decision maker by serving as a memory-jogging aid or by processing large amounts of information. The user (the clinician) is assumed to have the expertise to evaluate the advice being given by the DSS and determine whether that advice is suitable for the decision at hand.

Clearly, there will be situations when the DSS recommends a course of action which is beyond the expertise of the user to evaluate, for example a DSS that could advise an emergency telephone hotline counselor on the caller's risk of suicide. Should the counselor be permitted to use the DSS if she is unable on her own to make such an assessment or evaluate the quality of the assessment the DSS has made? Already expert systems have been shown to be as good as or better than humans in making diagnostic assessments. As the demand for quality healthcare increases and the need to contain costs continues, there will be increasing pressure to have untrained personnel using DSSs make decisions that go beyond their capability.

A related issue has to do with legal liability concerns when using a DSS. It is not clear whether the courts will view DSSs as simply tools to be used in professional practice and therefore subject to negligence or medical malpractice law, or whether they will be seen as medical devices or products and be subject to strict liability law. Thus it is not clear what liability the practitioner incurs if he or she uses a DSS. Interestingly, at such time as DSS use has become the standard of care in a given community, a practitioner could potentially be held responsible if he or she did *not* use a DSS and the patient was harmed.

Until liability issues are resolved, the prudent practitioner should use a DSS only if he or she understands the basis for the recommendations it makes and can determine that the DSS is valid for the decision-making task at hand. Thus, it is important that the DSS be able to give a clear explanation of its advice so the user can evaluate it. This does not relieve the developer of the DSS of responsibility for validating the advice a DSS gives. Research has shown that clinicians tend to accept erroneous advice if the explanations are good, whereas they reject correct advice if the explanations are weak or poorly expressed.

◆ ◆ ◆

We have concluded our discussion of decision support systems by looking to the future and trying to anticipate how DSSs will come to be used in behavioral healthcare. It is difficult to know exactly what capabilities DSSs will come to have and how they will be used in practice, since DSS technology is still in its infancy. But it is clear that we will see an increasing role for DSSs in behavioral health practice, and as that occurs it will be incumbent on managers and clinicians to ensure that DSSs are used appropriately and contribute to the quality of care.

Notes

P. 12, *U.S. Bureau of the Census:* Deitel, H. M., & Deitel, B. (1985). *Computers and data processing.* New York: Academic Press.

P. 12, *large financial institutions:* Silver, M. S. (1991). *Systems that support decision makers.* New York: Wiley.

P. 13, *decision support systems were born:* Silver, M. S. (1991). *Systems that support decision makers.* New York: Wiley.

P. 13, *relatively unstructured problems:* Gorry, G. A., & Scott Morton, M. S. (1971). A framework for management information systems. *Sloan Management Review, 13,* 55–70.

P. 13, *solve unstructured problems:* Sprague, R. H., & Carlson, E. D. (1982). *Building effective decision support systems.* Reading, MA: Addison-Wesley.

P. 13, *the essential characteristics of DSSs include the following:* Vogel, L. H. (1985). Decision support systems in the human services: Discovering limits to a promising technology. *Computers in Human Services, 1,* 67–79.

P. 14, *three basic components:* Holsapple, C. W., & Whinston, A. B. (1987). Artificially intelligent decision support systems—Criteria for tool selection. In C. W. Holsapple and A. B. Whinston (Eds.), *Decision support systems: Theory and application* (pp. 185–213). Berlin: Springer-Verlag; Sage, A. P. (1991). *Decision support systems engineering.* New York: Wiley.

P. 15, *help with treatment planning:* Modai, I., & Rabinowitz, J. (1993). Why and how to establish a computerized system for psychiatric case records. *Hospital and Community Psychiatry, 44,* 1091–1095.

P. 15, *predict future behavior:* Miller, M. E., Langefeld, C. D., Tierney, W. M., Hui, S. L., & McDonald, C. J. (1993). Validation of probabilistic predictions. *Medical Decision Making, 13,* 49–58.

P. 15, *making a psychiatric diagnosis:* First, M. B., Opler, L. A., Hamilton, R. M., Linder, J., Linfield, L. S., Silver, J. M., Toshav, N. L., Kahn, D., Williams, J.B.W., & Spitzer, R. L. (1993). Evaluation of an inpatient setting of DTREE, a computer-assisted diagnostic assessment procedure, *Comprehensive Psychiatry, 34,* 171–175.

P. 16, *specified problem area:* Waterman, D. A. (1986). *A guide to expert systems.* Reading, MA: Addison-Wesley; Gingerich, W. J. (1995). Expert systems. In R. L. Edwards (Ed.), *Encyclopedia of social work* (19th ed.) (pp. 917–925). Washington, DC: NASW Press.

P. 16, *organism is not group-D:* Buchanan, B. G., & Shortliffe, E. H. (Eds.). (1984). *Rule-based expert systems: The MYCIN experiments of the Stanford Heuristic Project* (p. 86). Reading, MA: Addison-Wesley.

P. 17, *structure of biological systems:* Caudill, M., & Butler, C. (1990). *Naturally intelligent systems.* Cambridge, MA: MIT Press.

P. 17, *psychiatric emergency room:* Somoza, E., & Somoza, J. R. (1993). A neural-network approach to predicting admission decisions in a psychiatric emergency room. *Medical Decision Making, 13,* 273–280.

P. 18, *state psychiatric hospital:* Davis, G. E., Lowell, W. E., & Davis, G. L. (1993). *M.D. Computing, 10,* 87–92.

P. 18, *evaluating past choices:* Simon, H. A. (1977). *The new science of management decision* (rev. ed.). New York: Harper and Row.

P. 20, *Although there are notable exceptions:* Beutler, L. E., & Williams, O. B. (1995). Computer applications for the selection of optimal psychosocial therapeutic interventions. *Behavioral Healthcare Tomorrow, 4,* 66–68; Barlow, D., & Barlow, D. (1995). Practice guidelines and empirically validated psychosocial treatments: Ships passing in the night? *Behavioral Healthcare Tomorrow, 4,* 25–29.

P. 23, *effectiveness of treatment:* COMPASS Information Services, 1060 First Avenue, Suite 410, King of Prussia, PA 19406, tel. 610–992–7070.

P. 24, *within the PsychPro system:* Psych Resources Group, Inc., 6 Devine St., North Haven, CT 06473, tel. 800–357–1200.

P. 25, *planning through practice guidelines:* Institute for Healthcare Quality, 8000 West 78th St., Minneapolis, MN 55439, tel. 800–241–4270.

P. 27, *provider-reviewer-payer continuum:* PsychAccess Care Delivery Systems, Community Sector Systems, 700 Fifth Ave., Suite 5500, Seattle, WA 98104, tel. 206–467–9061.

P. 28, *trigger treatment recommendations:* PATHware Inc., 316 Mooreland Rd., Kensington, CT 06037, tel. 203–225–8245.

P. 30, *patient care management strategies:* PKC Corporation, One Mill St., Box A8, Burlington, VT 05401–1530, tel. 802–658–5351.

P. 36, *strict liability law:* Shortliffe, E. H. (1987). *Journal of the American Medical Association, 258,* 61–66.

P. 36, *weak or poorly expressed:* Shortliffe, E. H. (1995). When decision support doesn't support. *Medical Decision Making, 15,* 187–188.

CHAPTER THREE

THE USE OF COMPUTERS IN THERAPY

Roger L. Gould

This chapter is about the use of computers as psychotherapeutic agents, a concept that is foreign to most therapists, anathema to many, and mystifying to most who have not used such programs.

The image of a computer as plastic, metal, wired, and impersonal is in strong contrast to a patient's positive expectation of a therapist as a warm, intelligent, caring helper experienced in the mysteries of the unconscious mind. When we consider how hard it is to understand the complexity of any single life, how impossible it is at times to get through a patient's resistance to change or fully understand the meaning of what is being said, and how difficult it is to interpret accurately and therapeutically what is not being said . . . how can we expect a computer to do what therapists manage to do?

The answer to these questions is simple. A computer, or more accurately, a computer program, cannot do what a therapist can do. A computer program cannot even "understand" natural language sufficiently well to reliably engage in the process, although much progress has been made in this area during the last thirty years and that element may soon be ready. But even when language understanding is available, the issue of human intelligence being of a different order and kind than machine intelligence will always be the basis for the gap between any program and a human therapist. That said, we can rest easy that therapists will not be recreated in purely electronic form.

However, therapists may still have to worry about being partially displaced in some circumstances. Computer programs can perform some functions that therapists cannot. Ken Colby expressed this quite well in 1980:

> The advantage[s] of a computer psychotherapist would be several. It does not get tired, angry, or bored. It is always willing to listen and to give evidence of having heard. It can work at any time of day or night, every day and every month. It does not have family problems. It does not try to perform when sick or hungover. It has no facial expressions of contempt, shock, surprise, etc. It is polite, friendly, and always has good manners. It is comprehensible and has a perfect memory. It does not seek money. It will cost only a few dollars a session. It does not engage in sex with its patients. It does what it is supposed to do and no more.

In addition to the above, computer programs can print accurate verbatim summaries that can be handed to the patient at the end of the session for review and homework so the therapeutic work can continue between sessions. When as therapists we stop worrying about being replaced or displaced, we can then begin to see what a powerful tool we have in our hands.

Do computers actually help patients do psychotherapeutic work? If so, are they effective? If effective, how do they do it? If therapists want to use such programs, which ones should they use, and with which patients? These are the questions we address in this chapter.

Early Efforts

The pioneers in the field, J. Weizenbaum and K. Colby, both demonstrated that the computer could deliver psychotherapeutic work defined as "to communicate an intent to help, as a psychotherapist does, and to respond as he does by questioning, clarifying, focusing, rephrasing and occasionally interpreting."

They used mainframe technology and a teletype-like machine. Patients typed in their input, the program responded, and this sequence was repeated for as long as the patient wished. The model behind the program was the interviewing technique of a Rogerian therapist or a stereotyped psychoanalyst. The attempt was truly to mimic specific aspects of human intelligence. It replaced the highly trained and highly skilled, theory- and experience-rich practitioner with a program that questioned and clarified—but did not utilize an explicit model of conflict or psychopathology or problem solving to inform that questioning and clarifying.

This was considered to be an artificial intelligence approach because the patient could type in anything (natural language) and the program utilized response rules to the natural language based on key words, sequences, and language structure as if it actually understood what was being stated.

This prototype was doomed to failure, however, because to carry it off would require a program that contained all of the experience, information, and judgment of a human being, not just the superficial language techniques that a therapist uses to intervene with a patient. Nevertheless, it was a noble experiment conducted in the early days of idealistic computing when artificial human intelligence was the holy grail. Weizenbaum abandoned this whole line of inquiry because he came to think it was morally incorrect to try to replace an empathic human relationship with a computer program. (Furthermore, he wisely concluded it was impossible to do it in the framework he was using.) His initial program, Eliza, is now available as a parlor game in the local software store.

The artificial intelligence approach of producing a program with full human knowledge has largely been abandoned and replaced by the more modest goal of creating expert systems. Colby has productively pursued his interest in the efficacy of the computer as a psychotherapeutic tool throughout his academic career, and in retirement he has produced a sophisticated natural language program expert system for PCs dealing with the topic of depression. He has built thousands of responses and response sequences of how he, as an expert, would reply to different kinds of typed-in entries, going far beyond previous superficial techniques and utilizing the implicit model of his own clinical thinking. His program is the best of its type, available to the general public as well as for professional use.

Although no true psychotherapy outcome studies accompanied these pioneering efforts, Colby and Weizenbaum did demonstrate that patients can accept the computer as a medium for thinking about personal problems, and that they do get some benefit out of a sustained period of thinking and sorting-out in response to the computer program. This reported benefit is consistent with the well-documented outcome benefits of something quite similar: sustained structured writing, as demonstrated by Lou L'abata. Sustained interior dialogue about a distressing issue is an implicit agency common to all therapies and can be mediated by a computer program that is designed to engage the user in an inner focus.

Think About What?

If a computer program is capable of helping a patient engage in prolonged inner dialogue, then questions arise: what should the subject matter of that dialogue be, and will different kinds of programs be necessary for different subject matters to cover the field of psychotherapy? When the focus is changed from free-form dialogue to learning how to master an important subject matter, a new way of using the computer is created. The computer is used for structured learning.

Although there were intermittent reports about using the computer for desensitization in the 1970s, the next major approach offering psychotherapy subject matter was reported by Morton Wagman in 1980. He developed the Dilemma Counseling System (which later became the commercial PLATO system). A dilemma is a decision-making conflict in which both or all solutions to a particular problem are accompanied by undesirable consequences. The principles of dilemma resolution are taught on the computer through a process that requires the user to formulate sample cases within the dilemma format. The program begins, in somewhat skeletal form, as follows:

> If I do action P, then unhappy consequence R will occur. And if I do action Q, then unhappy consequence S will occur. But I must do either action P or Q and therefore unhappy consequence R or S will occur.

Once the user has mastered the ability to reformulate a sample case into this format, he or she types in a personal situation and then reformulates it into this dilemma matrix. If that is done correctly, the user is then carried through a known route of extrication. The students who first used the program to work through their own personal dilemmas reported greater improvement than did the control group.

Although Wagman correctly puts his program in the category of psychoeducation rather than psychotherapy, it is an important milestone in this review. Wagman demonstrated the efficacy of a structured learning approach by starting with a model of the therapeutic work that had to be done by the patient and then designing a computer program that could help the patient do that work. It can also be argued that working through a dilemma is close to the core of psychotherapy. Even though the Dilemma Counseling System is a highly rational system for dealing with conscious problems, it also touches on the problems of reality testing and self-regulation that go deeper into the fabric of patients' lives.

While Wagman was developing his system, I was creating the Therapeutic Learning Program. This too starts from the point of view of the patient rather than the techniques of the therapist. It is founded on my theoretical and practical work in adult development. The subject matter is broad: changes, transitions, and movements through the life cycle. At its center is deciding on new or appropriate actions and the attendant developmental conflicts about taking action.

By 1980, the adaptational model of the Therapeutic Learning Program (TLP) was completely worked out in detail—prior to even the thought of a computer program. It was a model derived from my clinical experiences, my work in adult development, and the culmination of a project to create a learning model. As such, it was an experiential rather than highly abstract model. It was rich in detail and nuance because of its origin, yet structured by the explicit goal of translating that information into a learning model. As part of a learning model approach, we provided the patients with more responsibility for doing the processing of specific thought exercises, and with a workbook as a tool to guide them through the process. My central role as therapist was transformed into that of guide and facilitator as the workbook and the exercises became a more sophisticated and integrated program.

Moving from a paper-and-pencil structured program to a computer program seemed to be more of a natural next step than a major leap, with one exception. Our hope was that patients would use, and therapists would accept, the computer. As it happened, patients accepted the computer easily; approximately fourteen thousand have used it in treatment over the past fifteen years. However, therapists are just beginning to accept this and other computer-assisted therapy programs as a legitimate adjunctive tool for psychotherapy.

The Cognitive-Behavioral Approach

The first approach to using the computer as a psychotherapeutic agent was with natural language and artificial intelligence. The second was the structuring and elaboration of action dilemmas specific to a person's daily life. The third was the cognitive-behavioral approach, which formed the basis of several programs in the 1980s and early 1990s.

Some cognitive-behavioral programs are automated desensitization protocols for various phobias, the best known being the highly successful programs for agoraphobia by Isaac Marks in England. Even though the subject matter in his programs is not explicit decision making about how to conduct one's life on an ongoing basis, the programs do promote an implicit inner dialogue about the patient's deeper issues of life course with respect to coping with perceived danger.

The cognitive-behavioral approach focuses on a specified set of symptoms and stays within a purposely delimited sphere of the person's life. This approach is part of the basic strategy of this theoretical orientation, carried over into the computer program. Aaron Beck's cognitive therapy of depression represents the more cognitive end of the cognitive-behavioral spectrum. It begins with a focus on depressive symptoms and then moves into the patient's beliefs and deeper thought patterns and assumptions about life related to the depressive syndrome. There is a depth and delimitation of focus simultaneously.

P. M. Selmi created a computer program based on Beck's work and reported on a small sample. The program was judged to be as effective as a therapist for the treatment of depression. Jesse Wright and Beck have just announced a CD-ROM program for training and treatment, utilizing live-action video demonstrations. Effective programs have been built for phobias, depression, anxiety, sexual dysfunction, and the control of obsessive-compulsive symptoms.

In these programs, the patient characteristically works alone at a keyboard and follows a programmed set of instructions that would otherwise have been provided by the therapist. The therapist is consulted at the beginning (assignment to the program), at the end, and as needed in between. Marks tells how he discovered patients who were recovering from agoraphobia after reading the instructor's manual for desensitization treatment for this disorder. That was when he decided to put the manual on computer. Although his program has been refined over time, it is essentially a computerization of what a cognitive-behavioral therapist is taught to do to facilitate patients' gradual exploration of their fears through safe, controlled, and small action steps.

Other programs focus on self-regulation in the areas of eating, smoking, and drinking. Each of these programs specializes in a piece of the therapeutic enterprise and uses cognitive and behavioral approaches to help the patient learn and apply concepts, monitor behavior, and practice skills designed to increase competency in the area of focus. The programs are built on well-known and well-worked-out protocols focusing on what the patient has to learn and do to improve.

The preexisting highly structured and topic-delimited approach of cognitive-behavioral therapy is ideal for translation into a computer program. The rules are already explicit (in contrast to the practice of most psychotherapy, where the rules are implicit), and the process is perceived by patients as conducting therapeutic work. We will undoubtedly see many more of these cognitive-behavioral programs in the future, focusing on symptoms or disease entities.

How Do These Programs Work?

We have described three large-scale historical approaches to doing computer-assisted psychotherapeutic work. Now we look more closely into how these programs are designed and how they facilitate work.

These programs are all forms of mediated therapeutic communications. Some are delivered as stand-alone educational programs, while others are done under the supervision of a therapist as part of a total therapeutic program. A sparse published literature explains in depth how these programs work. Here I use observations about the Therapeutic Learning Program, especially the elements it has in common with other computer-assisted therapy programs, to illustrate how these programs can work to enhance patient care. From that base, we can speculate about the other designs and forms of delivery.

Therapeutic Learning Program

The Therapeutic Learning Program (TLP) is a ten-session computer course which helps participants define a problem, propose an action solution, and resolve their conflict about taking action. In each session the patient spends about one-half hour alone with an interactive computer program, receives a printout, and talks immediately thereafter with a therapist, either individually or in a group session. The printout is the basis for the discussion with the therapist and focuses the treatment process into a series of decisions. The decisions at each stage are made by the patient after discussion with the therapist, and the patient is then ready to go on to the next session. A typical decision would be to prioritize problems at the end of the first session in order to work on one problem at a time, and to prioritize action solutions at the end of the second session in order to focus on a particular action conflict.

The TLP is therapy conducted by a professional therapist. The goal is to remove symptoms through a change in perspective, which comes about through clarification and decision making. It is somewhat different from conventional forms of therapy inasmuch as it is short-term rather than prolonged. Also, interventions from the therapist are not provided through transference interpretations, but rather through help in distinguishing adaptations that were effective in the past from present realities, and rational from irrational thinking.

When the patient is working with the interactive program directly, she is really having a private, controlled, interpersonal relationship with the designer of the program. The program represents a condensation of years of therapeutic experience, designed into a very explicit model and then translated into a computer program. The intelligence of the designer-therapist is built into the program and available to the patient. Since other consultants have contributed their wisdom and experience to the program, the TLP can be said to contain the learning from over one hundred years of clinical experience. In this sense, the patient is having a phantom interpersonal conversation with a collective clinical other.

The TLP program has been designed to help the patient have a self-reflective experience, and in particular to create a "cleavage plane" between a rational contemporary part of the self and a conflicting part of the self dominated by an irrational past history. The participants in the TLP report that they very quickly forget about the program and computer because they become so intrigued with their own internal drama. Their emotions are stimulated, and they become inward-focused, self-absorbed, and involved in a very intense self-reflective training process. In this sense, the person is having a private experience in which the medium is largely obliterated from emotional consciousness. We use special programming techniques, particularly the use of patients' favored language patterns, to facilitate this self-reflective internal process.

So far we might summarize the process from the patient's point of view as beginning with a phantom interpersonal relationship with the program designer. It quickly leads to an articulated intrapersonal dialogue between facilitative and inhibitory aspects of the self as the patient considers an action-oriented decision that represents a new developmental behavior.

When the patient completes the interactive portion of the program at the end of each module, she receives a printout. The printout documents everything that was learned in the interaction, including all of the distinctions between rational and irrational thinking that the person discovered. The format of the printout is straightforward; its skeleton reinforces the model of learning and allows for the specifics of the individual user.

The printout also reflects the patient's words and choice of language. The most commonly reported experience from the user is, "That's exactly what I'm thinking, but I could never had said it more clearly or as exactly!" The program and the printout help patients become more articulate, focused, and clear thinking than they could possibly have been on their own in the same amount of elapsed time (about thirty minutes). In particular, the distinction between current perceptions and past distortions is clearly made. If it is not totally accurate, the therapist and patient can correct it in pen or pencil by crossing out what is incorrect and substituting what is more correct. This printout is a very important part of the process; patients frequently refer back to it in between sessions as well as use it as a discussion piece with their therapist.

In this document, the work to be accomplished by patient and therapist is subtly laid out so that the essential activities of the therapeutic relationship are helpfully contained. This serves several purposes. On the one hand it helps the patient think more clearly because she does not have to understand and articulate all her thoughts but only deal with that which is essential at a particular step in the process. It also gives the patient confidence that she can talk intelligently with a trained therapist without feeling overwhelmed by the therapist's education and experience. It helps to democratize the interpersonal relationship and convert the therapist from a potential magical guru into a teacher who can help with a specific learning task.

Because the patient only has to master one specific point in the process at the moment of interaction, the dependence of the patient on the therapist is diminished and her self-confidence is increased. This leads to less resistance and more open communication and revelation than would otherwise take place in unmediated communication.

For example, a therapist may have spent as little as ten or fifteen minutes with the patient in the first two sessions, yet have an almost complete working knowledge of all the things that are bothering the patient, how the major issues should be prioritized, what the symptoms are, the exact statement of the patient's perceptions, the patient's acknowledged inability to cope in specific areas, the ineffective patterns, a choice of multiple action options, ideal areas in which the patient needs to develop, exact action statements, and healthy motives for carrying out the intended action. It would literally be impossible for this much information to be gathered and shared without the use of such a medium as the computer program.

This medium makes the interpersonal relationship between the patient and the therapist different. The patient is better prepared, less dependent, looking for a different kind of help, and more articulate. The therapist is also different: face-to-face with a different kind of patient, with a less global responsibility, guided by the focus and the model, having a tool to help do some of the insight and clarification work, and having an infinitely greater amount of information available in a recorded and usable fashion than would otherwise be the case.

The therapist becomes a teacher and is relieved of the burdensome role of guru. However, the therapist still achieves the one important goal of ideal psychoanalytic communication: to demonstrate to the patient how her life is dominated by reified internal object-controlled irrational patterns.

This process of working on the computer, getting a printout, and having an interpersonal relationship with a therapist is repeated for each of the ten steps in the process. The patient gets deeper into her intrapersonal dialogue as the modules advance into deeper psychological issues. As the issues become deeper, that is, more emotionally powerful and related to earlier training patterns, the patient gets involved in more intense and emotionally cathected states of mind. Usually, in conventional unmediated treatment, this leads to a greater dependency on the therapist for guidance. But in the TLP, this does not occur because the patient becomes progressively more skilled in making distinctions about rational and irrational processes and is able to work with the programmed "lessons" as learning topics, without being overwhelmed.

As an example of the kinds of issues that are then dealt with, the question of one's negative self-esteem, the weakest and most vulnerable part of the psyche, is the subject matter for the whole second half of the course. When patients gain a new perspective on these deep fears, they become more independent and more anchored to their current time frame. They are then ready to leave the TLP course with a greater sense of control.

Cognitive-Behavioral Programs

Those cognitive-behavioral programs that are used in conjunction with a therapist will share most of the process characteristics described above, but in a slightly different way that reflects other goals and strategies.

Certainly all programs in this category mediate an internal dialogue during the time the patient is actually using the computer program. That dialogue will be about the subject matter. If the program is about desensitization of a phobia, the dialogue will be about fear.

The internal dialogue is indirect and implicit, but the actual work on the computer is concrete, specific, and oriented around taking "homework-assigned" actions that will prove to the patient that the fear sensation is not grounded in current reality. The patient follows a desensitization schedule upon which he must act that may be combined with relaxation exercises during the interactive program or off-line. To the degree that the patient experiences the phobic symptoms as sufficiently representative of his life problems, he will see the program as a substitute for the therapist and will have achieved a measure of self-empowerment. To the degree that the patient does not see the phobic symptoms as representative of all other immediate problems, the patient's dependence on the therapist remains and the shifting of the relationship described above does not occur. On the other hand, since symptoms are basically like pain centers, working on those pain centers directly and experiencing relief when applying the methodology is extremely rewarding and gives the user a heightened sense of self-mastery.

The period in between sessions is an important aspect of most cognitive-behavioral programs; it is when the patient practices what has been learned and monitors his progress. The patient's full participation in the practice prescription with the help of the expert system replacing the live therapist should lead to a heightened motivation to do the exercises. If the patient does not connect deeply with the contents of the program on a personal level, that motivation will be diminished.

This is where the design of an experience-near program becomes important. The patient, to be maximally motivated by the program, must not only have faith in the integrity and expertise of the program but must also feel that the program is about him or her. This can be difficult for some patients to do in a cognitive-behavioral program because for certain types of patients the strength of the program (well-structured protocols based on clear concepts of learning) can also be a weakness. For those who learn easily from a conceptual starting point, a well-written program will be experienced as related to them because they can easily translate from concept to personal experience. But if that is not easy for a patient, the difference between a program and a live therapist becomes apparent. A live therapist makes the translation for the patient and thereby makes the concepts come alive and the program relevant.

There is another difficulty. Current computer programs in cognitive therapy do not go as deeply into the life assumption structure as cognitive therapists do in actual practice. According to Beck, "Structural change extends beyond modifying the cognitive errors associated with the specific syndrome to changing the underlying organization of rules, formulas, and assumptions that misclassify events as threatening or upsetting." Current cognitive-behavioral computer programs do not yet go beyond the introduction and practice of the cognitive errors associated with the specific symptoms.

Despite these qualifications, the cognitive-behavioral structured learning programs promote most of the same patient processes that the TLP structured learning approach utilizes for therapeutic benefit. There is a shift in the relationship between therapist and patient from dependent to adult learner. The patient is provided with a set of concepts, an opportunity to practice those concepts, a printout, and new skills in making distinctions between rational and irrational thought processes in the content domain of the program. The programs also help the patient attend to and monitor their actions and observations over time.

Computer-Based Self-Help Programs

When programs are offered to the public without the intercession and supervision of a therapist, these same elements will be available for patients' learning and processing independently. However, no process studies have been reported to date that explain how self-help improvement occurs. Nevertheless, the outcome studies that have been done strongly suggest that many patients can improve substantially using these programs without the intervention of a therapist. That should not be too surprising, since many patients are aided by self-help books, learn anxiety-reduction techniques in classes, and change their behavior and outlook following deaths, rejections, and disappointments.

H. Eysenck suggests that depression is often abated within two years without treatment, while psychotherapy speeds up the self-healing process so that relief occurs in an average of six months. If psychotherapy is a specialized form of learning that accelerates and acts on a natural healing process, then self-help aides such as computer programs and books also fall into the same category. Which form of intervention or combination of interventions is best for which patients and under which circumstances is the real issue to study.

Understanding the Design Elements of a Psychotherapeutic Program

Understanding some of the more granular elements of psychotherapeutic programs may help the practitioner choose the type best suited for a particular patient.

The cognitive-behavioral programs all have several design elements in common. Concepts about the subject matter, dysfunction, or symptom complex are presented, and some type of simple feedback test is applied to be sure the patient understands what is being taught. Then exercises are used to help deepen the understanding. These exercises may begin with a hypothetical case example, and then invite the user to type in her own example. This sequence will be repeated for each concept constituting the learning in the subject matter domain.

A frequent addition to the design of these programs is the ability to monitor and report progress from session to session. Decision-based homework assignments are usually added to these cognitive-behavioral computer programs. The individual answers questions. An algorithm is applied to create a printout, which is basically a homework assignment asking the individual to make observations and answer more questions. This element is surprisingly powerful. When a therapist leaves a patient thinking about an issue at the end of a face-to-face therapeutic session, the therapist is asking the patient to do some continuing thinking work between sessions. This simple exercise does the same thing: it extends the therapeutic work into the intersession period and enables the patient to be a fuller participant in her own care. The important design is in asking the right questions to keep the work moving forward. The algorithm that generates the questions is usually quite simple.

This cognitive-behavioral element is best exemplified in Selmi's program, which uses Beck's method. Practitioners would choose this program for patients who have a well-defined clinical syndrome, especially when the symptoms pertain more to dysfunctional thoughts and less to immediate events or problems in the patient's life. The same comments apply to similar programs for anxiety and sexual dysfunction.

The "Life in Progress" Level

In contrast, a clinician might choose the Therapeutic Learning Program to carry out a short-term therapy approach based on problems in living, adaptation, and developmental considerations. To approach problems-in-living on a broad scale, different design elements are necessary than those used in the cognitive-behavioral model described above. First of all, the patient must be guided through a problem-solving sequence that starts with a very exact and precisely worded problem statement in an experience-near, rather than conceptual, language. The patient must be able to feel that it is his or her problem, not a problem from a catalog.

This is a very difficult programming task. Defining a problem in a real-life setting is not all that simple. If a person reports anger at his boss, is that the problem? Or is it the marital stress at home that puts him on edge before and after work? Or is the accompanying depression that leads to poor performance at work the problem? If any of these categories are determined to be the problem, are the category and subtype sufficiently developed so that we have enough properly framed information to begin to consider action options?

We address this question by having the computer program control the structuring of the problem statement to include all the essential elements. We connect the problem context and content to the psychological pain that drives the person to attempt change. We also point the client to the goal he or she hopes to achieve by successfully working through the problem. This is usually the satisfaction of some important but frustrated need.

For example, an employee is depressed; his performance is deteriorating; he complains about his authoritarian boss and a stressful home life. He already has several problems to describe and a number of frustrated needs to get on the table. By the time he finishes the second half of the first computer session, we have several potentially workable problems to choose from. He will be able to consider all of them in print even before starting the first session with the counselor.

One prototypical problem statement for our sample employee might be, "I'm having tension with my boss, who overpowers me and doesn't listen to me. This makes me feel crushed and depressed. This pain tells me I'm not getting respect and the opportunity I need to express myself."

If work is really the problem, then the employee with the perceived-to-be-authoritarian boss may truly have a difficult boss. On the other hand, he may instead just have a challenging employment situation complicated by a highly focused and demanding manager in a company that is downsizing and reengineering its operations.

The client has to consider whether his need for respect and self-expression is being frustrated totally by his boss, or by patterns within himself that he needs to change, or some combination of both. In either case, he is in the midst of an adaptational challenge.

It is easy to see that once one takes on the task of "thinking along" with the patient on a problem of living, the interactive software can quickly get into a level of complexity that is quite daunting. Once a problem is identified and probed and the final statement is produced, a new series of issues have to be sorted out before an appropriate action step can be agreed upon.

One of the problems we encountered in the creation of the TLP is that the concepts we use in psychotherapy do not readily lend themselves to prescriptions. Instead, they provide general guidelines. The linkage between these guidelines and specific prescriptions is provided by the intelligence of the therapist using her own life experience, common sense, and discriminant-thinking capacities. That is also the material used for interactive software programming in computer-assisted therapy. It cannot be derived solely from textbooks or formal training materials.

Therefore, when the practitioner chooses to have her patients use a computer-assisted therapy program, she is choosing to use another clinical intelligence to work with the patient on the same level that psychotherapy usually takes place. As long as the practitioner agrees with the clinical intelligence built into the program, then the practitioner has rented an auxiliary therapist self to carry some of the burden of treatment. If the practitioner does not agree with the model and the program, then obviously she should not use the program since it will only confuse the patient.

As new programs come on the market, it is important to evaluate them on the basis of their programmed clinical sense, the quality of their attempt to think along with the patient, their degree of acceptance of the real complexity of the human situation, and their engagement with the multiple meanings of common terms.

For example, *guilt* is a commonly used word and concept which has at least seven different meanings. *Fear of success* or *fear of failure* can be broken down into thirty-three different subvarieties. In order to ask the initial questions about any feeling of guilt or feelings of failure or success, one has to know explicitly what the patient is responding to. Therefore, one has to use hierarchical menus and several branches just to pinpoint the particular meaning of an answer. Once the meaning is derived, the response to the answer has to be created. This is a lot of work, but it has to be done if the computer is going to reflect accurately what the patient is thinking and respond with useful insights and follow-up questions.

Are Resistances to the Use of Computers in Psychotherapy Justified?

Although computer therapy and computer-assisted therapy programs have existed and been studied for over thirty years, very few examples have come to market. Most have been products of university research that have demonstrated efficacy on a small, scientifically valid sample but have not borne the test of everyday clinical usage on a large scale. The TLP has been somewhat of an exception, although it too experiences obstacles to widespread acceptance.

Ten separate studies have been completed over the last decade on samples totaling roughly 15 percent of the patient population who used the TLP. Each study supports the conclusion that the TLP can be an effective adjunct to a short-term therapy program and help complete a therapeutic episode in seven sessions, with significant symptom reduction and improved functioning. Favorable comparisons have been made to a panel of clinicians who did not use the program, and the most recent study done at UCLA compared patients who received ten face-to-face therapy sessions with patients who only used the TLP. Both groups did equally well at six-month follow-up. In addition, one study strongly suggests that generalized learning continues for at least three years and that 65 percent of the users keep their printouts that long for reference in dealing with future problems in living.

In addition to the studies on the TLP, outcome studies have been conducted on the major cognitive-behavioral computer programs. There are striking findings in three studies that parallel the UCLA TLP study. Marks has demonstrated that at six-month follow-up severely agoraphobic patients do as well on a self-administered computer program as they do with a therapist. Selmi and J. Greist have demonstrated that depressed patients do as well at six-month follow-up as with a cognitive therapist. Several self-administered smoking cessation programs demonstrated abstinence rates equivalent to well-run live programs.

Consequently, there is a growing body of evidence that computers not only offer strong adjunctive treatments to ongoing therapy but are actually powerful substitutes for many. The patient accepts and utilizes the computer. Furthermore, all of the satisfaction studies in the literature, and our own reported and unreported studies, confirm that patients across treatment settings like using the computer. They find it helpful and easy to use. They tend to be more honest in their replies and more forthcoming with sensitive information when they are comfortable with the arrangements for confidentiality.

Resistance

Despite a decade of active marketing, verified results, patient acceptance, and professional and public articles about the availability of the program, the Therapeutic Learning Program and others have not been widely accepted. Also, no competitors have entered the field. I have been understandably puzzled about this state of affairs. Here are my observations.

Other than the usual computer phobia and hesitancy to learn new technology, there does not seem to be any significant resistance to the use of computers in the mental health field for a number of important functions such as billing, data base creation, managing risk, reports, and filling out the necessary forms for intake. There seems to be very little resistance now to computerized testing, assessment, and scoring of tests. The Minnesota Multiphasic Personality Inventory (MMPI) broke ground and established a precedent twenty years ago that has been followed to the point where now such use of the computer is generally accepted.

The boundary of this acceptance is quickly established when one begins to talk about computers as an adjunctive device to the process of psychotherapy. Then resistance often becomes immediate and visceral. Rational and irrational statements are commingled. When I first began lecturing on computer-assisted therapy, I would present a detailed description of the process, which always included a therapist. The patient worked on the computer, got a printout, spent a full session with a therapist, and repeated this up to ten times with our TLP.

I would mention this, show a slide of it happening, and present it on a chart. At the end of every lecture, someone would always ask the same question: "How can you condone the use of a computer without a therapist?" At least half the audience were shaking their heads in agreement with the questioner.

After I explained again that there was always a therapist present and that the computer was a tool to be used by both the therapist and the patient, a tool that helped prepare the patient for the therapy hour, there was some sigh of relief. My professional reputation was only temporarily reclaimed, however, because I am quite convinced that the half-life of my factual explanation was less than twenty minutes. During the first couple of years I believed that the aforementioned popular image of the computer as a piece of cold metal and plastic was so strong, so anti-intuitive, and so unusual to most of the audience that image dominated information.

As computers became more common and ubiquitous, I believe that this factor diminished over the years. However, other factors remain strong or have become more evident. I believe there are five primary factors in resistance to the use of computers in therapy:

1. Sanctity of the therapeutic relationship
2. Financial threat
3. A loss of rigor and quality
4. Organizational resistance
5. Patient resistance

Sanctity of the Therapeutic Relationship. There is a strong phenomenological basis for some of this resistance because it is difficult for people to conceive of the computer being useful in an intimate relationship, especially when they visualize the computer coming between the two people.

This perception can be quite strong, but it is not consistent with the actual sequential process of how computer-assisted therapy programs are used. The patient sits at the computer and, with the aid of menus and a guided thinking process organized by a computer program, begins to think about and work through problems-in-living methodically. The patient then receives a printout of the results of the work session and a copy of that printout is given to the therapist. They then sit down and talk.

There is no computer physically between the two of them. Nor is the computer program standing between them mentally. Instead, the computer program stimulated the patient's thought and therefore empowered the patient with vocabulary, ideas, concepts, and a story line that he developed to be explored further with the therapist's help in the intimate, one-to-one therapeutic setting. Oftentimes, the printout is used as a springboard at the beginning or a summary at the end of the session, or both. Therapists report a heightened intensity in these sessions. Patients report an intense, quick bond with and strong appreciation for the therapist. In fact, therapists consistently get higher marks than the computer program in satisfaction surveys.

Another argument against the use of computers in therapy cites research findings about the strong correlation between positive outcomes and a trusting patient-therapist relationship. This argument asserts that no patient could actually trust a computer as he or she would a therapist or other human being. However, our studies have shown that patients trust the computer more in combination with the therapist, and therefore the program serves to enhance the therapeutic relationship. But what is not said, and what is probably the most important element of the argument, is the implicit belief that the relationship itself is therapeutic.

There are many theories as to how the relationship itself is therapeutic. It provides patients with a first-hand experience to which they must adapt and to which the therapist brings special qualities of empathy and care that foster trust. But if we switch the emphasis from trust to adaptation and learning, it can easily be argued that during the course of the relationship patients learn something about themselves and about new ways of looking at and resolving problems-in-living. Then trust is the mediating factor and learning is the therapeutic factor. The fact that learning takes place within the relationship is the therapeutic ingredient.

Until this is pointed out, therapeutic trust is taken out of context and elevated to be the only therapeutic factor. Learning can take place in many ways and through many experiences, sometimes directly with people at home and at work, other times mediated through newspapers, television, movies, novels, self-help books—and potentially through the most powerful self-help modality of them all, the interactive computer.

Financial Threat. Another layer of resistance for some therapists is rooted in their fear of managed care, which is sweeping the country and negatively impacting the financial well-being of many treatment organizations and private practices. These therapists, already feeling threatened financially and professionally, fear computer-assisted therapy programs might be used to replace them, unduly regulate them, or require them to do more work.

This is a mixture of rational and irrational concerns. On the rational side, it's certainly possible that some managed care companies would adopt a computer program as a tool for therapist and patient and also require the therapist to do more short-term therapy within the constraints of the model. This is something that has to be fought against.

On the other hand, efficiencies are required in the medical field; we in the mental health field are not exempt from that requirement. Brief therapy is here to stay, and computer-assisted therapy is an efficient way of making use of human resources in the face of a large and unregulated need for services. But given the nature of human beings, and the explicit nature of the computer programs, it seems very unlikely that computers will ever replace human contact. The computer should be seen as a tool to augment services otherwise limited by economic constraints.

A Loss of Rigor and Quality. The more subtle argument regards the issue of rigor. Therapists are not usually supervised after having completed training. There is very little quality control over our services, unlike the quality control and quality management of medical and surgical services. We have been exempt partly because psychotherapy is seen as an idiosyncratic art form, and because it is difficult to apply the appropriate standards to the process of psychotherapy (although standards are applied to the outcome of psychotherapeutic interventions). Consequently, it is easy for us to rely on our experience and reputation and not constantly upgrade our knowledge and skills. Along comes a computer representing a clear and crisp thinking pattern and a specific model with interventions on the screen and in the printout that have been carefully thought through and coordinated. The computer program is an exemplar of rigor. As such, it presents a challenge to any therapist who, in his own mind, has not been as explicit in his cognitive approach as he might otherwise be.

Other legitimate arguments have to be taken into account before computer-assisted therapy can be widely used. One concern is that the computer program might be too narrowly focused and, consequently, might mislead the patient; instead of benefiting from clear thinking on a broad scale, the patient might be limited by the scope of thinking available on the computer program. This is an important design consideration, one of the reasons that computer-assisted therapy is computer-assisted therapy rather than computer therapy (that is, the printouts and work on the computer are supervised and talked over with a therapist to guard against this mishap). In the hands of a responsible therapist, the computer program affords a powerful combination. It requires a higher degree of rigor from the therapist, who now has more information available and must be sure that the patient's understanding of all this information is optimized. This requirement guards against the potential danger that therapists will lose their edge by letting the program do the work.

Organizational Resistance. There is often organizational resistance to adopting a new program, including problems with the purchase and installation of the hardware itself. The perceived hassle of dealing with computer hardware and software, printers and printouts can diminish the value of the intervention program from the point of view of professional administrators or therapists if the move is not handled well.

I remember our first experience at Harvard Community Health Plan, with senior professors down on their knees under a table, midway through a group session, trying to fix a jammed printer. One very distinguished professor with an imposing presence and a good sense of humor found himself in a situation that he would laugh at in retelling but never wants to repeat again.

Patient Resistance. Last but not least is the resistance of the patients. In our experience there was very little resistance from the patients, so long as the therapeutic staff felt the program was useful and helpful. When that sense was communicated by staff, in any of a number of ways, the patients typically began their work on the computer with some trepidation but within moments felt comfortable. After completing the first session, with only a few exceptions they were ready to continue.

Exceptions came when patients were particularly eager to capture a listening ear and unburden the story of their pain and suffering. When that need was very intense at the beginning of therapy or when the patient had a particularly strong dependency pattern, he or she would often request not to use the computer. This request is always granted in our clinics since the computer program is optional from the points of view of both therapist and patient.

Future Possibilities

When computer-assisted therapy programs are used widely in the mental health field, the profession derives distinct benefits for itself, for practice within a managed care setting, and for practice with the general public.

Benefits for Our Profession

Since most computer-assisted therapy programs integrate a therapeutic model, method, and form of delivery, research on the all-important questions of effectiveness and efficiency is easier to mount and more likely to result in clear-cut outcomes than we are accustomed to in this field.

Because the psychological work is spelled out in detail and is in the framework of psychological work accomplished by the patient, measurement of progress in the process can be accomplished and systematically played against outcome measures.

Because the therapist's work is described in detail and related explicitly to each step of the process, this all-important variable can finally be isolated in a relatively simple manner.

Having a commonly held model and method makes training of staff easier. Having a computer program and a therapist manual as teaching aides increases the reliability and replicability of training. Quality control can more naturally become an extension of the training mission.

The computer program serves as its own quality-control monitoring device. At the end of a series of treatment sessions, patients can enter a summary of their learning and an evaluation of the program and the process of their learning.

Benefits for Practice in a Managed Care Setting

The TLP can be considered as a workhorse program in managed care settings, where resources are limited and demand for services is high. This can be done without sacrifice of quality or patient satisfaction.

The model of adult development and the concept of developmental work units help therapists who are committed to brief treatment explain the rationale for their work to critics, who claim that brief treatment is just a new way of short-changing patients from what is "always" necessary, that is, long-term treatment.

One of the outstanding problems of mental healthcare in a managed care setting is the large case load of patients assigned to each therapist. With too many people to keep in mind, it is easy to be overloaded and resort to coping mechanisms that diminish the quality of care despite the best of intentions. Many computer-assisted therapy programs lend themselves to intensive group work and large psychoeducational class formats. Both of these mechanisms help relieve the load while providing intensive, quality care to the panel patient. Computer-assisted therapy can keep focused and record detailed interactions, leaving the therapist free to do what he or she does best.

It is very difficult to look into the crystal ball and arrive at a plausible scenario for the use of computer-assisted therapy in the mental health field. We have described the benefits, but the resistances outlined above are still present to a large degree.

Fortunately, the demand side is changing rapidly. If managed care leads inexorably to the lowest possible price, then an oversupply of underemployed practitioners may bend to pricing pressures with the result being inferior care. Worse, computer programs will be used as cheap fillers. If, on the other hand, employers demand higher-quality care efficiently and effectively delivered, then computer-assisted therapy will have an important future.

Benefits for Patients

An estimated 25 percent of the adult population are in need of psychological services. Only 3–5 percent of the population receives services during the course of a year. Where can the underserved 20 percent of the population go for help? There are articles in the daily press about how people are using "chat rooms" and bulletin boards to find support and help in resolving problems in living. Medical support groups and AA groups use online services regularly. People who would not ordinarily become patients are eager to find self-help tools.

I have been asked repeatedly about when I will provide online, interactive software directly to the public. I now have an answer. We have had a self-help service on Prodigy since September 1995. I anticipate our service will soon be only one of many. This is not therapy. We will not enter into a therapeutic contract or take clinical responsibility, but we will provide software and support to people who want to learn how to solve problems, improve their relationships, make decisions about their life course, and mature their perspectives and values. When we encounter users who are symptomatic, we will assist them in reaching out for professional help in their community.

I anticipate that this kind of service will proliferate. Although we plan to provide high-quality professional services, I suspect the lure of riches will entice many who have only a profit motive. We hope to open up this media to provide primary prevention in a way that we have all hoped to provide since the early days of the community mental health movement but have been unable to provide because of the barriers of cost, distribution, and disinterest.

We may be able to prevent problems, work out problems that do not need professional help, and help those in need to get the professional care that therapists have been trained to provide.

Notes

P. 40, *the advantage[s] of a computer psychotherapist:* Colby, K. M. (1980). Computer psychotherapists. In J. B. Sidowski, J. H. Johnson, & T. A. Williams (Eds.), *Technology in mental health care delivery systems* (pp. 109–117). Norwood, NJ: Ablex.

P. 40, *pioneers in the field:* Colby, K. M., Watt, J. B., & Gilbert, J. P. (1966). A computer method of psychotherapy: Preliminary communication. *Journal of Nervous and Mental Disease, 142,* 148–152; Weizenbaum, J. (1966). Eliza: A computer program for the study of natural language communication between man and machine. *Communications of the Association for Computer Machinery, 9,* 36–45.

P. 41, *sustained structured writing:* L'abata, L. (1992). *Programmed writing: A self-administered approach for interventions with individuals, couples, and families.* Pacific Grove, CA: Brooks/Cole.

P. 42, *intermittent reports about using the computer for desensitization:* Binik, Y. M., Servan-Schreiber, D., Freiwald, S., & Hall, K. S. (1988). Intelligent computer-based assessment and psychotherapy: An expert system for sexual dysfunction. *Journal of Nervous and Mental Disease, 176,* 387–400; Binik, Y. M., Westbury, C. F., & Servan-Schreiber, D. (1989). Interaction with a "sex-expert" system enhances attitudes toward computerized sex therapy. *Behaviour Research and Therapy, 27,* 303–306; Chandler, G. B., Burck, H., & Sampson, J. P. (1986). A generic computer program for systematic desensitization: Description, construction, and case study. *Journal of Behavior Therapy and Experimental Psychiatry, 17,* 171–174; Chandler, G. M., Burck, H., Sampson, J. P., & Wray, R. (1988). The effectiveness of a generic computer program for systematic desensitization. *Computers in Human Behavior, 4,* 339–346; Hedlund, J. L., Vieweg, B. W., Wood, J. B., Cho, D. W., Evenson, R. C., Hickman, C. V., & Holland, R. A. (1981). *Computers in mental health: A review and annotated bibliography* (DHHS Publication No. ADM 81–1090). Washington, DC: U.S. Government Printing Office; Lee, B. S., McGough, W. E., & Peins, M. (1976). Automated desensitization of stutterers to use of the telephone. *Behavior Therapy, 7,* 110–112.

P. 42, *approach offering psychotherapy subject matter:* Wagman, M. (1983). A factor analytic study of the psychological implications of the computer for the individual and society. *Behavior Research Methods & Instrumentation, 15,* 413–419.

P. 42, *the Dilemma Counseling System:* Wagman, M. (1984). *The dilemma and the computer: Theory and research foundations.* New York: Praeger.

P. 42, *the commercial PLATO system:* Wagman, M. (1980). PLATO DCS, an interactive computer system for personal counseling. *Journal of Counseling Psychology, 27,* 16–30.

P. 42, *personal dilemmas reported greater improvement than did the control group:* Wagman, M. (1984). *The dilemma and the computer: Theory and research foundations.* New York: Gordon and Breach.

P. 42, *the Therapeutic Learning Program:* Gould, R. L. (1989). The Therapeutic Learning Program (TLP): computer-assisted short-term therapy. In G. Gumpert & S. L. Fish (Eds.), *Talking to strangers: Mediated therapeutic communication* (pp. 184–198). Norwood, NJ: Ablex.

P. 43, *automated desensitization protocols for various phobias:* Marks, I. M. (1991). Self-administered behavioural treatment. *Behavioural Psychotherapy, 19*(1), 42–46.

P. 43, *cognitive-behavioral spectrum:* Beck, A. T. (1979). *Cognitive therapy of depression.* New York: Guilford.

P. 43, *computer program based on Beck's work:* Selmi, P. M., Klein, M. H., Greist, J. H., Sorrell, S. P., & Erdman, H. P. (1990). Computer-administered cognitive-behavioral therapy for depression. *American Journal of Psychiatry, 147,* 51–56.

P. 43, *CD-ROM program for training and treatment:* Commercial announcement.

P. 44, *Effective programs [for a variety of] symptoms:* Selmi, P. M., Klein, M. H., Greist, J. H., Sorrell, S. P., & Erdman, H. P. (1990). Computer-administered cognitive-behavioral therapy for depression. *American Journal of Psychiatry, 147,* 51–56; Marks, I. M. (1991). Self-administered behavioural treatment. *Behavioural Psychotherapy, 19*(1), 42–46; Binik, Y. M., Servan-Schreiber, D., Freiwald, S., & Hall, D. S. (1988). Intelligent computer-based assessment and psychotherapy: An expert system for sexual dysfunction. *Journal of Nervous and Mental Disease, 176,* 387–400; Chandler, G. B., Burck, H., & Sampson, J. P. (1986). A generic computer program for systematic desensitization: Description, construction, and case study. *Journal of Behavior Therapy and Experimental Psychiatry, 17,* 171–174; Robertson, E. B., Ladewig, G. H., Strickland, M. P., & Boschung, M. D. (1987). Enhancement of self-esteem through the use of computer-assisted instruction. *Journal of Educational Research, 80,* 314–316.

P. 44, *Other programs focus on self-regulation in the areas eating, smoking, and drinking:* Schneider, S. J. (1986). Trial of an on-line behavioral smoking cessation program. *Computers in Human Behavior, 2,* 277–286; Schneider, S. J., Walker, R., & O'Donnell, R. (1990). Computerized communication as a medium for behavioral smoking cessation treatment: Controlled evaluation. *Computers in Human Behavior, 6,* 141–151; Colby, K. (1995). Personal communication.

P. 44, *programs focus on self-regulation:* Servan-Schreiber, D. (1986). Artificial intelligence and psychiatry. *Journal of Nervous and Mental Disease, 174,* 191–202; Schneider, S. J. (1986). Trial of an on-line behavioral smoking cessation program. *Computers in Human Behavior, 2,* 277–286; Schneider, S. J., Walker, R., & O'Donnell, R. (1990). Computerized communication as a medium for behavioral smoking cessation treatment: Controlled evaluation. *Computers in Human Behavior, 6,* 141–151; Slack, W. V., Porter, D., Witschi, J., Sullivan, M., Buxbaum, R., & Stare, F. J. (1976). Dietary interviewing by computer. *Journal of the American Dietetic Association, 69,* 514–517.

P. 44, *observations about the Therapeutic Learning Program:* Gould, R. L. (1989). The Therapeutic Learning Program (TLP): computer-assisted short-term therapy. In G. Gumpert & S. L. Fish (Eds.), *Talking to strangers: mediated therapeutic communication* (pp. 184–198). Norwood, NJ: Ablex.

P. 49, *threatening or upsetting:* Beck, A. T., & Rush, A. J. (1989). Cognitive therapy. In H. I. Kaplan & B. J. Sadock (Eds.), *Comprehensive Textbook of Psychiatry* (Vol. V, pp. 1541–1550). Baltimore: Williams & Wilkins.

P. 49, *outcome studies:* Jacobs, M., Christensen, A., Huber, A., & Polterock, A. (1995, April). Computer-assisted individual therapy vs. standard brief individual therapy. Computer-psychotherapy: Wave of the future? Symposium conducted at meeting of the 75th Annual Western Psychological Association Convention, Los Angeles, CA; Selmi, P. M., Klein, M. H., Greist, J. H., Sorrell, S. P., & Erdman, H. P. (1990). Computer-administered cognitive-behavioral therapy for depression. *American Journal of Psychiatry, 147,* 51–56; Marks, I. M. (1991). Self-administered behavioural treatment. *Behavioural Psychotherapy, 19*(1), 42–46.

P. 49, *an average of six months:* Eysenck, H. J. (1957). *Sense and nonsense in psychology.* New York: Penquin.

P. 50, *cognitive-behavioral element:* Selmi, P. M., Klein, M. H., Greist, J. H., Sorrell, S. P., & Erdman, H. P. (1990). Computer-administered cognitive-behavioral therapy for depression. *American Journal of Psychiatry, 147,* 51–56.

P. 50, *Beck's method:* Beck, A. T. (1979). *Cognitive therapy of depression.* New York: Guilford.

P. 52, *Ten separate studies:* Gould, R. L. (in press). Development, problem solving, and generalized learning: The Therapeutic Learning Program (TLP). In M. Miller, M. Hile, & K. Hammond (Eds.), *Mental Health Computing.* New York: Springer-Verlag.

P. 52, *Favorable comparisons: Managed Health Network* (1995). Private unpublished report.

P. 53, *the most recent study done at UCLA:* Belar, C. D., Dolezal-Wood, C., Snibbe, J. (1995, April). *A comparison of computer-assisted psychotherapy and cognitive behavior therapy.* Paper presented at the 75th Annual Western Psychological Association Convention, Los Angeles.

P. 53, *one study strongly suggests:* Klein, R. (1988). *The effects of implementation on program outcome: an evaluation of the Therapeutic Learning Program (TLP) at CIGNA Healthplan.* Unpublished doctoral dissertation, University of California, Los Angeles.

P. 53, *Marks has demonstrated:* Greist, J. H., Klein, M. H., & Erdman, H. P. (1978). Computer interviewing: Beyond data collection. In F. H. Orthner (Ed.), *Proceedings: The second annual symposium on computer applications in medical care* (pp. 227–230). Long Beach, CA: IEEE Computer Society.

P. 53, *follow-up severely agoraphobic patients:* Marks, I. M. (1991). Self-administered behavioural treatment. *Behavioural Psychotherapy, 19*(1), 42–46.

P. 53, *self-administered smoking cessation programs:* Schneider, S. J. (1986). Trial of an on-line behavioral smoking cessation program. *Computers in Human Behavior, 2,* 277–286; Schneider, S. J., Walker, R., & O'Donnell, R. (1990). Computerized communication as a medium for behavioral smoking cessation treatment: Controlled evaluation. *Computers in Human Behavior, 6,* 141–151.

P. 53, *satisfaction studies:* Gould, R. L. (in press). Development, problem solving, and generalized learning: The Therapeutic Learning Program (TLP). In M. Miller, M. Hile, & K. Hammond (Eds.), *Mental Health Computing.* New York: Springer-Verlag.

P. 53, *reported and unreported studies:* Gould, R. L. (in press). Development, problem solving, and generalized learning: The Therapeutic Learning Program (TLP). In M. Miller, M. Hile, & K. Hammond, (Eds.), *Mental Health Computing.* New York: Springer-Verlag.

P. 53, *Minnesota Multiphasic Personality Inventory:* Fowler, R. D. (1985). Landmarks in computer-assisted psychological assessment. *Journal of Consulting and Clinical Psychology, 53,* 748–759.

P. 59, *adult population are in need of psychological services:* Wells, K. B., Burnam, M. A., Rogers, W., Hays, R., Camp, P. (1992). The course of depression in adult outpatients results from the medical outcomes study. *Archives of General Psychiatry, 49,* 788–794.

P. 59, *adult population receives psychological services:* Wells, K. B., et al. (1992), *ibid.*

CHAPTER FOUR

CLINICAL ASSESSMENT AND OUTCOMES MEASUREMENT

Murray P. Naditch and Kevin L. Moreland

It could be said that American mental health practitioners have been concerned about measuring outcomes as far back as 1754, when Benjamin Franklin wrote about the first American general hospital. In 1773, the first American psychiatric hospital opened its doors, in Williamsburg, Virginia. Today the concern has reached new heights with the confluence of a number of events. The payer revolt against high healthcare prices sweeping our nation over the last decade has resulted in massive changes in how healthcare is being delivered, and in the emerging need on the part of both payers and providers to demonstrate the value of that healthcare. At the same time, the wave of sociotechnical change moving through the postindustrial world promises new decision support models in behavioral healthcare that will provide new opportunities. These new models will accelerate change in the content, organization, and delivery of mental health services. The results will have profound impact on payers, providers, and consumers.

This chapter briefly reviews the history of both mental health outcomes measurement and computer-assisted psychological measurement (CAPM); it also

Note: Thanks are due to Albert Farrell, Grant Grissom, Barry Schlosser, and Bruce Vieweg for providing information about their systems. Thanks are also due to Dr. Schlosser for his insightful comments on Table 4.2.

discusses how changes in computer-based outcome measures may impact behavioral health therapy.

A Brief History of Computer-Assisted Psychological Measurement

Methods for measuring the outcomes of contemporary mental health treatment and computer-assisted psychological measurement technology developed along parallel but separate tracks until recently.

Formal reports of the outcome of psychotherapy date back to the 1920s. These early reports were crude, involving therapists' subjective estimates of the degree to which their clients had improved. The early reports were also academic exercises that had no apparent influence on client care. Such was indeed the case until very recently. Psychological measurement also was crudely automated in the 1920s, when a Hollerith electromechanical card sorter came into use to score the Strong Vocational Interest Blank.

Neither psychotherapy research nor automated assessment changed during the thirties, but both fields experienced the beginning of rapid changes at the end of the 1940s. The rate of publication (if not the quality) of treatment outcome studies quadrupled between 1945 and 1950. During that same period it became possible to score a questionnaire that could be used for outcomes measurement—the Minnesota Multiphasic Personality Inventory (MMPI)—using an analog computer.

Early Efforts

The pace of change accelerated in the fifties. In 1952 a British psychologist, Hans Eysenck, shocked the field by claiming that psychotherapy was not efficacious. That same year witnessed the introduction of the first modern psychiatric drug, the antipsychotic medication chlorpromazine. These events generated improvements in outcomes measurement because psychotherapists were determined to prove Eysenck wrong, while psychopharmacologists needed to demonstrate the efficacy of their new medications. Research reports began to appear in which outcomes were measured from the perspectives of clients and independent observers in addition to therapists. Researchers also began to develop multidimensional measurement tools that were both reliable and sensitive to change.

The 1950s saw two lasting changes in CAPM. The first was the advent of optical mark-reading equipment, which eliminated cumbersome and error-prone keypunching of answers.

The second significant change in CAPM during the fifties was the development, at the end of the decade, of the first computer system to assist in the *interpretation* of a psychological test. That system, developed at the Mayo Clinic, is still in operation, generating about ten brief statements, mainly describing current psychiatric symptomatology and designed to help physicians decide whether a mental health consultation is needed. The Mayo system emphasizes treatment *planning* rather than treatment *outcomes*. Our view is that the ideal outcomes measurement system includes tools that can be used for both functions.

In 1962 researchers documented that some clients *deteriorate* as a result of psychotherapy. Shortly thereafter Donald Kiesler noted that psychotherapy researchers tended to treat clients, therapists, therapies, and outcomes as if they were uniform. He pointed out that researchers were asking "Does psychotherapy work?" when they should have been asking "Which treatment delivered by which therapist will produce desired outcomes for which clients?" In July 1961, when Fort Logan Mental Health Center opened its doors, data on the first client were entered into the first comprehensive, computerized "information system for clinical and administrative decision-making, research, and evaluation". The routine computerization of all data at Fort Logan surmounted an enormous logistical obstacle hampering outcomes measurement. While this was going on, computerbased test interpretation systems became both more common and more elaborate.

Rapid Progress

In the 1970s Hans Strupp, one of the deans of psychotherapy research, asserted that "[a] truly adequate, comprehensive picture of an individual's mental health is possible only if . . . behavior [society's interest], affect [the client's interest], and inferred psychological structure [the therapist's interest] are evaluated. . . ." That same year CAPM was revolutionized when Psych Systems, Inc., developed the first microcomputer-based system. Earlier in the decade the same group had developed the first system with which clients interacted with the computer.

Early in our careers, clinicians could be heard to argue that "statistical significance is not the same thing as clinical significance." In other words, one can design an outcomes study in which statistics show changes in clients, but those changes are inconsequential. That complaint was mooted in 1984 when Neil Jacobson and his colleagues introduced statistical methods for determining when clinically significant change has taken place.

The biggest change in CAPM in the eighties was in hardware. At the beginning of the decade National Computer Systems began to offer a service wherein responses to psychological tests were entered into a terminal in a clinician's office, transmitted to a central computer, and within a few minutes, test results were transmitted back to the clinician's office. This same technology is now used to maintain centralized outcomes data bases while providing clinically useful information to mental health professionals all over the country. We return to this point later in this chapter.

Advantages of Computerization

One impetus for the development and implementation of computer-assisted outcome measurement systems has been the need to address cost and methodological problems inherent in paper-and-pencil systems:

- High costs associated with printing and inventorying questionnaires, entering clean data, and training staff to administer questionnaires
- Problems in data accuracy related to lost or inadequately completed forms
- Difficulty in maintaining adequate staff motivation and compliance
- Difficulty in obtaining patient compliance because of the paperwork burden at intake
- Lack of real-time usefulness of outcome information because of turnaround time
- Problems associated with integrating outcome data with other clinical information and processes

Computer-Assisted Outcomes Measurement Systems

In the mid 1980s a panel of experts developed criteria for use in developing, selecting, or using outcomes measures. These criteria are paraphrased in Table 4.1. We invite you to use these criteria to evaluate the outcomes measures you read about in this section, as well as others that you now have or will encounter.

After you have determined which measures would be useful in your setting, consider the criteria we propose in Table 4.2 in evaluating the computer implementation of an outcomes measurement system.

We now discuss outcomes measurement systems designed for computer implementation. There are many other excellent systems that we do not cite as examples here, because they are primarily assessment rather than outcome measurement systems or because they are outcome systems not yet computerized.

CASPER

Computerized Assessment System for Psychotherapy Evaluation and Research, or CASPER, is an excellent basic system for the individual practitioner who is not

TABLE 4.1. CRITERIA FOR DEVELOPMENT, SELECTION, OR USE OF OUTCOMES MEASURES

Applications	Methods and Procedures	Psychometric Features	Cost	Utility
1. Assesses characteristics relevant to the target group (e.g., inpatients)	2. Easily taught 3. Facilitates comparisons among clients (e.g., norms available) 4. Uses multiple respondents (e.g., clients, clinicians) 5. Provides information about therapeutic process	6. Reliable 7. Valid 8. Sensitive to treatment-related change 9. Insensitive to extraneous factors (e.g., accountability pressures)	10. Low cost	11. Easily understood by nonprofessionals 12. Uncomplicated interpretation making feedback easy 13. Useful in clinical services (e.g., provides information useful in treatment planning) 14. Compatible with clinical theories and practices

accustomed to formally tracking the therapeutic progress of his or her patients; it lacks the built-in data management and reporting functions that are handy for institutional administrative purposes. Currently this program will run on (all but the most ancient) microcomputers using the DOS operating system, that is, "IBM-compatibles"; an upgrade to the nearly universal Windows operating environment is planned for 1996. Although CASPER has been under development for over a decade, the authors are still calibrating the system. Therefore, they are willing to make it available free of charge to sites that are willing to assist in its pilot testing by providing data that can be used to help validate it.

The heart of CASPER is an online interview completed by the patient. The interview includes 122 questions linked to sixty-two target complaints. The 122 questions tap eighteen complaint categories ranging from physical symptoms to dissatisfaction with finances. Clients rate both the severity of complaints and the extent to which they wish to focus on them in treatment; the length of time they have had a given complaint also is assessed. Inspection of the categories makes it clear that CASPER maps common complaints subsumed under DSM–IV and many other potential treatment foci. Moreover, it is clear that CASPER is likely to be responsive to the outcome measurement of pharmacotherapy, as well as psychotherapy.

TABLE 4.2. CRITERIA FOR EVALUATION OF THE COMPUTER IMPLEMENTATION OF AN OUTCOMES MEASUREMENT SYSTEM

Input	Hardware	Software	Output	Cost
1. Quick 2. Easy 3. Accurate 4. Multiple methods (e.g., touch screen, optical scanning) 5. Multiple modes (e.g., on-line, paper-and-pencil)	6. Minimal required hardware 7. Compatible with other widely used applications software 8. Compatible with other widely used hardware 9. Easily maintained 10. Upgradable 11. Support easily accessed	12. Does not require specialized installation procedures 13. Compatible with other widely used applications software (e.g., database, billing) 14. Can be configured to meet local needs 15. Upgradable 16. Support easily accessed	17. Brief 18. Easily understood 19. Easily accessed	20. Low cost

Note: This table provided courtesy of Barry Schlosser.

When CASPER is used to track the course of treatment, the patient can respond to the intake interview or to a shorter interview based on the target complaints he or she endorsed initially. The latter approach is particularly useful when the clinician wishes to measure progress in treatment at short intervals. The shorter interview can be completed on the computer or via an individualized paper-and-pencil form generated by the computer.

During treatment, patients rate how much each target complaint has been focused on and how severe it is. They also rate their own overall functioning. In a departure from the intake interview, patients describe their experience of the therapeutic process by rating the degree of understanding, concern, and genuineness the clinician conveyed during the most recent session. Clinicians can rate a patient's progress using either the patient's target problem list or their own. In addition to rating the patient's overall functioning, the clinician rates motivation, resistance, and likableness during the most recent session. These procedures are changed only slightly at termination and follow-up, at which times patients and clinicians are asked to rate how each target complaint has changed during the course of treatment and to provide three global ratings of the effect of treatment.

Details about how to contact the developers of CASPER and the other systems described in this chapter may be found in the notes at the end.

Clarity Health Assessment System

Built around a psychological model of health, as opposed to a medical model of illness, the Clarity Health Assessment System (CHAS) comprises a modular family of scales designed for tracking the progress of outpatient treatment.

The Clarity Well-Being Scales (CWBS) measure subjective health, and the Clarity Distress Scales (CDS) measure psychopathology along the same six dimensions: physical, emotional, mental, social, life satisfaction, and life direction. The system includes a measure of patient factors that bode for successful treatment. The patient measures used at intake currently comprise two hundred items, but it is anticipated that further research will soon reduce that number. Until field testing is completed the system will be exclusively paper-based, with intake patient answer sheets mailed in for processing. Clinicians can complete a brief measure designed to flesh out the data provided by the patient-report scales.

Progress in treatment can be tracked in two ways. Well- being and distress can be tracked comprehensively using a twelve-item instrument consisting of the strongest items from the CWBS and CDS until score changes indicate that it would be useful to obtain the more detailed assessment afforded by the full-length measures. Alternatively, outcomes can be measured by having patients complete only those subscales of the CWBS and CDS that deviated significantly from the community average at intake. The latter method of tracking treatment progress may require the patient to respond to as few as half a dozen items. In addition to providing data on their well-being and distress, patients may complete a brief scale describing their experience of the psychotherapeutic process, covering areas that have been linked to positive outcomes. A similar scale is available for clinicians.

Clinical/Management Information System

The Missouri Institute of Mental Health has been a hotbed of mental health computing since the 1960s. Most recently their staff has put together the Clinical/Management Information System (C/MIS) for tracking and evaluating the treatment of seriously mentally ill patients. Like CASPER, the C/MIS system will run on all but the most primitive DOS-based microcomputers. Copies of C/MIS are routinely made available to not-for-profit agencies, but system support is not available.

C/MIS data provided by the patient covers eight areas, including an admission questionnaire (demographic data), financial resources questionnaire, medical history questionnaire, social work assessment, St. Louis Symptom Checklist

(SLSC), Missouri Alcoholism Severity Scale (if indicated; twenty items), FACES Quality-of-Life Scale, and the Customer Satisfaction Questionnaire (CSQ–8). The system is flexible, employing several data-entry methods. The first three "questionnaires" mentioned are actually computer-mediated interviews: the computer prompts an interviewer with questions and the interviewer keyboards the patient's responses. The patient usually interacts directly with the computer to provide the other information, though an interviewer is employed if need be (for example, if the patient cannot read). Outcomes data can be collected using paper-and-pencil versions of the symptom checklist, alcoholism scale, quality-of-life scale, and CSQ–8. The patient outcomes battery currently comprises 141 items, including the alcoholism checklist. The system will soon be upgraded to include a brief assessment of the patient's status, in key life areas such as employment and housing, that can be completed by anyone with relevant knowledge of the patient. A sixty-four–item assessment of the patient's symptoms and functioning that is meant to be filled out by the patient's significant other is available as an option.

Upon admission, clinicians rate all patients on the Brief Psychiatric Rating Scale (BPRS) and the Global Assessment of Functioning (GAF) scale of the DSM–III–R. Clinicians complete the BPRS at follow-up, along with a simple five-point rating of improvement. The BPRS includes only eighteen items, tapping broad symptom categories ranging from anxiety to unusual thought content, so the demands on the clinician's time are minimal. The system was developed with the goal of collecting follow-up data quarterly and at discharge; however, nothing in the system's design precludes tracking patient progress more or less frequently.

COMPASS

COMPASS was designed specifically for the concurrent assessment of outpatient psychotherapy. However, the developers report it can also be used to assess outpatient pharmacotherapy for nonpsychotic patients. It is currently being expanded for use with inpatients.

The flexibility of the COMPASS system has recently increased markedly. Originally, paper-and-pencil questionnaires were mailed to a central site for processing and reports were mailed back to users. Now data gathered prior to a treatment session can be faxed and the results transmitted back to the clinician before the end of the session.

COMPASS questionnaires are completed by both patients and clinicians. Naturally, during their initial consultation patients provide demographic information and enumerate their presenting problems. They also respond to items tapping their motivation for treatment. COMPASS developers dealt with the lack of consensus about outcomes measurement by basing the system on an empirically supported phase model of psychotherapy outcome. According to this model, psychotherapy first causes an upsurge in patients' morale; then their symptoms can be remediated; and finally, when symptoms have remitted, patients can get on with the business of developing a career, taking care of their families, and so forth. Thus, COMPASS requires patients to respond to questions about their sense of well-being, psychological symptoms, and current life functioning. This initial assessment has 111 items.

Clinicians' resistance has been minimized in part by calling on them to make only seven brief ratings. The clinician provides a rating of the patient's life functioning in each of the aforementioned six areas and provides a global assessment of the patient's lowest level of current functioning on a scale similar to the GAF scale.

As treatment proceeds, the patient provides an indication of well-being, symptoms, and life functioning at the fourth session and every six sessions thereafter. In addition, the strength of the therapeutic alliance is assessed by having patients respond to items tapping their perception of the clinician. This assessment comprises eighty-three items. The clinician rates the patient's life functioning and global adjustment at those same sessions. Comparison of COMPASS scores to norms for similar patients at various stages of treatment allows COMPASS users to identify patients who are not improving or who have achieved a level of functioning characteristic of a nontreatment population.

To further minimize clinicians' resistance to COMPASS, the developers insist that it be used in managed care in a collaborative, nonpunitive manner. They believe the reports produced on individual patients should be used to alert clinicians and case managers when treatment is not progressing as well as the system's norms suggest it should so that they can consult, professional-to-professional, about how the treatment plan might be usefully altered.

Outcome Questionnaire 45.1 (OQ–45.1)

The OQ–45.1 is even more basic than CASPER and, like CASPER, is a good starting place for the individual practitioner who is not accustomed to formally tracking the therapeutic progress of patients. However, it is also meant for hospital and managed care settings. It is currently in use in many treatment facilities, including Intermountain Health Care Center for Behavioral Efficacy in Salt Lake City, Utah. Plans call for it to be incorporated into the outcomes measurement program of Human Affairs International, a national managed behavioral healthcare company.

The OQ–45.1 is a patient report questionnaire with forty-five items assessing three areas of functioning: subjective discomfort, interpersonal relationships, and social role functioning. Michael Lambert, one of the instrument's developers, concluded from his long experience in mental health outcomes measurement that these three domains were the most crucial.

In 1991 researchers at Intermountain Health Care Center concluded that instruments commonly used to measure outcomes of mental healthcare were too expensive, too time consuming, and too difficult for clinicians to understand—and relatively insensitive to change, to boot! At that point Lambert and his colleague at Brigham Young, Gary Burlingame, set out to develop the OQ–45.1 to tap the three areas of functioning mentioned previously.

The OQ–45.1 can be implemented on microcomputers in the Windows operating environment. Licensing fees are minimal. Contact information is included at the end of this chapter.

RES–Q

Researchers at Strategic Advantage, Inc. (SAI) developed TQM Advantage in 1987 as a paper-and-pencil system to measure clinical outcomes and match patients to the treatments most effective for them. This system was implemented in more than three hundred treatment sites, most of which were in inpatient free-standing adult and adolescent mental health and chemical dependency treatment centers. The RES–Q (Reliable Electronic Survey Questionnaire) system was developed in 1994 to address methodological problems SAI found in the course of implementing a paper-based system on such a large scale. RES–Q contains a number of innovative components, which are described below.

RES–Q uses an electronic questionnaire, based on the fifty-three-item Brief Symptom Inventory, that eliminates problems and costs in maintaining an inventory of questionnaires and in entering data. Electronic delivery facilitates branching questionnaire logic, thereby shortening and tailoring questionnaires. Errors related to incomplete and illogical responses are eliminated. When patients do not provide acceptable responses, self-administered entry is replaced by a clinical interview format. Reports delivered on the screen can be printed as needed.

RES–Q data can be entered via telephone, keyboard, or mouse, or with a touch screen in a full multimedia format. In that format, voice and video accompaniment extends use of the system to less literate, more confused, and sicker patients.

The narrator interacts with an animated character who raises points of resistance the patient may be experiencing. RES–Q also uses patient incentives at the end of each section of the instrument, including maps showing the patient how far she has come, positive feedback, and other reinforcing devices.

The RES–Q architecture also facilitates increased flexibility in making changes to the instrument. The electronic system can modify, add, or delete items throughout all system sites by way of electronic connections.

Data collected in each terminal are transmitted to a central data base, reports are calculated, and completed reports are downloaded by the originating terminal. The national data base—which contains approximately forty-six thousand patient cases at the time of this writing—is used to calculate national norms and empirically risk-adjusted outcome norms. Empirically risk-adjusted norms are used to compare the effectiveness or efficiency of therapists, programs, locations, or plans when these entities may not have patients of comparable difficulty.

With paper-and-pencil-based systems, outcome reports were calculated periodically from batched data. Aggregated outcome reports were delivered to clients two or three times a year. That methodology had two inherent user interface problems:

1. End users required both aggregated and individual patient outcome information at the point at which they were making decisions.
2. The format of outcome information was constructed more from a researcher's perspective than a clinical or management user's.

RES–Q provides online information as needed and has restructured presentation of outcome information so that it is more congruent with the management and clinical decision-making processes. SAI is currently conducting pilot tests in which RES–Q is combined with Charter Medical Corp.'s Critical Treatment Path practice guideline system at inpatient treatment sites in four U.S. cities. The combined system is expected to have the effect of converting paper-based guidelines, based on expert judgment, into dynamic tools that will empirically validate the efficacy of recommended treatment paths as well as continue to differentiate these paths.

Future Trajectories

Behavioral healthcare rides the same wave of information-driven sociotechnical change that is carrying the rest of the postindustrial world. Data base creation, integration, access, and software applications that provide computer-assisted decision support models create major new opportunities; they also unravel the status quo, resulting in the downfall or realignment of dominant institutions and players. This can be seen in the declining influence of such seemingly immutable institutions as the Soviet Union, General Motors, and national broadcast networks such as CBS and NBC. In our field, we witness the decline of professional authority, as in the diminished decision-making authority of physicians.

In behavioral health, as in the rest of medicine, formerly independent data bases are being combined into integrated clinical information systems. Development of computer-assisted decision models that take advantage of access to these data will have profound implications on the quality and efficiency of care and the nature and structure of the players in the behavioral healthcare arena.

Computer-Assisted Decision Making Will Transform Clinical Practice

A major catalyst for transformation will be access to computerized decision support systems that will enable decision makers to explore the effectiveness and efficiency of treatment options.

Computer-assisted decision making based on large outcome data bases will be used to support both individual patient and aggregated benefit and contracting decisions.

Treatment-effectiveness decision support models can be applied to patients by treatment-matching decisions that examine the effectiveness and efficiency of alternative treatment scenarios. Decision makers will be able to choose the providers, programs, and treatment paths that are most effective and efficient. As in industrial quality control, decision makers with access to process and outcome information will be able to eliminate waste and rework.

One effect may be emergence of more individualized treatment programs, matching patients to services that are projected to be most effective for them, just as manufacturing plants are beginning to do shorter and more differentiated computer-driven production runs based on customer needs. This trend is evident in widely scattered industries, from automobile manufacturing to jeans. As this process—made possible by access to large integrated data bases and computer decision models—becomes more widespread, it will have profound implications for existing concepts of inventory and distribution. It is not unreasonable to expect similar changes in healthcare as decision makers can more precisely match patients to providers and treatments.

From a payer perspective, this will mean

- Benefit programs and triage access rules based on decision support tools that provide likely treatment outcome scenarios for specific types of patients
- The ability to choose, contract with, and hold accountable only those providers who demonstrate effective and efficient patient-centered care

From a provider-organization perspective, this will mean the ability to

- Assess populations, or individual patients, in terms of probable outcomes and the resource needs to provide those outcomes, creating more scenarios in which providers will choose to assume risks based on projected outcomes and costs
- Match patients to the combinations of care levels, programs, and therapists likely to provide the most effective and efficient outcomes

From an individual clinician's perspective, this will mean the ability to

- Use scenario modeling to estimate the effectiveness and efficiency of levels of care and specific treatments
- Assess patient progress during treatment based on expected progress for specific types of patients, with decision support related to changing the course of, or concluding, therapy

And as access to outcome-based decision support models becomes available to patients and their family members, consumers will have more information on

- When treatment is warranted, what to expect
- How to assess treatment and provider options

Consider an example of how these scenarios could be realized. A patient is having behavioral problems and encounters the treatment network through a visit to a general practice physician, a telephone call to a managed care organization, or a scheduled visit to a behavioral healthcare provider. At the first encounter, the patient would be asked to provide information directly into a computer system at a terminal or through a telephone keypad. The questions asked of the patient, the patient's family, or an observer provide a decision support model with the information it requires to generate alternative outcome scenarios.

Questions in this initial encounter consist of psychosocial characteristics that have been found to relate to treatment response, and baseline information about the variables to be measured again later to determine treatment outcomes.

For each decision maker, and at each decision point, users can estimate the effects of various treatment paths and providers for a particular type of patient, based on a combination of the patient's psychosocial characteristics and available treatment options.

SAI, for example, is moving toward providing actionable information by collecting and reporting on data mapped within a hypothesized causal model. Such a model is shown in Figure 4.1. Data collected and analyzed using this type of model can provide decision-driven information at four points:

1. At triage, determining which care level and treatment center will produce the most effective and efficient treatment
2. At intake, matching the patient to the therapist and the specific treatment program that will be most effective and efficient
3. During treatment, deciding whether the treatment plan should continue, terminate, or be redirected
4. At termination, deciding what additional care is projected to be most effective

This type of information can also be viewed from an aggregate perspective, providing outcome information about treatment effectiveness of various portions of the system for different types of patients, along with general rules about the effectiveness and efficiency of various treatment combinations and providers for different types of patients.

The same logistic regression model used to risk-rate outcome measures can also be used in a gaming-theory context to develop a simulation, to predict the recidivism rate of a particular patient at intake. Consider the tree diagram shown in Figure 4.1 as an example.

From a decision maker's perspective, knowing a patient's score on the five factors represented can be used to predict a recidivism rate that varies from as low as 1 percent (for patients who have not had any prior mental health hospitalization or partial hospitalization, were not recommended into treatment by their psychiatrist, did not have financial problems related to their mental problems, and had low initial phobic anxiety scores) to 51 percent for a patient who presented positive on each of these measures.

Note how closely the actual scores correspond to the predicted scores using this model, shown in Figure 4.2 for all 912 patients tested. This model indicates a range of projected recidivism rate for each patient prior to therapy. A more comprehensive model-in-progress indicates how much the recidivism rate can be expected to change as the result of therapeutic interventions for each patient. These early models will probably look like stone-age artifacts in a few years, but they are useful in illustrating one approach to making outcome information actionable in terms of specific clinical decisions.

New Paradigms for Development of Scientific Knowledge

The type of scenario-based decision support system postulated in the last section provides knowledge in the form of decision support based on empirical findings

FIGURE 4.1. SIMULATED PROBABILITY OF REHOSPITALIZATION[1]

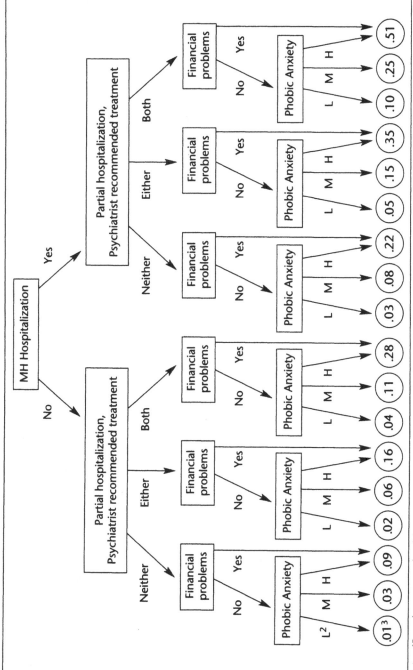

Notes: [1]Based on a sample of 912 patients from SAI's adult mental health national data base.

[2]Brief Symptom Inventory (BSI) Phobic Anxiety T-Score: Low = 30, Medium = 55, High = 80.

[3]Probability of rehospitalization within six months.

Source: Strategic Advantage, Inc. © 1995. Reprinted by permission.

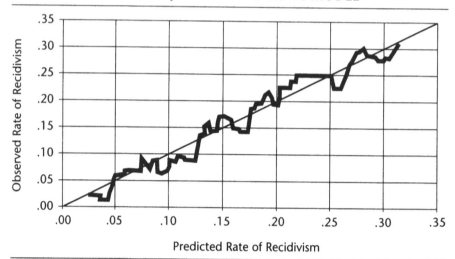

FIGURE 4.2. OBSERVED VERSUS PREDICTED RATE OF RECIDIVISM FOR RISK ADJUSTMENT LOGISTIC MODEL[1,2]

Notes: [1]Each point represents result of moving averaging on 200 patients.

[2]Based on a sample of 912 patients from SAI's adult mental health national data base.

Source: Strategic Advantage, Inc. © 1995. Reprinted by permission.

from a large integrated data base. It also builds cumulative knowledge by using the results of each new patient to continuously evolve the empirically based models underlying the decision support algorithms. Our lack of cumulative scientific knowledge about how to match patients to procedures stems largely from the fact that researchers use different measures and methods and are not iteratively testing consistent questions. Emerging computer technology creates a research situation in which hundreds of treatment sites with a continuous flow of patients can use the same measurement instruments and procedures; this provides an opportunity for generation of cumulative scientific knowledge.

More patients moving through the system will enable the models to make more accurate predictions with a smaller number of predictor variables, thus reducing the amount of information required from patients.

Emerging networks in which a large number of clients complete common instruments entered into a large data base provide opportunities to both deliver and empirically evolve

- *Psychological tests* in which test development time is reduced because of the ability to examine reliability and validity, add or delete items, and retest in real time

- *Computer-assisted therapy* with matching of patients to programs, empirical evaluation of results, and differentiation of computer-assisted treatment pathways for specific types of patients
- *Dynamic, empirically driven practice guidelines* by empirically testing the efficacy of pathways for different types of patients, and adding more differentiated decision rules as more patients move through the system

In each of these tasks, the system that delivers the service is also testing and differentiating the underlying models, providing continuous improvement. The underlying empirical testing and evolutionary portion of the program is invisible to nonscientific research users, and continuous small changes in items and elements can be made automatically and seamlessly throughout the system.

There are other applications that would share these elements but add an additional factor: a new and untested function in the evolution of empirically based cumulative scientific knowledge. For lack of a better name, let us call it "group thought." Shared thinking has always been an element of the research process, with scientists publishing papers and presenting papers for colleague response. The emergence of computer-based communication networks, such as the Internet, provide the opportunity for interchange of ideas that are not only quantitatively but also qualitatively different because of the possibilities for worldwide access—a richer brew through which inquiring minds can ferment scientific ideas.

In addition to being asked the questions driven by constructs already in the theoretical model, suppose that respondents were also asked to suggest additional variables that they thought affected their behaviors but were not reflected in questions in the existing model. If these questions were screened and operationalized by researchers, added to the model, and empirically tested, a new paradigm for scientific theory building would be introduced that could have interesting, evocative, and unforeseen consequences.

Shift of Power and Decision Making Directly to Consumers

The decline of the decision-making authority of physicians has taken place in the context of payer organizations that are rebelling against the high cost of medical care, and providers who are unable to demonstrate adequately that they provide the most effective and efficient solutions to specific patient problems. In addition, information that was previously available only to physicians is now becoming available to consumers in the form of computer-based decision support programs telling consumers how to respond to symptoms.

This trend will accelerate because it results in medical-cost savings to managed-care organizations. Giving members computer-driven medical decision support systems will result in more self reliance and less utilization of traditional medical care.

Imagine a scenario in behavioral health in which consumers respond to structured inquiries about their symptoms and histories and can review the potential outcomes of alternative treatment approaches.

Consumers will have more information than therapists do now about anticipated results of varying treatment options, altering both the manner in which treatment is prescribed as well as the range of potential treatments and providers that consumers and their families may consider.

Inclusion of More Alternative Approaches to Treatment

Emerging economic and technological forces create incentives and opportunities for a realignment of what are considered acceptable and reimbursable care options.

Healthcare systems that combine capitation with compulsory outcomes create a strong economic incentive for providers to use innovative and alternative approaches to treatment, if these methods can be demonstrated to be cost-effective for some types of patients. Payers and managed care companies who only a few years ago would not pay for partial hospitalization programs are now beginning to pay for home care, acupuncture, homeopathic, and other treatment approaches that have long been considered outside the mainstream. These approaches have been shown in some cases to offer lower-cost alternatives to traditional treatments while having positive outcomes. These trends will accelerate as consumers gain access to computer-based decision support tools that examine the effectiveness of a broadening range of alternative treatments.

The use of outcome data to determine cost-effective interventions will also result in an increased emphasis on prevention. Prevention efforts will be further accelerated by decision support models for prevention. Provider and payer organizations will use these models to examine the return on investment of preventive strategies, and encourage consumer use of illness-prevention approaches.

Tendency to Underestimate Scope and Speed of Change

After an obscure amateur inventor named Gutenberg combined his interests in hand printing stamps and development of a better wine press, the resulting printing press eventually came to upset the entire existing social and political order. This occurred even though there was no infrastructure for making paper or distributing literature, and almost no one knew how to read.

Today's emerging information and communication revolution will also have far-reaching effects on the existing social and political order, profoundly affecting everything from the way we conceive of education (change from going to school to lifelong computer-assisted instruction) to the nature of representative government (away from a system originally based on sending representatives to Washington because people back home could not gain access to information about issues).

Is it unreasonable to think that these changes will be as far-reaching and profound in behavioral healthcare? In healthcare, as in other areas of industry, technological change will outstrip people's ability to absorb and accept what it offers. The emerging changes in behavioral healthcare will challenge payers to reevaluate benefits structures, consider wider treatment options, and enter into partnerships with providers based on demonstrated value. Clinicians will be challenged to use clinical information systems and make changes in their practice patterns. Consumers will have access to new kinds of information and take more responsibility for their own health. Researchers will accept new paradigms and learn new disciplines.

As in the diffusion of any innovation, there will be innovators, early and later adapters, and laggards. The nature of these changes is inexorable and profound; they are overtaking and transforming the rest of our society very rapidly. The natural resistance to change on the part of people with vested interests will probably result in a rapid separation of those behavioral healthcare organizations with and without the knowledge base associated with these emerging technologies. We hope what will emerge from the other side of a reconfigured industry will be more knowledgeable and self-aware consumers, more effective treatment paths, and a more effective and efficient healthcare system.

Notes

P. 63, *opened its doors, in Williamsburg, Virginia:* Dain, N. (1971). *Disordered minds: The first century of Eastern State Hospital in Williamsburg, Virginia 1766–1866.* Williamsburg, VA: Colonial Williamsburg Foundation.

P. 63, *moving through the postindustrial world:* Toffler, A. (1990). *Power shift.* New York, Bantam Books.

P. 64, *outcome of psychotherapy date back to the 1920s:* Huddleson, J. H. (1927). *Military Surgeon, 60,* 161–170.

P. 64, *their clients had improved:* Bergin, A. E. (1971). The evaluation of therapeutic outcomes. In A. E. Bergin & S. Garfield (Eds.), *Handbook of psychotherapy and behavior change: An empirical analysis.* New York: Wiley.

P. 64, *treatment outcome studies quadrupled between 1945 and 1950:* Bergin, A. E. (1971). *ibid.*

P. 64, *the antipsychotic medication chlorpromazine:* Klerman, G. L., Weissman, M. M., Markowitz, J., Glick, I., Wilner, P. J., Mason, B., & Shear, M. K. (1994). Medication and psychotherapy. In A. E. Bergin & S. L. Garfield (Eds.), *Handbook of psychotherapy and behavior change.* New York: Wiley.

P. 64, *in addition to therapists:* Schjelderup, H. (1955). Lasting effects of psychoanalytic treatment. *Psychiatry, 18,* 109–133.

P. 64, *reliable and sensitive to change:* Wittenborn, J. R. (1955). *Manual: Wittenborn Psychiatric Rating Scale.* New York: Psychological Corporation.

P. 64, *mark-reading equipment:* Moreland, K. L. (1987). Computerized psychological assessment: What's available. In J. N. Butcher (Ed.), *Computerized psychological assessment: A practitioner's guide.* New York: Basic Books.

P. 65, *interpretation of a psychological test:* Fowler, R. D. (1985). Landmarks in computer-assisted psychological assessment. *Journal of Consulting and Clinical Psychology, 53*(6), 748–759.

P. 65, *some clients deteriorate as a result of psychotherapy:* Bergin, A. E. (1971). *op. cit.*

P. 65, *"decision-making, research, and evaluation":* Wilson, N. C. (1974). An information system for clinical and administrative decision-making, research, and evaluation. In J. L. Crawford, D. W. Morgan, & D. T. Gianturco (Eds.), *Progress in mental health information systems: Computer applications* (pp. 205–230).

P. 65, *systems became both more common and more elaborate:* Fowler, R. D. (1985). Landmarks in computer-assisted psychological assessment. *Journal of Consulting and Clinical Psychology, 53*(6), 748–759.

P. 65, *[the therapist's interests] are evaluated:* Strupp, H. H., & Hadley, S. W. (1977). A tripartite model of mental health and therapeutic outcomes. *American Psychologist, 32*(3), 187–196.

P. 65, *first microcomputer-based system:* Fowler, R. D. (1985). Landmarks in computer-assisted psychological assessment. *Journal of Consulting and Clinical Psychology, 53*(6), 748–759.

P. 65, *to the clinician's office:* Moreland, K. L. (1987). Computerized psychological assessment: What's available. In J. N. Butcher (Ed.), *Computerized psychological assessment: A practitioner's guide.* New York: Basic Books.

P. 66, *paper-and-pencil systems:* Naditch, M. P. (1994, May–June). Shifting to a new paradigm to measure clinical outcomes. *Behavioral Healthcare Tomorrow,* pp. 1–5.

P. 66, *using outcomes measures:* Newman, F. L., & Ciarlo, J. A. (1994). Criteria for selecting psychological instruments for treatment outcome assessment. In M. E. Maruish (Ed.), *The use of psychological testing for treatment planning and outcome assessment* (pp. 217–248). Hillsdale, NJ: Erlbaum.

P. 66, *CASPER:* For further information about CASPER, contact Albert D. Farrell, Department of Psychology, P.O. Box 842018, Virginia Commonwealth University, Richmond, VA 23284–2018; Internet:afarrell@cabell.vcu.edu.

P. 66, *sixty-two target complaints:* Farrell, A. D., & McCullough-Vaillant, L. (in press). Computerized assessment system of psychotherapy evaluation and research (CASPER): Development and current status. In M. Miller, M. Hile, & K. Hammond (Eds.), *Mental Health Computing.* New York: Springer-Verlag.

P. 66, *under DSM–IV:* American Psychiatric Association. (1994). *Diagnostic and statistical manual of mental disorders (3rd ed., rev.).* Washington, DC: Author.

P. 69, *the Clarity Health Assessment System (CHAS):* For further information about CHAS, contact Barry Schlosser, Clarity Health Assessment Systems, Inc., 197 East Ave., Norwalk, CT 06855; Internet:barrychas@aol.com.

P. 69, *Clarity Well-Being Scales:* Schlosser, B. (1990). The assessment of subjective well-being and its relationship to the stress process. *Journal of Personality Assessment, 54*(1&2), 128–140.

P. 69, *successful treatment:* Orlinsky, D. E., Grawe, K., & Parks, B. K. (1994). Process and outcome in psychotherapy—noch einmal. In A. E. Bergin & S. L. Garfield (Eds.), *Handbook of psychotherapy and behavior change* (4th ed., pp. 270–376). New York: Wiley.

P. 69, *since the 1960s:* Sletten, I. W., Ulett, G. A., Altman, H., & Sundland, D. (1970). The Missouri standard system of psychiatry (SSOP): Computer generated diagnoses. *Archives of General Psychiatry, 23*(1), 73–79.

P. 69, *(C/MIS):* For further information about C/MIS, write to Bruce W. Vieweg, Director of Information Systems, Missouri Department of Mental Health, P.O. Box 687, 1706 East Elm St., Jefferson City, MO 65102.

P. 69, *mentally ill patients:* Hile, M. G., & Hedlund, J. L. (1989). Development of a management information system for a purchase of service setting. *Computers in Human Services, 5*(3&4), 71–82.

P. 70, *COMPASS:* For further information about COMPASS, contact COMPASS Information Services, Inc., 1060 First Ave., Suite 410, King of Prussia, PA 19406.

P. 70, *for nonpsychotic patients:* Grissom, G. R., Howard, K. I., Malcolm, D. J., & Brill, P. L. (1993). *Integra's COMPASS system: Developmental history and usefulness.* Radnor, PA: Integra, Inc.

P. 71, *phase model of psychotherapy outcome:* Howard, K., Lueger, R. J., Maling, M. S., & Martinovich, Z. (1993). A phase model of psychotherapy outcome: Causal mediation of change. *Journal of Consulting and Clinical Psychology, 61*(4), 678–685.

P. 71, *OQ–45.1:* For further information about the OQ–45.1, contact Curtis Reisinger, Executive Director, IHC Center for Behavioral Healthcare Efficacy, 36 South State St., 21st Flr., Salt Lake City, UT 84111–1486.

P. 72, *mental health outcomes measurement:* Lambert, M. J., & Hill, C. E. (1994). Assessing psychotherapy outcomes and processes. In A. E. Bergin & S. L. Garfield (Eds.), *Handbook of psychotherapy and behavior change* (pp. 72–113). New York: Wiley.

P. 72, *RES–Q:* For further information about the RES–Q system, contact Murray P. Naditch, President and CEO, Strategic Advantage, Inc., 300 Clifton Ave., Minneapolis, MN 55403.

P. 72, *such a large scale:* Naditch, M. P. (1994, May–June). *op. cit.*

P. 73, *institutions and players:* Toffler, A. (1990) *op. cit.*

P. 79, *evaluation of results:* Naditch, M. P. (1983). PLATO STAYWELL: A behavioral medicine microcomputer program of health behavioral change. In R. E. Dayhoff (Ed.), *Proceedings of the Seventh Annual Symposium on Computer Applications in Medical Care* (pp. 363–365). Baltimore, MD: Computer Society Press.

P. 79, *cumulative scientific knowledge:* Blalock, H. M. (1969). *Theory construction: From verbal to mathematical formulations.* Englewood Cliffs, NJ: Prentice-Hall.

P. 81, *innovators, early and later adapters, and laggards:* Rogers, E. (1995). *The Diffusion of Innovations.* New York: Free Press.

PART TWO

MANAGEMENT

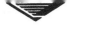

CHAPTER FIVE

EASING THE TRANSITION FROM PAPER TO COMPUTER-BASED SYSTEMS

Larry D. Rosen and Michelle M. Weil

It is clear just from scanning the contents of this book that technology is here to stay in the mental health profession. However, most clinical staff are not yet "techno-savvy." We believe that this is due in part to global attitudes and beliefs about technology as well as the way that clinical staff are introduced to technology. There are more and less effective ways to introduce technology. This chapter describes attitudes toward technology and details a proven model for successful implementation.

In early 1995 we interviewed a random sample of over two hundred clinical psychologists in California. This comprehensive interview, the first of its kind, examined how psychologists are integrating technology into their mental health practices. The results of this study were poignant and telling. One result stood out among all others:

> Although nearly three-quarters of all psychologists use computers in their practice, most use them only for word processing.

Nevertheless, mental health practitioners need to be "technologized" and to learn to use all technological modalities. Many managed care and insurance companies (Medicare, for example) are now beginning to implement electronic transmission of data. Some experts have guessed that this transition will be complete within five years; others have predicted ten to fifteen years. Regardless of the time frame, experts agree that mental health practitioners *need* to technologize.

Clinicians do need to be able to process words, of course. But they also need to maintain financial data, communicate with managed care and insurance companies, collect and analyze outcome assessment data and process treatment updates, summaries, and other relevant information for their mental health "business." Our recent interview data support the conclusion that although psychologists have been given the keys to start new machines, they need to make serious headway lest they become stalled on the on-ramp to the information superhighway. For example, we found that

Only one-fourth of all psychologists have ever scored a
psychological assessment by computer.
Only 11 percent have administered a psychological assessment by computer.
Only 3 percent have billed an insurance company electronically.

These results suggest that psychologists have not reached the information age. However, they *do* suggest that mental health professionals are not very different from the general population. Recent surveys by MCI, Associated Press, *Newsweek*, Louis Harris and Associates, Gallup, and the Times Mirror Center for the People and the Press have all corroborated that business executives in particular and the American public in general are not rushing to use technology. This chapter addresses avoidance and presents our model for successful introduction of technology. This model is based on over a decade of research on people's psychological reactions to technology.

We first present a picture of the behavioral, attitudinal, and organizational barriers that prevent mental health practitioners from gaining technological competence. Following this, we consider a model for avoiding these barriers and ensuring successful technological implementation. This model is generic and applicable to the implementation of *any* technology in *any* system. It facilitates bringing a personal computer into the home as simply as it eases the transition from paper to computer in a large corporation. It is based on recognizing barriers to successful implementation and taking steps to remove those barriers before beginning the entire process of technologizing.

Attitudinal and Behavioral Barriers to Technology

Our research has consistently shown that there are underlying psychological reactions to the initial introduction of any new technology. Figure 5.1 depicts one

FIGURE 5.1. ATTITUDES AND BEHAVIORS TOWARD TECHNOLOGY

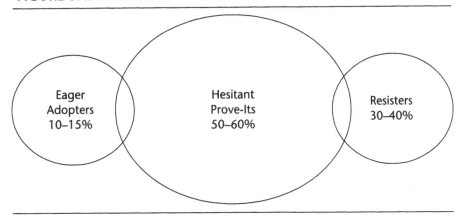

perspective of this phenomenon. As seen in the overlapping circles, there are three types of reactions.

Eager Adopters

The Eager Adopter is a first-wave user of technology. He is the first one to buy *any* new technological gadget. Often, while others are fretting over the purchase of their first personal computer, the Eager Adopter is on his fifth or sixth and drooling at the newer and faster computers that seem to arrive daily.

From a psychological point of view, the Eager Adopter views technology as fun and challenging. He *enjoys* playing and tinkering. Perhaps the Eager Adopter's most important defining characteristic is that he has a sense that even if he does not understand something the answer will eventually be available. When a problem arises—and new technology does have its problems—the Eager Adopter knows that he can either figure out the answer or find someone who can. In fact, the Eager Adopter *expects problems,* and when a problem arises he does not feel that he is the cause or that it is his responsibility. It is simply normal routine; he is convinced that an answer is close at hand. In fact, for the Eager Adopter, finding the answer can be fulfilling and satisfying.

Our research has shown that only 10 percent of psychologists are Eager Adopters. A recent MCI study found 12 percent of business executives to be Eager Adopters, while a marketing study in Ohio found 22 percent of their consumers fell into this category. Our study of consumer response to the notion of the coming information superhighway found 15 percent of Americans could be classified as Eager Adopters.

Hesitant "Prove Its"

The most common response posture to new technology is the Hesitant "Prove It." This group comprises over half of the population (54 percent in our study of psychologists, 59 percent in MCI's study of business executives, 65 percent in the marketing study, and 48 percent in our information superhighway study) and is characterized by both behavioral and attitudinal responses to new technology. Hesitant Prove-Its will choose to wait until any new technology is "proven" before venturing to try it. They want all of the bugs worked out of anything technological before they purchase it.

The Hesitant Prove-It has some discomfort and resistance to technology, as tacitly expressed in the recurring question, "Why do I *need* it?" If you can show this person how something new will make life easier, she is willing to consider it.

On a psychological level, the Hesitant Prove-It *knows* that technology has problems. In fact, she is certain that technology has *lots of problems*. However, she may personalize any glitch and assume responsibility for the problem. Unlike the Eager Adopter, however, the Hesitant Prove-It believes that the answers to these problems may not be available readily. We have seen Hesitant Prove-Its who have turned their personal computers into wonderful plant stands (with a cloth draped over it to hide it from view) because they could not get it to work and did not feel they could find someone to help them. The Hesitant Prove-It may internalize problems that occur with technology, often saying: "It must be my fault!" and "I must have done something wrong."

The Hesitant Prove-It does not feel that technology is fun. She feels that it is work better left to "professionals." This is why in discussions with psychologists we find so many who had an office computer that sat idle while financial billing information was sent to an outside service, at a hefty monthly charge.

Resisters

Resisters avoid technology. They do not want technology, no matter what you try to say or do to convince them. Not only is technology *not fun* for these people, but they are *sure* that it is not for them. They believe they will not be able to do it. They do not always let on that they feel this way; they simply avoid technology. Whenever a technological problem arises, the Resister is *certain* that it was his fault. Problems with technology are taken as severe blows to the Resister's self-esteem and self-confidence. Resisters have difficulty asking for help because they feel foolish, stupid, and embarrassed. They are sure that *they* made the mistake.

Nearly all Resisters are technophobes, and many Hesitant Prove-Its are as well. Technophobia is another dimension of the attitudinal barriers to technological success. Technophobes form a substantial portion of the population; estimates from our research and hundreds of other researchers in the field place this group at anywhere from 25 percent to over 50 percent. A 1993 study of one thousand American adults by Dell Computer identified over 55 percent to be technophobic. MCI's study found that 49 percent of business executives were either cyberphobic (defined as feeling intimidated by the information superhighway concept) or resistant to technology. Our recent California interview study found 54 percent of psychologists to be technophobes.

When we began using this research paradigm in the mid 1980s we used to label this entire group "Computerphobes." Our focus then was on university students' reactions to the introduction of personal computers on college campuses. By the end of the 1980s we changed the label to Technophobes to encompass aversion to the inundation of all forms of technology. We consider Technophobia as present when there is evidence of one or more of the following:

- Anxiety about present or future interactions with computers or computerized technology
- Negative global attitudes about computers and technology, their operation, or their societal impact
- Specific negative cognitions or self-critical internal dialogues during computerized technology interaction or when contemplating computerized technology interaction

Figure 5.2 displays data about the prevalence of technophobia among different groups. As can be seen in this figure, results from eleven studies of nearly three thousand American university students have shown that 35 percent of them are technophobic (with 25 percent highly so). Slightly more secondary school teachers were technophobic, but most of these were mildly so. Strikingly, over half of a large sample of elementary school teachers were technophobic, with 30 percent being highly afflicted. This is particularly troublesome, given results from an earlier etiology study which demonstrated that (1) one of the greatest causes of technophobia was a negative or uncomfortable attitude in the introducer of technology and (2) many people now learn about computers from their elementary school teachers.

When a Technophobe is faced with technological interaction, the primary response is *avoidance,* if possible. In an unpublished study examining coping styles, we found that all Eager Adopters and many Hesitant Prove-Its used either a problem-solving or support-seeking coping style in dealing with everyday problems, while Technophobes used an avoidance coping style.

As shown in the definition above, technophobia can be manifested by a variety

FIGURE 5.2. WHO IS (UN)COMFORTABLE WITH TECHNOLOGY?

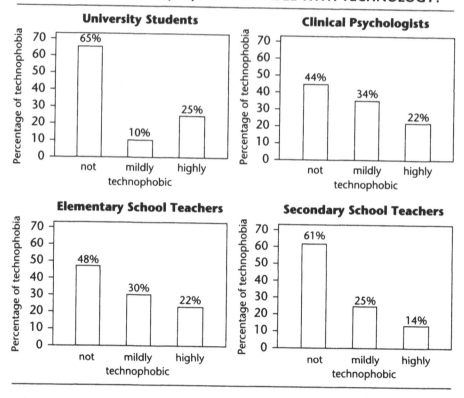

of reactions to technology. In our work, we have identified two predominant types, the Anxious Technophobe and the Cognitive Technophobe. Each avoids technology whenever possible and each feels uncomfortable when forced to use technology, but the reactions are decidedly different. The Anxious Technophobe exhibits classic stress/anxiety reactions, including sweaty palms, heart palpitations, etc., when faced with either actual technological interaction or even with imagined interaction. The Cognitive Technophobe shows few outward signs of distress. However, internally, the Cognitive Technophobe is bombarding herself with negative self-statements ("I will never be able to learn this!" "I'm sure that everyone else can figure this out but me!" "I'm so stupid." "I'll probably push the wrong button."), leaving little room for confidence-building cognitions. Both avoid technology.

Table 5.1 displays the results of the etiology study mentioned earlier, where we asked people to recall their earliest experiences with computers and indicate which of a list of thirty feelings they experienced. For each group, the adjectives

TABLE 5.1. FEELINGS EXPRESSED BY EAGER ADOPTERS, HESITANT "PROVE ITS," AND RESISTERS

Most common feeling adjectives for Eager Adopters, Hesitant "Prove Its," and Resisters during their first computer experience (ordered from most often selected to least often selected; adjectives checked by at least 30 percent of the group)

Eager Adopters	Hesitant "Prove Its"	Resisters
Excited	Uncomfortable	Frustrated
Amazed	Uncertain	Nervous
Eager	Awkward	Awkward
Great	Eager	Uncertain
Successful	Excited	Amazed
Relaxed	Amazed	Dumb
Frustrated	Dumb	Overwhelmed
Pleased	Hesitant	Upset
	Upset	Uncomfortable
	Annoyed	Hesitant
	Frustrated	
	Self-Conscious	

Source: Adapted from Weil, M. M., Rosen, L. D., & Wugalter, S. E. (1990). The etiology of computerphobia. *Computers in Human Behavior, 6,* 361–379. Reprinted by permission of the authors.

checked by at least 30 percent of the group are ordered in Table 5.1 from most often selected to least often selected. The differences between the groups is profound and telling. While the Eager Adopters felt excited, amazed, eager, and entirely positive about their first computer experience, the Hesitant Prove-Its felt a combination of uncomfortable, uncertain, and awkward, yet at the same time eager, excited, and amazed. The Resisters' and Technophobes' first computer encounter was experienced as frustrating, awkward, uncertain, and approached nervously. It is clear that these groups have very different attitudes toward technology.

This description of attitudinal and behavioral reactions to technology provides a ready explanation for the limited integration of technology into the mental health profession. The behavioral and performance ramifications of the Hesitant Prove-Its, the Resisters, and the Technophobes are seen clearly from numerous studies of the integration of technology in the business world:

- Resistance
- Poor performance when forced to use technology

- Decreased productivity
- Decreased job satisfaction
- Diminished morale
- Increased absenteeism and attrition
- Costs to businesses in millions of dollars in inefficiency, stress-related workers' compensation claims, and decreased productivity

Organizational Barriers to Technology

How an organization approaches technology—whether multinational corporation or small group mental health practice—can hamper the successful implementation of technology through fractured organizational philosophy, poor technological planning, and poor staff training.

Fractured Organizational Philosophy

Technology is usually introduced into an organization via a top-down mandate from management. Recipients of the technology (the end-users, in business terms) may be the last to be consulted, if they are informed of the changes at all. With little understanding of the psychological reactions that surround technological innovation, management often plans little or no transition time, which exacerbates the negative psychological reactions.

What discriminates between successful and unsuccessful technological implementation? We recently published the results of an extensive comparison of technological adaptation of twenty-three countries around the world. Relying on our own data, collected from 3,392 university students and published data on the level of technological infusion and acceptance, we discovered major and definable features highlighting countries that have successfully technologized and those that have not. These differences are precisely what predict the success of *any* organization's adaptation to technology.

Several countries that we studied have comprehensively integrated technology, including Israel and Singapore. Although vastly different politically, these two countries showed similarities in organizational philosophies. In both countries, the government has both mandated and supported the early introduction of technology. As early as the primary grades, students use computers funded by the government. Teachers receive extensive computer literacy training as part of their general teacher training. Teachers are confident introducers of technology and value it. In both countries the political structure *values, supports, and accepts* technology as good for the entire country. Interestingly, both countries are very homogeneous in terms of personal values, cultural identity, and religious affiliation. This homogeneity may help to promote a strong cultural acceptance of the transition to technology. Overall, only 10 percent of the students in each country were technophobic.

Contrast these "organizations" with two others: the United States and Japan. In our study, over one-third of American university students were found to be technophobic, and for Japan the number was a staggering 60 percent. Why? From an organizational standpoint, each result makes sense. To look first at the United States, we know that consumer technology is rampant. Nearly everyone owns some high-tech household devices, including a VCR, microwave, television set, digital clock, etc. As early as 1983, 100 percent of our elementary and secondary schools had computers for instructional use. Yet one-third of the American university students in our recent study were technophobic.

What went wrong? First, even though computers are *available* in every school, teachers are not adequately trained to use them. In fact, in a study of nearly six hundred public school teachers we found that one-third to two-thirds of the teachers were not using computers personally or with their students because they lacked confidence, felt victimized by the technology, and felt inadequately prepared. Second, there are no governmental expectations and support for technology. It is not even clear which level of government (federal, state, local) should support technology—a societal lack of clarity that retards growth. Third, there is no financial support for the integration of technology in education. Schools often have outdated, broken equipment and little or no funding to upgrade or even make needed repairs. Fourth, there is no inherent "organizational" value for technology. Until recently, the federal government's stance on technology was, at best, neutral. In the late 1980s and early 1990s, President George Bush stated publicly that he *never* used computers—and he was applauded by most of those in power. It was not until 1988 that California mandated that teachers show evidence of coursework in computers. However, this only pertained to "clearly" credentialed teachers (many teachers are still working on credentials) and did not include those previously credentialed. To date, however, there is still no overall organizational philosophy on technology and no consistent technology plan.

Most people are quite surprised by the large number of technophobic students in Japan. In fact, from an organizational perspective, it makes perfect sense. For a variety of cultural reasons, including a strong sense of the "common good" and a denial of the independent learning that computers promote, the Japanese government has historically kept computers out of elementary schools. In addition, even though computers are available in secondary schools, the teachers for the most part are not able to operate them. When asked why she did not use computers with her third-grade students, one mathematics teacher stated "class time is too precious to use on machines." Recently, however, the Ministry of Education has determined that Japanese students are falling behind technologically and has planned to spend $2.6 billion to place twenty-two personal computers in each primary school and forty-two in each secondary school by the year 2000. This infusion of funds is in addition to plans to change teacher training programs to include computer literacy and operation. These expenditures, plus other Japanese government policy and funding changes, indicate a new organizational valuation of technology and are sure to lead to successful integration of technology into the Japanese educational system and, most likely, Japanese culture over time.

These four macro examples—Singapore, Israel, Japan, and the United States—can serve as models for technological integration in organizational systems of any size. The lessons learned indicate that

- The organization must value technology.
- The organization must support (physically and financially) the early introduction of technology.
- The organization must value a comprehensive technology training program.
- The introducers of technology must be competent and confident.

Poor Organizational Planning

Four potential roadblocks arise when an organization plans to introduce technology:

1. The organization has no cognizance of the actual need for technology.
2. The organization has no awareness of staff attitudes toward technology.
3. The organization fails to develop motivation or desire in the people who will use the technology.
4. The organization fails to pretest the technology.

With technological change happening so rapidly, many organizations determine their technological needs by reacting to a perceived need to keep up. They have little idea what technology is needed or what it can do. They read doomsday reports about how they are being left behind and decide that they must act *now*. Unfortunately, they often act without clear objectives or plans to fund the technology. Worse yet, when they plan for coming technology they fail to plan for the future.

For example, a small independent practice association (IPA) with which we recently talked had decided that they needed to put in a network computer system that would link all of their practitioners and the local hospital computer system. They allocated money to pay for the system but did not allocate funds for training their staff, for upgrades, or for repairs. These expenditures could amount to between one-fourth and one-half of the actual purchase price of the systems!

What happens so often is that one member of an organization decides that it is time to join the technological revolution. After inadequate planning, research, and consultation with the people who will actually *use* the technology but who have no strong belief in the value that the technology will add to the organization, the implementation process begins. Such a plan is destined to fail.

An essential foundation for any effective technological implementation plan is an awareness of staff attitudes toward technology. With 25–50 percent of the people guaranteed to be technophobic and up to 90 percent either resistant or waiting to have the value of technology proven, ignoring these attitudes is inviting failure. As part of our early research, we did a pilot study at a local aerospace company. As it happens, this aerospace company was offering free, three-day workshops (eight hours daily) for all staff on a volunteer basis. Over sixty staff members volunteered for this intensive training. We tested them before and after their workshops and found that 30 percent were more technophobic after their workshop! For these people, the workshop created increased anxiety and discomfort and was not likely to yield much training value. Matching staff attitudes and teaching methods can lead to greater success.

The Hesitant Prove-Its make up over half of the population. These people are not antitechnology, nor are they always technophobic. They are, however, in need of *motivation* and a *reason*. If you can give them a personally compelling reason for introducing the technology, they can become excited and turn into your biggest advocates. Attitudes can be shifted and motivation created when the technology is personalized.

Finally, organizations should pretest any new technological system. Regardless of the sophistication of the technology, any system is bound to have problems. For all but the Eager Adopters, these problems bring discomfort, self-doubt, and resistance. Remember, when a computer system crashes a Resister takes it personally. Organizations can avoid this barrier by providing adequate pretesting of any and all systems with a variety of potential end-users.

Poor Technological Training

All technology requires staff training. Someone must design and implement that training. All of our work indicates that the introducer of technology is perhaps the single most critical ingredient in successful implementation. Potential roadblocks include the introducer's attitude, the style of introduction, the method of instruction, and faulty time line expectations.

First and foremost, the attitude of the introducer has a strong effect on the attitudes of the staff. A "techie" who is too comfortable and eager with technology is likely to impact the learners negatively. You know the type. They spout jargon at a rate comparable to an auctioneer's. When asked how to make the computer do a particular action, this introducer is likely to answer by leaning over, pushing a few buttons, and saying, "See . . . this is easy!" Unfortunately, the learner not only does not *see* anything but internalizes more discomfort and self-doubt.

A second training issue concerns the style of introduction. Technology training must be personalized to the needs and the psychology of the learners. About 90 percent of all people do not feel that technology is particularly fun to implement. When we train people to use technology, we stress that the learning environment should be fun and full of play and exploration. Too often, training takes place in an evaluative atmosphere with time pressures and performance expectations. If you try to teach someone to use a word processing program to write a paper that is due at the end of the day you are likely to create a situation that will lead to frustration and discomfort.

In addition, trainers often err on the side of providing too much information too fast. In the aerospace study mentioned earlier, the three-day, eight-hour-per-day workshops clearly provided too much too fast, and many participants suffered. Technology trainers *must* anticipate problems. Participants *will* have their reactions to the technology training. They can feel overwhelmed and easily shut down. You may deliver a beautiful training workshop, but there is no guarantee that the Hesitant Prove-Its, the Resisters, or the Technophobes will be psychologically capable of paying attention and absorbing the material.

Finally, many technological training programs provide an optimal time line rather than a practical one. There is no time included to deal with attitudinal issues. Thrusting these people into a technology workshop without first attending to their underlying issues only dooms the workshop. The Resisters and Technophobes watch the Eager Adopters accepting the technology and feel more separate, intimidated, and frustrated. The Hesitant Prove-Its will keep listening to hear why they need it. Without that critical motivation, they cannot and will not learn.

Thus several major organizational obstacles stand in the way of successful technological implementation. The organizational philosophy concerning both the value of the technology and the psychology of that technology can provide major barriers to its successful implementation. Lack of planning, particularly planning for a variety of reactions to technology, can stymie a technology program before it even begins. Lack of attention to these issues in designing a training program can breed resentment and frustration and lead to poor performance.

A Model for Successful Implementation of Technology

Figure 5.3 describes a model we devised for successful technological implementation. This model takes into consideration a vast array of research on how people react to technology, borrowing liberally from psychology, business, and education.

This model depicts the entire process as being housed under an umbrella of *systemwide support* and *systemwide values*. This suggests that organizational support needs to permeate *all* levels of the implementation process. There needs to be clear, visible, ongoing encouragement from those in charge. They must be willing to listen and be committed to success. They must be willing to change what is not working at any point in the process and go to any lengths (including offering incentives, as some have done successfully) to facilitate the implementation process. And those in charge must actually use technology as well.

As Dorothy Leonard-Barton of the Harvard Business School and William Kraus of General Electric so aptly stated:

> Overt resistance to an innovation often grows out of mistakes or overlooked issues in an implementation plan. Tacit resistance does not disappear but ferments, grows into sabotage, or surfaces later when resources are depleted. Because the advocates of change have such a clear view of an innovation's benefits, resistance often catches them by surprise. The worst thing a manager can do is shrug such resistance aside on the dual assumption that it is an irrational clinging to the status quo and that there is nothing to be done about it. Clinging to the status quo it may indeed be—but irrational, rarely. And managers can do something about it. . . . The higher the organizational level at which managers define a problem or a need, the greater the probability of successful implementation. At the same time, however, the closer the definition and solution of problems or needs are to end-users, the greater the probability of success. Implementation managers must draw up their internal marketing plans in light of this apparent paradox.

Needs Assessment

The first step in the model is a *needs assessment*. The system (whether it be a corporation or a small group practice) needs to examine what technology is *really* needed. To do this requires examination of two questions:

- What are your technological needs?
- What technology is currently available to meet those needs?

FIGURE 5.3. A MODEL FOR SUCCESSFUL TECHNOLOGICAL IMPLEMENTATION

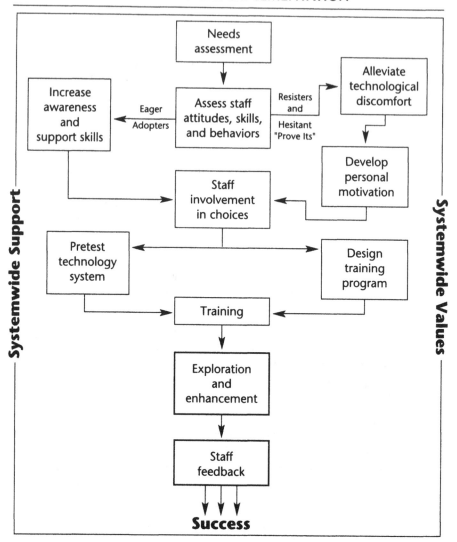

Your technological needs may not be clear. If you do not know what you need (or, perhaps, why), the most direct approach is to ask. Ask colleagues in similar organizations what they are using; ask about their projected needs. Ask them to show you what technology they use. Read the literature; attend conferences; ask lots of questions. Ask if the system is easy to use. Ask about its comprehensiveness. Will it do what you need it to do now, easily? Is it likely that it will still do so some years in the future?

The second question involves careful investigation. When you see what technology is available, you will face a myriad of choices. It is important to remember that technology advances quite rapidly. When a flashy new system is put on the market, this does not necessarily make your system obsolete. Do you really need the top of the line? It depends on the tasks you need to do now and those you think you may need to do in the future. Your system does need to be flexible; it should grow with your needs. You need to ask questions. If you think that you may need something different in the future, build this into your technology plan.

Another important aspect of a needs assessment is an assessment of training and support needs. Plan not only for the purchase of technology (hardware, software, etc.) but for the training of all staff and for their continued support. Some experts suggest that this training and support may add up to 50 percent of your technology budget, but the benefits far outweigh the costs.

For successful needs assessment, collect information from experts as well as end users and give careful consideration to your current needs as well as ongoing or long-term needs.

Assess Staff Attitudes, Skills, and Behaviors

You should determine which of your clinical staff are Eager Adopters, Hesitant Prove-Its, and Resisters. Technophobes should be identified early on. Straightforward measures are available to aid this process. For example, we have developed and normed three measures—Computer Anxiety Rating Scale, Computer Thoughts Survey, and General Attitudes Toward Computers Scale—to provide a three-dimensional representation of attitudes, reactions, and behaviors toward technology. Each measure includes twenty Likert-scale items, and the entire set can be completed in ten to twenty minutes. Armed with this information, you can enhance your future training by designing training to accommodate your staff's true needs.

Treating Technological Discomfort

Resisters and Hesitant Prove-Its need assistance in removing their preconceived technological discomfort. Most of all, they must be told that they are not unusual or alone and that overcoming their discomfort is important to the successful implementation of technology and to their ease in using it. By and large, Resisters, Hesitant Prove-Its, and particularly Technophobes feel that they are the only ones who experience discomfort, and they are often afraid to admit it.

This discomfort is not difficult to remove. As part of a three-year grant from the U.S. Department of Education's Fund for the Improvement of Postsecondary Education, we developed a straightforward program to eliminate technophobia.

This program required no more than five hours and showed a 92 percent success rate in working with nearly two hundred university students. Based on sound psychological principles, it demonstrated enhanced performance and improved attitudes and behaviors over a rigorous longitudinal evaluation. In short, it showed that technological discomfort is easily overcome.

Developing Personal Motivation

Once you have taken the essential step of alleviating their discomfort, next you can help Resisters and Hesitant Prove-Its develop a personal motivation to learn technology. Some are motivated by organizational needs, such as time savings, increased effectiveness, or company desires. Others need a more personal motivator, which may be as simple as keeping their jobs or seeing how technology will help make their work easier.

Technology has gotten much easier to use over the past decade, with point-and-click methods replacing arcane typewritten commands. Often just showing someone how easy it is now to use a computer system may be motivational. However, this motivation needs to be personal. It is the hook that will catch the person's attention.

For example, we just recently made it possible for an eighty-one-year-old woman, who had never touched a computer, to get hooked on the Internet. We did this by showing her, in a few brief minutes of pointing and clicking, how to locate vast amounts of information and pictures about her favorite topic: Mexican archeological ruins. All it took was finding a personal motivation.

Increasing Awareness and Support Skills

You cannot ignore the Eager Adopters. Let them know that not everyone else is as excited as they are and that others do not share their fun and enjoyment at embracing computer problems. Once an Eager Adopter recognizes the psychological reactions that others are having, he can be a valuable asset. We recommend that a psychologically aware Eager Adopter can make a good addition to a training team, or a good buddy for another coworker.

You should also assess critical performance skills. For example, if keyboarding is to be a required skill, make sure that each person can touch-type at a minimal level of competence.

Staff Involvement in Choices

Next, it is time to involve the staff in your technological choices. A technology plan that does not allow the end users to assist in the choices that affect their lives is doomed to resistance. Ask the staff what would make their lives easier. There needs to be a fit between the organization's needs and the staff's style and needs.

We have seen companies that, without staff consultation, installed complicated company management computer systems with many bells and whistles, only to find out the hard way (by lack of staff use) that a simpler system would have sufficed. Even though a vendor may encourage you to buy a system that has enough power to leap tall buildings in a single bound, your staff may want and need something much less powerful and complicated.

Pretesting the Technology

Pretesting the technology is important before beginning training. Make sure that the technology does what the developer claims before you ask your staff to begin training. It is useful to have a selection of users from among all types (Eager Adopters, Hesitant Prove-Its, and Resisters) and at all system levels (from management to end users) try the technology first. Then use their feedback to adjust your training.

At this point in the process, it is important to assess your future technological support. People often need help with technology immediately, or else they begin to doubt their abilities. This means that the software itself should provide good online help as well as a useful, simplified, jargon-free manual. An online tutorial may be helpful for some people, too.

More important is human help. Make sure that your vendor has available telephone assistance (an 800 number is a nice feature). Before you buy, try calling your vendor for help with a problem; in this test run, see if the support is timely, considerate, and understandable. At the same time, you need to plan the help that you will give *after training is completed*. Will you designate a support person? How will your staff reach this person? One idea is to set up a help desk, with a physical location in the building and a telephone staffed during business hours. When the help staff are out working with computer problems, they carry a beeper to stay connected at all times. Just the knowledge that help is available is a help itself!

Training

There are thirteen key issues to be addressed in your training sessions:

1. *Time*   Sessions should be short and focused, with hands-on practice.

2. *Content*   Sessions should cover a single concept at a time and be practical and immediately useful.

3. *Hands-on*	Hands-on practice should be introduced early and often. It builds early success, motivation, and confidence.
4. *Hardware*	Teach on the same equipment that is to be used to foster transfer of learning more effectively.
5. *Help*	Show all sources of help (manual, online, help desk) early in the process.
6. *Match*	Match training to pretested levels of skills, knowledge, and psychological style (Eager Adopter, Hesitant Prove-It, or Resister).
7. *Learning style*	Vary the teaching modality. Some people learn best through visual presentation, others through auditory channels, and still others through tactile (touch) lessons.
8. *Predict problems*	Computers have problems and may crash for no apparent reason. Prescribe this to the trainees and discuss the meaning and cure. It is amazing how many people feel that turning off the computer is not an option.
9. *Assumptions*	Do not assume any preknowledge. Ask!
10. *Modeling*	Research has shown that modeling is an excellent training method. Have someone demonstrate first, and then have the trainee perform the task with the trainer close by for assistance.
11. *Assist*	If a problem arises, the trainer should tell the trainee what to do and let him do it himself. Pressing keys for someone is no help at all.
12. *Guided exercise*	Guided exercises (with pictures of the computer screen mixed in with the text) work well with novices.
13. *Summary*	Summarize information frequently to solidify learning.

The trainer is the key ingredient in the training process. The trainer *must* understand the "psychology of technology." She must be calm, non-evaluative, and not arrogant. It is a mistake for any trainer to say, "See, this is easy!" This intimidates anyone who is having a negative reaction to the technology. The trainer should also keep the training as free from jargon as possible. New terms must be introduced with explanations in simple language.

Ongoing psychological support is also critical to training. A psychologically aware trainer predicts symptoms of discomfort at the beginning of the training and provides learners with time to discuss these feelings and build positive coping styles. This trainer describes potential problems and difficulties and provides suggested ways of handling them psychologically as well as technically. Finally, the literature shows that humor can help with technology training.

Exploration and Enhancement (E and E) Time

Many training programs fail to include sufficient time or resources for staff to master the material. E and E time *must* be an ongoing part of any training program. There needs to be time dedicated to exploring the technology by pushing buttons to see what happens (and to see what bad events do not happen). This "play time" is critical to mastering both the technology and the psychology. It enhances the learning process while providing time to apply coping mechanisms to deal with any discomfort. Do not expect staff to explore on their own time. Structure it into the system introduction and let employees know that they are expected to explore (play with) the new system.

Our applied research has shown that discomfort around technology does not simply depart forever. Rather, people learn to combat the discomfort with positive coping styles. Building these coping mechanisms takes time. This E and E time must be sponsored and supported by the "system." It must be structured into the training and work environment without the fear, or reality, of additional work pressures. E and E time is what makes training successful.

Staff Feedback

Throughout the training the staff must feel comfortable in providing feedback about what is making sense and what is not. A viable, successful training program must build in time for the trainees to provide feedback to the trainer about the training and to others in the organization (managers, programmers, support staff) about their experiences with the new system. This feedback should then be incorporated into the training to show continued system value and support for the psychology of technology.

◆ ◆ ◆

The technological era is rapidly sweeping through the mental health profession. Clinical staff have balked at these changes, because of their attitudes toward technology and the way they have been introduced to technology. In this chapter we have applied more than a decade of research on the psychology of technology to the successful transition from paper to computer. We have detailed the attitudinal and behavioral barriers as well as the organizational barriers that inhibit successful adaptation to technology, and we have provided a proven model to guide the transition. Using our implementation model should help you avoid these barriers and lead to early and continued success.

Notes

P. 87, *sample of over two hundred clinical psychologists:* Rosen, L. D. (1995, July/August). Psychologists relish computer opportunities, survey shows. *The National Psychologist,* pp. 14–15.

P. 87, *transition will be complete within five years:* Geraty, R. (1994). Vision 2001—Behavioral Informatics. *Behavioral Healthcare Tomorrow, 3*(1), 64.

P. 87, *others have predicted ten to fifteen years:* Harriman, M. (1994). Open networked, integrated, multimedia, client/server behavioral healthcare. *Behavioral Healthcare Tomorrow, 3*(1), 17–21.

P. 88, *For example, we found:* Rosen, L. D. (1995, July/August). Psychologists relish computer opportunities, survey shows. *The National Psychologist,* pp. 14–15.

P. 89, *15 percent of Americans could be classified as Eager Adopters:* Rosen, L. D., & Weil, M. M. (1995). Adult and teenage consumer users of technology: Potholes on the information superhighway? *Journal of Consumer Affairs, 29*(1), 55–84.

P. 91, *we used to label this entire group "Computerphobes":* Rosen, L. D., Sears, D. C., & Weil, M. M. (1987). Computerphobia. *Behavior Research Methods, Instrumentation, and Computers, 19*(2), 167–179.

P. 91, *one or more of the following:* Rosen, L. D., & Weil, M. M. (1990). Computers, classroom instruction, and the computerphobic university student. *Collegiate Microcomputer, 8,* 275–283.

P. 91, *eleven studies of nearly three thousand American university students:* Rosen, L. D., Sears, D. C., & Weil, M. M. (1992). *Measuring technophobia. A manual for the administration and scoring of three instruments: Computer Anxiety Rating Scale (Form C), General Attitudes Toward Computers Scale (Form C), and Computer Thoughts Survey (Form C).* Dominguez Hills: California State University, Computerphobia Reduction Program.

P. 91, *technophobic, with 30 percent being highly afflicted:* Rosen, L. D., & Weil, M. M. (1995). Computer availability, computer experience, and technophobia among public school teachers. *Computers in Human Behavior, 11*(1), 9–31.

P. 91, *from an earlier etiology study:* Weil, M. M., Rosen, L. D., & Wugalter, S. (1990). The etiology of computerphobia. *Computers in Human Behavior, 6,* 361–379.

P. 92, *results of the etiology study:* Weil, M. M., Rosen, L. D., & Wugalter, S. (1990). The etiology of computerphobia. *Computers in Human Behavior, 6,* 361–379.

P. 93, *studies of the integration of technology in the business world:* Craig, J. S. (1994). Managing computer-related anxiety and stress within organizations. *Journal of Educational Technology Systems, 1993–1994, 22*(4), 309–325; Frude, N. (1991). Psychological aspects of the new technological age. In A. Ager (Ed.), *Microcomputers and clinical psychology: Issues, applications and future developments* (pp. 195–214). New York: Wiley.

P. 94, *twenty-three countries around the world:* Weil, M. M., & Rosen, L. D. (1995). The psychological impact of technology from a global perspective: A study of technological sophistication and technophobia in university students from twenty-three countries. *Computers in Human Behavior, 11*(1), 95–133.

P. 95, *in a study of nearly six hundred public school teachers:* Rosen, L. D., & Weil, M. M. (1995). Computer availability, computer experience, and technophobia among public school teachers. *Computers in Human Behavior, 11*(1), 9–31.

P. 95, *"class time is too precious to use on machines"*: White, M. I. (1991, Fall). Higher education: A comparative examination. *The NEA Higher Education Journal, 7*(2), 5–18.

P. 96, *to include computer literacy:* Gross, N. (1992, April 6). A PC boom in Japan's classrooms. *Business Week,* p. 89.

P. 99, *Leonard-Barton . . . and William Kraus . . . so aptly stated:* Leonard-Barton, D., & Kraus, W. A. (1985, November–December). Implementing new technology. *Harvard Business Review, 63,* p. 108.

P. 101, *measures are available to aid this process:* Rosen, L. D., & Maguire, P. D. (1990). Myths and realities of computerphobia: A meta-analysis. *Anxiety Research, 3,* 175–191.

P. 101, *we have developed and normed three measures:* Rosen, L. D., Sears, D. C., & Weil, M. M. (1992). *Measuring technophobia. A manual for the administration and scoring of three instruments: Computer Anxiety Rating Scale (Form C), General Attitudes Toward Computers Scale (Form C), and Computer Thoughts Survey (Form C).* Dominguez Hills: California State University, Computerphobia Reduction Program.

P. 101, *straightforward program to eliminate technophobia:* Weil, M. M., Rosen, L. D., & Sears, D. C. (1987). The computerphobia reduction program: Year One. Program development and preliminary results. *Behavior Research Methods, Instrumentation, & Computers, 19*(2), 180–184.

P. 102, *working with nearly two hundred university students:* Rosen, L. D., Sears, D. C., & Weil, M. M. (1993). Treating technophobia: A longitudinal evaluation of the computerphobia reduction program. *Computers in Human Behavior, 9,* 27–50.

CHAPTER SIX

COMPUTERIZATION IN GROUP PRACTICES

Peter S. Currie

The overriding change occurring in the behavioral health industry is the shift from a cottage industry of independent autonomous providers to organized systems of care. The private practices that flourished in the 1980s have been truncated by managed care in many areas of the country. The forces of supply and demand have worked against the private practitioner as the average length of treatment comes under control and the selection process trims the number of preferred providers being utilized by managed care to a smaller and smaller pool.

The Industrialization of Behavioral Healthcare

Managed behavioral care is not the only factor in the industrialization of behavioral healthcare. Changes in medicine as a whole have foretold what is now happening to behavioral healthcare. Physicians have been driven into organized IPAs and medical groups, which in turn have been acquired by practice management companies. These companies, many of which are publicly traded, have served as leading examples for recent attempts by other companies to adopt similar models for acquiring and consolidating behavioral health providers in order to form organized systems of care. With the economic power of publicly traded companies focused on "rolling up" providers into new delivery systems, the future of the cottage industry of private practice is in doubt.

Acquisition fever hit behavioral health only recently, as we are but a small piece of the healthcare industry and are often overlooked. With the restructuring of healthcare into organized systems such as medical groups well under way, behavioral health is now undergoing a wave of pruning, acquisition, and consolidation. Many provider networks are not only closed to new entrants but are also being downsized. Organized group practices have become a hot property as companies making acquisitions seek an advantage by gaining a working delivery system that already covers a specific geographical region. These groups have also established contracts with payers and produce revenues and earnings that are particularly valuable to publicly traded companies seeking to acquire groups. There appears to be much competition to buy up the largest groups across the country, but some companies are also making offers to small groups and solo practitioners.

Managed behavioral care organizations (carve-out companies) are attempting to stay ahead of the curve; they could be challenged by the growth of these emerging provider organizations and large groups if they do not develop a strategy for partnering with organized provider groups. Costly utilization review and case management functions performed centrally within these MCOs are now seen as excessive overhead that depletes the MCO's earnings and, with shrinking margins, may even sink the MCO ship altogether. The mature provider group is seen as a more efficient model for managing aspects of the behavioral health delivery system that have previously been handled within the MCO. The mature group can perform the functions of utilization management, case management, and quality improvement and thereby accept capitated (risk) contracts just as the medical groups have done for years.

The movement to performance-based contracting such as capitation is under way, and this is fueling the development of fully functional group practices that are capable of managing themselves. Consequently MCOs are evolving, streamlining their operations by emphasizing their regional and national marketing expertise while partnering with groups in various ways to off-load most of the expensive case-management, quality-improvement, and utilization-review functions. Some of the largest MCOs have adopted a more aggressive strategy of acquiring groups, thereby building their own staff model or integrated delivery system. MCOs that previously prided themselves on their large network of individual providers are evolving rapidly toward developing preferred contracts with organized provider groups. This strategy is intended to help them remain competitive by reducing costs and simultaneously increasing the accountability and reporting requirements of their providers.

Another looming trend that is creating new challenges for both providers and carve-out companies is the movement toward integrating behavioral health within organized healthcare as part of completely integrated delivery systems. The boundaries between medicine and behavioral health appear to be dissolving as the incorporation of behavioral health services is being recognized as desirable, especially in such areas of healthcare as disease management. The position of behavioral health in these integrated systems of care is apt to vary widely based on the relative importance that the behavioral health providers have in these settings. The advantages of continuity of care seem clear, but the most powerful motivator for integration is still an economic one. Often the reality has been that medical groups seek to include behavioral health services primarily to retain the behavioral health capitation dollar and to enhance profits rather than to actually develop behavioral health departments that enhance the quality of the healthcare they provide. This unfortunate profiteering has backfired for medical groups and HMOs that have not focused on the quality of the behavioral health services they provide. Many employers have carved out mental health and chemical dependency services to the MCOs. Having experienced this, many medical groups and HMOs have begun to develop strategies to "carve back in" the behavioral health component. Fueling this trend is the emergence of disease management, an integrated approach to managing the high-cost/high-risk population. Behavioral health is crucial to disease management, as many diseases are caused or aggravated by human behavior. Strategic health education and behavioral intervention in concert with medical treatment promises to be a very desirable combination.

Accusations of profiteering shoot back and forth between providers, carve-outs, insurers, and medical groups. Objectively, each group within our industry often lacks a true appreciation of the functions and roles of the others. Purchasers of healthcare no longer trust marketing propaganda and are demanding accountability. Report cards and other outcome measures are becoming powerful tools to demonstrate performance. To manage today's contracts, with their emphasis on accountability, information systems have become one of the most important and essential ingredients for survival and growth. Information systems are rapidly becoming the infrastructure of established and emerging group practices. Groups are now recognizing that information systems are the key to their ability to grow and survive. Only with sophisticated systems can a group manage performance-based contracts and step up to the demands for accountability that all payers now require.

Information systems promise to level the playing field within our industry by enabling providers and MCOs alike to produce the outcomes and accountability the purchasers of healthcare are demanding. With the right information systems, provider groups will be capable of moving up in the "food chain" by being able to provide managed care accountability along with the direct clinical services which purchasers want. Rather than seeing this evolution as threatening and fighting the growth of provider groups, many MCOs are evolving to partner in various ways with emerging provider groups. With this nondefensive response, mutually beneficial alliances are being formed and the status of the provider is becoming enhanced because of the increasing capabilities found in group practice.

Information Systems: The Essential Infrastructure of the Group Practice

Information systems for behavioral health are in their infancy compared with other industries such as manufacturing. Consequently, groups that have been looking for systems to automate their work flows and provide the accountability their payers want have not been able to find appropriate solutions. The practice management packages that were specifically tailored to behavioral health have not had the functionality required to manage capitated accounts. Medical practice management packages were typically able to handle the high volume and capitation management needed by medical groups, but these systems required significant customization to fit the work flows specific to behavioral health.

On the other hand, there were separate utilization review packages, outcomes packages, and other pieces of the needed system specific to behavioral healthcare, but no comprehensive system that would provide the whole integrated solution that behavioral healthcare groups required. The market, although seemingly large when viewed from within, was not significant enough to attract the larger software development companies to build new systems to fit our needs.

Consequently, a handful of existing practice management companies in our industry began to add on to their systems to approximate the functionality we needed and take advantage of the pent-up demand for information systems to manage behavioral group practices. Despite these efforts, information systems for the behavioral group practice are far behind the systems available to almost any other industry in America. Most groups are still searching for more adequate software packages and spending considerable money modifying existing systems to try to keep up with their growth and automate their work flows.

The Stages of Computerization of the Group Practice

Just as group practices evolve in stages, groups also develop their information systems in stages. A group's pattern of developing and acquiring new information system functions mirrors their growth and complexity. Furthermore, a group's resources are usually tied to its size, and new systems can only be afforded when resources allow. Consequently, most groups add information system functions in stages according to their current developmental needs.

First Stage

The vast majority of groups that begin the process of computerization start with the "back office." The billing and financial management of the group is usually the first priority. Most groups select an existing "legacy" system that is proven to perform the traditional functions of a group practice. A *legacy system* refers to software packages running within hardware configurations that have been well established and do not rely on state-of-the-art technology. There are relatively few practice management systems specifically designed for behavioral health that have the network capabilities, the functionality, and the robust design needed in the growing group practice. More often the larger groups choose from among the proven medical practice management systems that were primarily designed to handle the high volume of the medical group. These systems are moderately expensive as information systems go, $5,000–$100,000 depending on the functionality included and the size of the installation. They are often legacy systems that lack state-of-the-art features. Nevertheless, they are established, have proven themselves over time in medical groups, and are consequently seen as a stable base upon which to build or interface the unique functions required in a behavioral group practice.

A requirement that adds to the cost of the system is the capitation management component of the system. Most mature medical practice systems can handle taking in capitation and tracking the incurred but not reported costs (IBNR). This is adequate for a group that simply needs to be able to operate under capitation from a payer. However, larger groups need the increased capability of a capitation management system designed to manage the payment of capitation or other performance-based payment methods to providers. This more complex functionality is required when the group seeks to pass on incentives to providers within the group. Such full-function capitation systems add considerably to the expense of the system and also must interface with the fee-for-service billing module within the system. The following are the typical functions of an information system that is designed to automate the nonclinical functions of the group, often referred to as the front- and back-office functions:

- Fee for service billing with electronic capability
- Capitation management
- Claims adjudication
- Appointment scheduling
- Authorization management

- Patient registration and enrollment
- Payer and benefit registration
- Payer-specific accounting and reporting capability
- Customizable report generator

Second Stage

The second stage in computerizing the group practice involves automation of the clinical functions of the group practice. This focuses on the development or search for a suitable computerized patient record (CPR). Ultimately, outcome research will be drawn from the rich data generated within the clinical record. Pre- and posttreatment measures will be incorporated within the information system's CPR.

The CPR is needed to learn from, and improve upon, the treatment processes used in treatment. Measuring the outcome through surveys of patients' functional status or other stand-alone outcome measures does not tell us which treatment processes are the best predictors of the desired outcome. We can continuously improve our treatment standards by capturing the processes of treatment in a consistent, scientifically sound fashion within the CPR. This is accomplished by being able to apply statistical techniques such as factor analysis in crunching the data gathered within the CPR. To be useful, the data from individual patient records is downloaded to the system server, where it is stored in a "data warehouse" and made available for analysis. In a group setting this data can be used for in-house applied research that has immediate value to the group and its providers. As the CPR becomes more widely used, groups can pool their data into larger data warehouses to enable larger populations and more diverse clinical processes and interventions to be studied.

Other clinical oversight and review functions have been developed by MCOs over the past ten years. These systems perform such functions as utilization and case management. As the group practice becomes increasingly responsible for these managed care functions under capitation and other performance-based contracts, the functions have to be integrated with the group's information system.

Groups are now recognizing the value of the CPR and are exploring ways to automate their clinical records in order to standardize their recording and measurement of clinical processes. As the best of these efforts are realized, we anticipate that good CPR packages will become available on the market. With the current emphasis on accountability in healthcare, the CPR is a very valuable tool because it provides the accountability payers want. Furthermore, the integration of clinical management functions with the CPR provides a comprehensive solution. The second stage of computerization of the group practice includes the addition of the following clinical functions to the group's information system:

- Provider credentialing and peer review
- Clinical records
- Utilization review with external interface with payers
- Case management with external interface with payers
- Risk management (clinical protocols and procedures, appeals, and grievance functions)
- Quality improvement monitors and reporting
- Outcome research analysis and reporting

Third Stage

The third stage of computerization of the group practice focuses on the incorporation of expert decision support systems. These expert systems are capable of containing multiple assessment protocols that, when utilized to assess a patient, result in a recommended critical pathway or treatment plan. Currently, such systems are used at some MCOs to guide utilization and case management processes. This technology is currently being used in other industries to improve diagnostic and decision-making processes. Expert decision support systems can be a tremendous tool to help groups establish protocols and standards of care in order to stabilize their clinical processes.

There are valid objections to relying on an expert system to provide clinical judgment. Expert systems that are used to dictate a diagnosis or treatment plan to the clinician are potentially dangerous. The clinical judgment of the trained and experienced clinician who has face-to-face contact with the patient should not be overruled by a computer system. In addition to jeopardizing the quality of care, there would also be considerable liability for a group employing such a computerized clinician substitute. However, just as we have seen how the creative use of virtual reality is highly effective in the treatment of anxiety disorders, expert decision support can also be a highly valuable tool if implemented properly.

Expert systems that are "hard coded," and therefore not easily updatable or customizable, are quickly outdated. The system must be designed to incorporate new clinical information and continuously update the protocols and decision trees based on the latest outcome data. Such a system is "table driven," allowing the user to customize and update the protocols without having to use a computer programmer to make such updates. With a well-designed expert decision support system, competent clinical experts map the decision trees they use in assessing specific groups of patients. The critical factor is the ability to use the outcome data, combined with established standards of care, to modify and improve our protocols. Revisions to the protocols are made as we identify which treatment processes are likely to produce the most positive change in a given population of patients. By design, table-driven expert decision support systems can be easily modified by clinical experts to allow truly continuous quality improvement.

Implementing the computerization of clinical practice is much more challenging than automating the business and financial aspects that fall within the scope of practice management systems. The CPR needs to be clinically designed to fit the clinical work flow required within the group. This often differs from group to group, and ease of user customization is critical if the introduction of a CPR is to be successful. CPR systems with hard-coded screens modifiable only by a computer programmer should be avoided. Table-driven screens that allow the user to directly update the system to match the group's evolving delivery system are more desirable.

Even more difficult is incorporating an expert decision support system. Clinicians have been taught to think and use their experience when assessing and treating a patient, and no expert system can replace this fundamental function of the clinician. However, in addition to areas of expertise, every clinician has limitations in experience and knowledge. An expert system should incorporate the cumulative expertise of the provider group while supplementing the knowledge limitations of each individual provider. The computer-entered knowledge base is translated into an assessment tool (differential decision tree) and treatment protocol (critical pathway). For this technology to be used within the group, it must be easily customizable to include the expertise of the clinicians within the group. If providers have contributed to the development of clinical protocols, they are more likely to use the expert decision support system. Furthermore, the treatment recommendations of an expert decision support system must always be considered as guidelines, not as absolute rules. Clinical decisions are still made by the clinician with the expert decision support as a guide.

Direct Connectivity Between Provider Group and Payer

Payers are actively seeking ways to electronically connect with their providers. Similarly, provider groups see this trend as an opportunity to cooperate with these efforts in order to preserve and expand their relationships with these payers. Payers and providers have already begun linking electronic systems to transmit referrals, authorizations, encounter data, claims, and clinical reports. This connectivity has resulted in new concerns about confidentiality and electronic methods of interfacing.

Data Privacy

Security becomes a particular concern of providers when they are asked to send information to the payers via fax, modem, or telecommunication system. Providers remain legally bound to maintain their patients' confidentiality, and the chances of a security breach increase whenever clinical information is transmitted from one location to another. Although maintaining security within a group with multiple offices in a wide area network can challenge the group to make sure their systems have adequate security measures, the challenges increase when they are sending information out of their network to their payers. Many clinicians legitimately resist electronic hookup because they envision hackers or other unauthorized individuals will obtain confidential clinical information.

Security measures need to be in place particularly when groups enter the second phase of computerization, in which detailed clinical records are captured within the system. The paper method of reporting to payers is expensive and obsolete, and most payers are moving to some form of electronic data interchange with providers. Consequently, concerns over maintaining informational privacy and confidentiality must be addressed. Clinicians can no longer simply refuse to participate in electronic forms of communication; rather, they need to insist on adequate security measures. It is becoming apparent that a properly secured information system is far superior to the old paper file in protecting confidentiality and in maintaining the integrity of the data placed in these records.

Most systems offer basic security measures involving security code identification to access the system. This form of security is found on many off-the-shelf software products. Unfortunately, this basic and inexpensive form of security is inadequate alone to secure a patient record, particularly when the sensitive clinical data is being transmitted from one location to another. Identification codes are often not kept confidential, and the potential for unauthorized access exists. Furthermore, a simple security code does not provide adequate protection during transmission of the data, which is when it is most vulnerable to unauthorized access.

An improvement upon the basic type of security code is the addition of ID card security. This level of security is similar to the type of identification required by banks. The likelihood of unauthorized access is minimized by the addition of an ID card. However, this extra step in the security process is costly and has not been adopted by many of the systems being used in behavioral healthcare.

Security can also be enhanced by other widely used methods. An essential method for any user that is transmitting clinical data electronically is *encryption*. Encryption is the process of encoding the data in an unreadable format. The unreadable information is then secure while it is sent to its destination. Once the information has arrived, the authorized recipient system reverses the encryption and the information sent is presented in a readable format. This process helps prevent unauthorized access to confidential clinical information during transmission from one system to another, while the data is most vulnerable.

Other methods often found in more sophisticated software packages are read/write limitations and audit trails. Read/Write limitations refer to the program's built-in security system, to specify which users within the organization can read or view what specific data and what these users can write or document within the system. This is a very important feature for group practices that have various types of users on the system. Nonclinical staff such as billing clerks or receptionists require access to the practice's management functions of billing and appointment scheduling, but they do not need to read the clinical data within the Computerized Patient Record. Similarly, a provider may be authorized to read or view the billing information but not write in, or modify, this part of the system. Also, the integrity of the clinical record can be enhanced by placing write limitations on the clinical documentation, whereby new documentation is date stamped. If a clinician wishes to change a previously completed document, the system records the new entry as an update and preserves the integrity of the original document. In this way a treatment plan can be updated throughout treatment while preserving the historical integrity of the successive treatment plan iterations. Audit trails add to the security of the system by automatically recording the identity of the user who accesses the system. Audit trails can be used to trace who accessed the system and what they did within the system. Trails are also used to trace and report any unauthorized access to the system.

Interface Compatibility

Once the provider group is satisfied that the system they will use has sufficient security measures to be used to link with outside payers and managed care organizations, they need to evaluate the feasibility of such connectivity. Ideally, the provider's and the payer's systems should be capable of interfacing. However, not all systems were built to operate in an open (platform- and hardware-independent) environment. Consequently, the provider group needs to investigate which systems their payers are using and choose systems that are reasonably compatible. Practice management system vendors should be able to identify what it takes to create the direct connectivity desired between the provider's and the payer's systems.

Many provider groups are making their system choices based on the systems used by their payers. This decision to "follow the leader" has merit for many groups that expect to benefit from the research-and-selection process undertaken by MCOs. The difficulty is that these groups experience immediate pressure to automate in order to remain competitive. They cannot wait for consensus to be reached among their payers as to what systems they will use. Furthermore, many MCOs still consider their information systems proprietary and have not made efforts to standardize their systems. Many see their particular system as their competitive edge, used to differentiate them from the other MCOs. Consequently, provider groups will find it difficult to select a system that is compatible with all their payers' systems.

There is also an inherent danger in simply adopting the payer's system as the group's system. The functions of the group differ in many ways from the functions of the MCO. More and more, the groups serve a variety of payers, from behavioral health carve-out companies to medical groups and HMOs. As the group's book of business expands, the need for a fully functional system that has the capabilities to administer all of the managed care functions becomes more critical. Groups can borrow functions such as case management, utilization management, and claims adjudication from the established MCO systems. Nevertheless, groups must also design or select systems that provide the specialized functionality of the group's clinical delivery system. Groups must balance the efficiencies gained by following the leader (incorporating MCO compatible systems) with the need to match the selected information system to the group's own application (the group's clinical delivery system).

The emergence of telecommunication systems that provide connectivity between the provider's practice management system and the payer's system is not new. However, the scope of the information that can be transmitted is expanding, from claims to clinical reports to outcome data. Providers have reacted to the advent of sending clinical data via the Internet or other telecommunications vehicle as a dangerous assault on the confidentiality and informational privacy rights of our clients. On the other hand, visionaries argue that the potential gains of gathering the rich clinical data within the CPR, to create computerized warehouses for health research, outweigh the potential violations of a patient's right to informational privacy. This legitimate debate has unfortunately been tainted by the impatience of some providers and MCOs alike who produce so-called outcome research primarily for marketing purposes. "Outcomes" data is in danger of becoming another discredited marketing ploy, made up of manipulated and unreliable data. To prevent this damage, scientific standards of applied research need to be emphasized in development of the information systems we employ. Health psychology is a specialized science, as is the larger field of health or medical research. Ideally, the provider group's systems that gather the clinical data within the CPR should be designed by clinicians and health researchers and not by marketing departments.

The Quest for Standardization
Versus the Encouragement for Innovation

In recent years there has been a great deal of attention to the standardization of the data we gather. This is based on the pragmatic need to make sure the data we collect and report on are useful, as we seek to compare and draw generalizable conclusions. Also, the drive to standardize the data we gather is based on the research principle that parameters and controls are necessary to isolate the variables that are producing the outcomes we find. Standardization is necessary to reduce the waste that occurs when information is gathered repeatedly in different ways by different companies resulting in noncomparable data.

MCOs are recognizing the benefit of agreeing on a single method in performing certain functions such as credentialing. In the past, the credentialing process involved each MCO's independently performing a unique assessment of their provider's qualifications. Providers would be credentialed by multiple payers simultaneously, resulting in an incredible waste of resources. Many MCOs are coming to the conclusion that there is little competitive advantage to be gained from continuing to use their unique credentialing process, and they are exploring a standardized credentialing process they can all agree upon and share.

Similarly, there is an effort to standardize the CPR. The intention is to have clinicians gather information in a consistent format which can then be tapped for research and quality-improvement efforts.

Minimum data sets and other elements of standardizing data collection are not conducive to innovation, particularly in the clinical processes of the group practice. For this reason, the CPR and expert decision support systems should not be hard-coded into a standard, unalterable form. Rather, such clinical information systems need to be table-driven, allowing the group practice to continuously update and refine their clinical information systems to match the evolving clinical delivery system the group creates. Specific reports and standard data sets can always be drawn from such a table-driven CPR. This reporting can be done in a format that satisfies specific payer or research needs. The quality improvement that can be gained from a clinical information system that empowers innovation by allowing groups to easily modify its screens and data fields need not be lost due to standardization. Clinical innovation requires that the group practice not simply adopt the MCOs' systems but rather modify such systems or even develop new systems to interface with the existing ones. The provider's expertise and perspective should not be overlooked when systems are being developed.

Group Practice Economics:
The Cost/Benefit of Investing in Information Technology

The fact that we have to borrow practice management systems from medicine and try to adapt such systems to a behavioral health application is indicative of our relative lack of technology. This fact has led some of the group practices to the "bleeding edge" of developing systems themselves. Groups struggle with the decision to wait until some vendor develops a stable system that approximates their needs, or else plunge into the risky venture of being the first group to develop the ideal system using state-of-the-art technology. Most groups wisely shy away from developing systems from scratch and search for at least a basic system with which to begin. Since there is no complete solution available from any of the vendors, most groups are combining components of existing systems with customized modules to approximate their needs. Most start with a proven practice management system and set out to create custom additions, particularly in the areas of clinical information functions.

The incorporation of technology and systems into a group practice is very challenging, due to the limited resources available to these groups. Group practices typically lack the capital necessary to go out and buy a complete system. Rather, most groups add systems out of necessity as they grow beyond their outdated methods. Groups cannot always wait until they want to invest in new systems. The demand from payers for accountability and outcomes has driven many groups to attempt to acquire systems before they can afford them in order to be attractive to payers.

The overwhelming force that drives groups to select increasingly sophisticated and expensive systems is their own growth. It has been estimated that once a group reaches fifty thousand covered lives or twenty providers, a practice management system becomes essential. Once the group reaches one hundred thousand lives or forty providers, the system usually has to be replaced or expanded to accommodate the increasing complexities of the growing group. As the group exceeds 250,000 lives or eighty providers, the information system requirements start to look like those of a combination of an MCO and a large medical group. So large a group needs its own information system department and system manager to keep up with the maintenance and growth requirements.

Those groups that grow rapidly face major challenges in how to keep up with their information systems needs. They must differentiate the essentials from the luxuries in the options they consider. Groups should look down the road when acquiring their base practice management system. The system should be robust and scalable. Scalability is critical if the group wants to avoid dumping their system altogether when they reach a critical size. *Scalability* is the system's ability to handle increasing volume and complexity as the group grows to regional, multiple-site coverage that may require expansion of the hardware configuration from a local area network (LAN) to a wide area network (WAN), and to the addition of larger file servers. The openness or ability of the system to interface with other systems is also important in selecting a basic practice management system. The group will need to expand the functionality of their system to include addition of a CPR and eventually other specialized components, such as expert decision support systems, that the original vendor will not supply. Consequently, ease of interfacing the base system with other add-on systems becomes very important down the road.

The cost and complexity of acquiring and building needed information systems often appears overwhelming to a group practice. Some groups are seeking the economies of scale and expert knowledge provided by larger MCOs, management service organizations (MSOs), or other companies that have entered the practice ownership or management business. These consolidators often provide information systems and other management services to multiple groups, thereby spreading out the cost of the system. The group does not base their decision to join with these larger organizations solely on the affordable information systems they supply. Rather, the groups see the information system supplied by the larger practice management organization as one of the benefits to be weighed against the potential disadvantages of becoming part of a larger consolidated delivery system. Regardless of the legal structure that accompanies such partnering, the group becomes a part of the larger entity by virtue of its dependency on the centrally supplied information systems.

Virtual Groups: Information Systems as the Infrastructure of Provider Groups

As technology is applied to the industrialization of the behavioral health industry, the possibilities for how we combine to form new delivery systems multiply. One concept adapted from the business community is the formation of "virtual group practices." The concept involves the use of sophisticated information systems to form the infrastructure of the group's delivery system. Practice management software combined with a CPR and other system components can be installed in various settings, such as private practice offices, hospitals, structured outpatient programs, and multidisciplinary clinics. Providers linked through such an infrastructure can be combined to form cohesive delivery systems without having to exist under the same roof. IPAs and "groups without walls" that failed in the past due to a lack of cohesive infrastructure could be revised and become viable. The key to the success of the virtual group is the ability to combine a set of providers, services, and programs into a delivery system that best suits the needs of the population the virtual group is formed to serve. The strength of this new way of designing our delivery system is the group's ability to reformat itself rapidly to service a particular population while maintaining consistently high-quality service. This is made possible by the information system that ties all the components of the virtual group together.

The critical advantage in the virtual group's ability to respond to changes in payer demands and the needs of the populations they serve is based on using information technology that stabilizes and quantifies the clinical processes and services. Once the group is able to identify which clinical processes are most effective given a set of symptoms and presenting problems (clinical protocols or standards of care), the information system can guide and record the treatment process through the CPR. When innovative interventions are tried, the CPR can capture the resulting outcomes so that treatment protocols can be improved. Providers with expertise and superior outcomes in a particular area can be identified and their expertise mapped into improved protocols that become available to the other providers within the group via the expert decision support system.

Information systems used within a group of providers as described above can facilitate "real-time continuous quality improvement (CQI)." The CPR is designed so that the clinical processes, or specific factors that help define the clinical processes, and corresponding patient responses or outcomes can be captured at the point of service delivery. This is a powerful advance over reliance on retrospective outcome measures alone. The CPR can then provide the clinician with feedback on the patient's progress and provide suggestions from the expert protocols within the information system. This use of outcome data and treatment protocols can benefit the patient directly: real-time CQI.

The CQI loop is made possible because the clinical data gathered within the CPR is downloaded to the system's server, where complex analyses can be done on the quantified clinical data. The group can then study its population, clinical procedures, and outcomes. The results of such ongoing research can be fed back to the clinicians in reports and revised treatment protocols. In order to be truly useful, the CPR must have a data warehouse capability, allowing the group to gather data from all of its clinicians. This rich data is then available for extensive ad hoc research and analysis.

The value of such a system to a broader population can be enhanced by cooperative relationships between groups that share their clinical data in a common warehouse. Behavioral scientists can perform further research with such data warehouses, utilizing a much larger population. The incorporation of information technology within the group practice, to gather data at the point of service delivery, is a powerful and revolutionary advance in the way we can use outcome research to improve the care we provide. Information technology promises to bring applied research into the clinical practice, where it can continuously shape and improve the services provided to our patients.

◆ ◆ ◆

Industrialization of the behavioral healthcare industry is reshaping managed care and provider organizations alike. There is an immediate need for information systems that can interconnect diverse behavioral health payers and providers. Previous definitions and boundaries between payers and providers have become blurred. Group practices are responding by reengineering the way they think and practice, just as the rest of healthcare and the broader business community have done.

The behavioral healthcare industry has just begun to independently design its own systems. A few pioneers developed practice management software packages in the 1980s. Since then, a handful of vendors have sought to build comprehensive systems for behavioral health applications. Mostly, we have adapted systems originally built for medical groups and HMOs. These systems can only take us part way, as clinical design by behavioral healthcare professionals is needed to map the unique work flows and clinical processes of behavioral healthcare delivery systems. The current focus for the group practice should be to acquire or develop a CPR that can be interfaced with existing practice management systems. The CPR is the heart of the information system for emerging group practices, as it will be the source of the outcome data they will need in this age of accountability and reform in healthcare. The next challenge will be the addition of expert decision support systems to the group's CPR. Ultimately, the goal is to have a system that will not simply manage the financial and administrative functions of the group practice. Rather, a comprehensive system will require a sophisticated, clinically designed CPR that gathers and downloads clinical data into the system's warehouse. The data is continuously analyzed and reported back to the clinicians to facilitate real-time CQI.

The behavioral healthcare industry is in the midst of sweeping changes. The emergence of group practice is at the center of providers' efforts to reengineer their practices. Information technology offers the tools for providers to successfully reinvent their delivery systems and manage the treatment they provide. Information technology is the connective tissue that can integrate these group practices and link them with the other sectors of the evolving behavioral health industry.

CHAPTER SEVEN

COMPUTERIZATION IN COUNTY AND COMMUNITY MENTAL HEALTH CENTERS

Tuan D. Nguyen and Gary Olsen

Despite the fact that national healthcare reform did not proceed as envisioned by the Clinton Administration, its mere proposal initiated reform momentum in many states. Already more than six states have obtained Sect. 1115 waivers to apply managed care concepts to the Medicaid portion of their healthcare system. Other states are actively planning to redesign components of their health delivery systems. As a consequence of these reforms, most behavioral health organizations serving publicly funded clients face tremendous tasks in redesigning their data processing and information dissemination systems to meet the new business functions.

This chapter highlights principles and functionalities that are critical for successfully meeting these requirements in changing information systems. We use examples drawn from two community mental heath centers (CMHCs) that are at different stages of redesign, reformulation, and implementation of their information systems. These examples serve to illustrate the feasibility as well as the challenges facing any attempt to modify and enhance informational capacity to meet the additional reporting requirements stemming from major managed behavioral healthcare redirection.

Concurrent Business Concerns

Behavioral healthcare organizations can only realize the goals of managed care when they are able to implement, integrate, and operate within several complementary business mandates. These mandates are to manage costs, manage benefits, manage care, and manage outcome. Information system features needed to support each business mandate are reviewed in this chapter. A note of caution, however, is in order. Historically and typically, these four principal managed care capabilities have been developed sequentially, in phases, by private managed healthcare organizations. However, it is clear that their development must now occur rapidly and concurrently within public and semipublic behavioral healthcare organizations for these entities to survive the competitive challenge posed by the private sector.

There are three reasons for rapid information system redesign in CMHCs and related organizations:

1. The need to fast track care integration at the clinical level to reduce overhead cost
2. Emerging government (state and federal) initiatives to privatize services
3. The fundamental conceptual change from a fee-for-service paradigm to the managed care approach, which is often operationalized as capitation

The Need to Integrate Care at the Clinical Level

It is estimated that managed care organizations now spend about 17 percent of their budgets to monitor providers, and providers spend 15–22 percent of their budget to develop and maintain systems to meet the demands of MCOs. These levels of overhead cost are probably exceeded in publicly funded or publicly operated programs. Such high operational overhead (or indirect) cost can be drastically reduced only when care management is integrated efficiently and seamlessly at the clinical level. This state of affairs happens when the processes for determining the quality of care, its appropriateness, and its effectiveness are built into care delivery itself, rather than maintained at some upper, remote rung of the bureaucratic ladder.

Attaining clinical care integration requires integrating information domains to support decision making at the point of service—integration that can be enhanced dramatically by improved information technology. Thus, it is generally expected that automation will play a critical role in this move toward greater cost-effectiveness. Capitation-based financing will further require advanced information systems that allow care providers and managers to have quick access to accurate data on costs, as well as the ability to track specific patient use and key treatment outcomes.

The Trend to Privatize Public Healthcare

A second reason for needing a rapid organizational and information system redesign is in emerging state and federal initiatives to downsize government services by privatizing them wherever practical. Traditionally, behavioral healthcare organizations that served publicly funded consumers—community mental health centers, state hospitals, etc.—relied almost exclusively on public funds to carry out their missions. Public funds, in turn, were almost exclusively targeted at supporting publicly funded providers. These carve-out situations have been and are being actively rethought by state legislatures and local (usually county) governments.

Community mental health centers and related agencies, never having had to compete in order to serve publicly funded clients, lack the organizational and informational experiences necessary for competition. While many centers have some capacity for unit cost computation and rate setting for their various services, most have not been required to deploy—nor have they voluntarily developed—necessary managed care capacities, such as routine computation of cost by episode of care for different target populations. Consequently, the typical center often lacks many basic information capacities that are necessary to compete as a care provider or as a care manager when it contracts out its services.

Fee-for-Service Versus Capitation Management

The third reason for a rapid organizational and information system redesign is the fundamental conceptual change from a fee-for-service paradigm to the managed care approach, often operationalized as capitation. In the fee-for-service paradigm, more service is better fiscally for the service provider, since more services draw down more revenue from public funding sources or the insurance companies. By contrast, when care is to be managed using a fixed amount of finances to cover a fixed number of covered lives, the focus shifts to providing only what is appropriate, with the definition of *appropriate* varying from payer to payer. Some payers (typically insurance companies) establish limits on service or care coverage for each enrollee or illness condition. Other payers expect the provider to monitor and deploy services within the confines of capitated (preallocated) premiums, without a priori limits per "enrollee."

This fundamental conceptual shift requires basic shifts in managerial as well as clinical decision making. For example, issues of treatment efficacy (that is, effectiveness relative to cost) and severity-adjusted outcomes have become more salient and critical to the successful operations of behavioral healthcare delivery. These emerging decision-making parameters require retraining of staff, who will often be inclined to resist such distasteful notions as "capitation," "preauthorization," "rationing," "service packaging," and "practice standards." They also challenge information system staff to repackage the information delivery processes so as to maximize the organization's ability to perform the new functions.

Two CMHC Examples

Before we discuss the design and implementation principles associated with the four managed care business mandates (manage cost, manage benefits, manage care, and manage outcome), it is helpful to provide glimpses into the organizations and information systems of the CMHCs from which many of our examples are drawn.

One center, Valley Mental Health of Salt Lake City, Utah, incorporated many managed care features in the design and implementation of its new information system in 1991. While it still maintains fee-for-service and cost-of-service arrangements with many funding partners, Valley Mental Health has been Medicaid-capitated since 1991. This Medicaid capitation contract accounts for over half of its operating budget.

The other example center is the Mental Health/Mental Retardation Authority of Harris County, Texas. The Harris County Center upgraded its information technology capacity in 1992 to modernize its information technology and capacity. Organizationally and informationally, it has not had to contend with the rules and regulations of capitated funding, since it remains strictly a fee-for-service provider, even for Medicaid covered services. However, the center's management is well aware of the need to prepare for managed care requirements and mandates.

In using these two centers as examples we intend to show how most centers, even if different from each other in terms of revenue streams and reimbursement constraints, do in fact face similar reengineering challenges and information system changes when they move into the managed care environment.

Information System Capabilities of the Two Centers

The Harris County Center is responsible for a three million person catchment area, employs 1,586 individuals in a variety of occupations, and provides almost two million direct and indirect services to about twenty-nine thousand different consumers annually. Its service system covers the full array of "core" mental health and mental retardation services, from crisis intervention to housing assistance for persons with mental disabilities. The only exception is acute inpatient services, which are provided by the University of Texas under a separate state funding stream.

The Harris County Center is reasonably equipped in terms of data processing capacity and infrastructure. A configuration of over 1,000 connections is built around a cluster of three minicomputers, including 450 terminals, 560 PCs, and

80 Macintoshes. While they are spread over forty-eight locations in the 1,078 square-mile area of Harris County in the greater Houston area of Texas, these peripherals are connected through high-speed data connections to the core financial and clinical data bases.

The Harris County Center's software applications include two major business and clinical data systems. A major project is under way to build a client/server-based data warehouse that brings together data from the two applications and integrates them with other smaller data bases to facilitate data analysis and information processing without negatively affecting the routine data processing tasks.

In addition to the goal of improving consumer and service tracking, the Harris County Center's data system was also intended to maximize fee-for-service Medicaid billing and reimbursement. On this score, the system has literally paid for itself by allowing the agency to increase its Medicaid collection from $300,000 in fiscal year 1992 to $4.5 million in fiscal year 1995.

While Valley Mental Health provides only mental health services, it is considered a large provider, with forty decentralized sites for residents of Salt Lake and Summit counties in Utah. Its staff of over eight hundred is responsible for opening 9,100 new cases annually, maintaining an active caseload of 12,500 at any given time and providing services to 16,300 unduplicated consumers. Its information system recorded 1.1 million hours of outpatient and case management activities and 103,221 consumer days.

Valley Mental Health service sites are networked to its central computer configuration using high-speed communication lines and frame relay technology or direct connection. This infrastructure supports 105 simple access terminals, 254 personal computers, and 80 attached printers at this writing.

The information system at Valley Mental Health is composed of a patient management component and a financial management component. The financial component is third-party proprietary software, while the patient management component has been designed and programmed in-house. Data from both components are easily combined to meet reporting purposes.

Generic Mental Health Data Capabilities

Reviewing the content of any mental health information system since the mid 1970s reveals that its set of core data elements has remained fairly stable. Many states and CMHCs, including our two examples, have incorporated into the design of their data systems the federal guidelines published in the *Data Standards for Mental Health Decision Support Systems*. These guidelines provide a basic philosophy and data set for data system development. With the advent of managed care, however, this recommended data set must be reevaluated in terms of its comprehensiveness for new service delivery and management functions.

Turning to our example CMHCs, their information systems contain modules that capture clinical, fiscal, quality assurance, service and program monitoring, and research data. Some differences can be found between the centers in terms of how data elements are aggregated or integrated to provide information for management and decision making. Managed care, however, requires their information systems to incorporate additional management and clinical information capabilities. Here as in other CMHCs, the majority of informational capacity expansions and additions relate to service efficacy, treatment outcome, and effectiveness management.

It is exactly this expansion of information capability—in contrast to simply increasing data processing capacity or upgrading the data processing technology—that facilitates a CMHC's ability to excel in the managed care environment. Data processing involves the timely, efficient, reliable, and consistent gathering, transfer, and storage of data. Information capability is in manipulating, integrating, and reporting data in ways that make them directly relevant to decision making. As is often the case, there is a paucity of information even though data abounds. For example, clinical charts for many CMHC consumers are usually inches-thick while the chart data is so difficult to extract and integrate that clinical decisions are often made without taking into consideration the wealth of gathered data.

When information system development focuses on information processing rather than data gathering, the tasks for information system staff actually become somewhat easier in the short run; much can be achieved immediately by creatively relating and integrating existing data elements and involving the center's staff intimately and extensively in this effort. In general, this effort requires that a center address the following critical information system challenges:

- Ability to amalgamate data elements into indicators (cost, efficiency, risk, outcome, etc.) and decision-relevant statistics (rates, trends, profiles)
- Ability to establish information routing pathways and capacities that allow timely access by key decision makers irrespective of whether they are service providers or managers
- Ability to maintain closer relationships between data in the computerized system and data in the clinical chart
- Ability to formalize and standardize methods for assessments and treatment planning

In the remainder of this chapter, we discuss in greater detail how each of these information system functions can be developed for each of what we consider the four phases of managed care: managed cost, managed benefits, managed care, and managed outcome. Examples from our two CMHCs are used to illustrate the principles that should be observed when developing and implementing these information capabilities. For each phase, we first offer a conceptual definition, then a summary of its main informational features, and finally a description of how such features can be developed.

Information Features in the Managed-Cost Phase

For purposes of this discussion, cost management is defined as a provider organization's ability to determine its service costs and to establish billing rates. Cost is the monetary value of a service unit, for example, a procedure or a service package. A billing rate, on the other hand, is the amount one charges the recipient or payer for the service rendered. From an information system standpoint, the critical factors to be supported in the managed-cost phase include (1) the ability to gather data regarding staff time deployment, salient consumer and service statistics, operational expenses (such as personnel, utilities, supplies) and fixed expenses (property, plant, equipment) and (2) procedures that combine them to establish unit-of-service costs.

Differences Between Cost Data and Billing Rate Data

CMHCs do not usually have to pay close attention to the difference between cost and billing rate. This is because in the traditional fee-for-service approach to claiming and paying for services based on procedures or time, a center recuperates its expenditures by first billing some payers (for example, insurance companies, Health Care Financing Administration [HCFA], etc.) using billing rates that the payers impose. The remainder of the expenditures that are not so covered are then charged against state and local funds.

When billing reimbursements, state funds, and local allocations are not sufficient to meet its actual or planned expenses, a center would normally reduce programs or staff. But by and large, one-to-one relationships between expenses and service units are not routinely examined. In other words, service statistics are rarely matched against expenditures within the context of different programmatic, organizational, or demographic parameters. For example, in Texas the community mental health and mental retardation centers enter into a "performance contract" with the state Department of Mental Health/Mental Retardation. This contract requires separate (although parallel) reporting of effort and output on the one hand and expenditures on the other hand. These centers usually manage their billing and budgeting activities solely toward the "revenue maximizing goal" (to be discussed). Thus, until recently most Texas centers could not easily compute accurate costs per program, per consumer, per episode of care, per diagnostic or problem groups, per ethnic or age category, etc.

Because they are usually derived from full-year statistics, billing rates are rarely adjusted either seasonally or organizationally. However, adjustments to the rates may sometimes be allowed by payers to account for significant geographic variation or variation in cost of living over time. For example, in some states, after a Medicaid reimbursement rate is set for some procedure (e.g., an outpatient visit), the rate is indexed on the cost of living in the geographic area served by the CMHC. In other instances, cost-of-living adjustments are made to rates derived from the previous year's data in order to reflect current economic conditions.

In Utah, the state Medicaid office (HCFA), the state Department of Mental Health, and the counties that fund the mental health centers each conduct cost and organizational audits in order to assess the centers' responsible use of public funds. Consequently, Valley Mental Health has developed the capacity to provide cost analyses that are congruent with each funder's particular requirements, specifically regarding allowed and disallowed activities. The Harris County Center is subject to a similar Medicaid cost determination and auditing process. As would be expected, both centers are always faced with the problem of how to recover those costs which are disallowed. Both centers have also had to pay close attention to how to make up for reimbursement rates that fall short of true cost.

Variations in Cost

Cost, unlike reimbursement rates, can vary from one period to the next (from one month, one quarter, or one year to the next) depending on variation in expenditure and productivity. Per-unit cost also varies from site to site or program to program depending on staffing, service mix, or level of program utilization by consumers. Unfortunately, because they are accustomed to the fee-for-service methodology, CMHCs rely almost exclusively on payers to dictate the per-unit rates, which are incorporated into the automated or manual billing modules. Centers often do not go through rate-setting exercises, not to mention complicated cost-estimation processes. Those few centers that cost-analyze their services in order to set rates do not do so often enough, or with enough detail.

Even if billing or reimbursement rates come close to the service unit cost, it is more often the case that they fall short of true cost. The rate-estimation approach mentioned above contains inherent inaccuracy. For example, a center may set a centerwide rate of $15 for a fifteen-minute medication visit. But the cost of such a visit may be higher or lower depending on where it is provided and the level of staff productivity. Failure to take into account these variations can lead to sizable errors in cost estimates that jeopardize an agency's competitive stance, particularly when it negotiates reimbursement rates or basic capitation financing.

Expanding from Fee-for-Service

In the fee-for-service environment, a CMHC sets "revenue goals" for fee-for-service funders. For example, the Harris County Center sets an annual, agency-wide goal of $4.5 million of Medicaid revenue for fiscal year 1995 and apportions this amount to its programs as budgeted revenue. The revenue from each service provided then accumulates toward that goal. Reaching and actually surpassing the goal is considered desirable and an indication of positive growth. A similar reasoning led the Texas State Legislature to set a goal of $27.8 million in additional Title XIX (Medicaid) reimbursements for its community-based mental health and mental retardation programs for fiscal year 1996. Thus, the centers must draw down that amount from Medicaid in order to maintain their current service level. To the extent that the centers fail to do so, services must be reduced or other funding sources must be found to make up for the "deficit." It remains to be seen how the centers in Texas will fare when the federal government places a cap on Medicaid funding.

In sharp contrast to the fee-for-service model are capitation and other methods of at-risk financing. These models are rapidly becoming favored cost-containment strategies among funders moving into the managed care approach. Such funders are looking to set maximums on their reimbursement dollars, either per episode of care or for a set of covered lives (that is, eligibles) or both. In a capitation situation, a CMHC is faced with a fixed revenue amount per eligible member per month that is expensed as services are provided. Instead of monitoring how much revenue it is *accumulating*, a center must monitor how much is "left" of its resources before the contract year ends.

Thus, in the managed cost environment, simply having cost data or cost analyses is not enough. A center must also be prepared to undertake financial management practices that bear little resemblance to billing and budgeting practices under the fee-for-service model.

Need to Accommodate Multiple Payer Types

Another challenge facing any CMHC in the new managed care environment is the fact that while some of their funding streams may be capitated, others are not. The information system challenge is thus to be able to accommodate multiple payer types (fee-for-service, specialty contracts, etc.) and provide management with cost and revenue information to effectively monitor each funding stream.

Valley Mental Health has a billing module that not only can distinguish between funding sources (fee-for-service, specialty contracts with specific billing requirements, and capitated services) but can also bill them accordingly. This capacity has greatly increased the efficiency of the billing process, saved a significant amount of staff time, and helped improve cash flow.

The Information Technology Implications

How, then, does a CMHC lay the foundation for a successful cost management system? As mentioned earlier, most CMHCs have the basic financial, consumer, staff, and service data. What is needed first and foremost is a commitment to develop and implement information processing procedures that routinely produce the service statistics and cost analyses. The technical approaches undertaken at our example centers to arrive at cost data are by no means novel. Many practical manuals exist to help agencies with the nitty-gritty cost computation process.

At both of our centers, the intent to automate a comprehensive cost analysis process led to the assignment of a cost center (or procedure) code to all services, including nonbillable activities. Cost center codes are intended to facilitate the aggregation and reporting of the service data for per-unit cost-analysis purposes. Every service record in the data base also includes consumer and staff identification codes. These codes enable the computer programs to link a service to its consumer and its provider. The data are then easily combinable with client, staff, payroll, and operational budget data when performing cost analyses.

Cost analysis is done semiannually at Valley Mental Health and will be done monthly at the Harris County Center. The process begins by aggregating all similar services across the center's continuum of care in order to determine the per-unit costs. These per-unit costs are then adjusted for cost-of-living increases, or by specific service location, professional discipline, or particular provider as the case may be. It is also possible to compute cost per anticipated plan of care, per actual episode, or per consumer by aggregating the costs of the services associated with each respectively.

Valley Mental Health also maintains a running total of services and costs for each consumer episode (from admission to discharge) in its information system. This summary information facilitates regular calculations of episode costs and can be analyzed by numerous consumer variables (diagnosis, race/ethnicity, etc.). It is then possible to combine these cumulative cost data with outcome data when the latter become available in order to produce cost-outcome information.

Despite their mundane features, costs are critical for CMHCs in the new behavioral healthcare paradigm. In the movement to privatize or outsource care and services, public funds go to those providers that can best compete in the marketplace. While service quality, treatment effectiveness, and consumer satisfaction play a major part in that competition, the bottom line will most likely continue to be cost because of the severe shortfall in funding and the fierce competition for scarce public dollars. A center that cannot accurately determine its costs and variation in costs in a timely manner, and then analyze those costs from a variety of perspectives in order to manage them effectively, will surely lose the competitive race.

In order to facilitate and reinforce the paradigm shift, information systems have to make reliable cost information available to intake workers, care planners, clinicians, and utilization reviewers. This apparently simple requirement in fact offers formidable challenges, for it implies significant investment in additional training as well as hardware and software. For example, the computer access capacities currently in existence at our example centers (two terminals for every three employees at the Harris County Center and three for every five at Valley Mental Health) have to be expanded. Additionally, faster, more timely, and more user-friendly access for more users requires the expansion of computing and data communication capacity. Increased access by more users also leads to greater demand on information system staff to create additional, customized reports from and "views" into the data bases. Furthermore, mobile computing will soon become necessary as home healthcare practices gain ground with the behavioral healthcare industry (as they have with other healthcare sectors); this will require even further technological enhancement.

Implications for Human Resource Development

Information system capacity alone, however, is not sufficient to achieve a fully operational and effective cost management system in a CMHC. As is often the case in other functional areas, new information system features often impose, necessitate, or motivate behavioral changes in the work force. These changes must in turn be reinforced and sustained through systematic training and skill development.

Thus, as cost management processes are implemented, there must be a corresponding increase in staff's understanding of the fundamentals of healthcare economics, among which are the center's cost-finding and rate-setting procedures. Without this understanding, there cannot be truly informed decision making, wherein both staff and consumers consider cost issues when planning the utilization of service.

At a minimum, staff must know how their ways of spending time impact the center's costs. In a capitated contract, staff must also realize how a referral to external agencies incurs a cost to the center and depletes available funds to serve other consumers. Furthermore, every package of planned services carries with it a cost, and staff should be able to determine easily the relative costs of alternative packages. Valley Mental Health will soon include cost training as part of its employee orientation and training. Its time-deployment reference manual contains a section entitled "How You Spend Your Time Affects Cost." Both of our example centers also plan to distribute more widely the results of their cost analyses.

The conceptual shift from providing to coordinating and managing services—from "more is better" to "provide what is needed"—will take some time to accomplish at both centers. Most CMHC staff are too well indoctrinated in the fee-for-service mentality, since performance expectations have been largely and frequently based on this mode of thinking. Only after cost analysis procedures are well developed, implemented, refined, and understood by all staff can a mature cost management system occur and be integrated with other phases described in this chapter for optimal service delivery management.

Information Features in the Managed-Benefits Phase

Benefits management is defined here as a center's ability to obtain, implement, and monitor various payer-allowed and disallowed services or service limits. In some instances, the center has to implement these limits itself in order to ensure adequate and equitable resource availability to its covered lives. It is not unlike trying to stretch the availability of scarce drinking water during a drought so that at the end of the dry season there is still sufficient water for all concerned. Managed care has exponentially raised the emphasis on, and in most instances the requirement for, benefits management.

Operational Implications of Benefits Management Systems

For a CMHC, the critical factor in benefits management is the ability to determine what the benefits are for each consumer or group of consumers. This is easy when a consumer has private insurance, because benefits are usually spelled out in the enrollee's coverage. It is not so easy when services are to be covered by other funds. Worse yet is when a consumer's needs for services far exceed her benefit coverage.

Valley Mental Health has expanded its information system to include capabilities to track each consumer's private insurance limits or Medicaid regulations (for example, a 168-hour cap on day treatment), benefits effective dates, method of accumulation (hours or days), and the corresponding maxima and copay requirements for various services. The information system at the Harris County Center is also set up to track the most basic form of benefits management, namely, whether a consumer is eligible for Medicaid or insurance coverage. This information system is also set up to bill only "authorized" services. This feature, although it is not truly a benefits management function, can later be modified to flag inappropriate claims submitted to the agency by its contractors for payment.

Benefit Packaging in the Publicly Funded Sector

Besides Medicaid, financial support for CMHCs also comes from county and state funds. These state and county funds are often used to augment services paid by other funders (such as Medicaid match). They are typically earmarked for broad and ambiguous purposes, such as "the medically indigent" or "the severe and persistently mentally ill." Consequently, funding in the public sector is generally not tied to a well-defined and specific benefits package, such as maximum number of inpatient days or lifetime number of outpatient visits, etc. Instead, more general "eligibility" criteria are used to define access, with decisions regarding the level, duration, and intensity of service or care usually being left to "clinical judgment."

For example, the definition of the "priority" mental health population in Texas is so broad that the Harris County Center faces an eligible pool of persons three times the caseload it now serves. Yet, its state funding is at the 25th percentile of all Texas centers, and Texas ranks near the bottom nationally in terms of per capita mental health funding.

Eligibility Criteria and Benefits Guidelines

Benefit definitions usually vary from one capitation or contract model to another. For example, one managed care plan may define inpatient psychiatric benefits in terms of number of hospital days per episode while another may define them in terms of number of days per lifetime. Thus it is critical that the information system make it possible for intake workers, service planners, clinicians, and utilization reviewers to refer to these benefits definitions on demand and for each consumer.

Valley Mental Health accommodates this requirement by making the information available online as part of the fee record. This benefits management feature is not yet salient for the Harris County Center since the center as yet has only a negligible number of consumers with insurance coverage. However, both centers realize that they cannot ignore or underestimate the necessity for this capacity. Both realize that it will be a challenging task to document benefits (that is, entitlement to types and amount of services) when a capitation system is imposed on the non-benefits-specific population whose services are covered by county and state funds.

Managed care financing in the form of capitation, however, will present a new set of problems and issues for the CMHCs since there are currently no well-established guidelines for determining eligibility for treatment or well-defined standards of care in the public sector. Recently, realizing that the agency cannot meet the demand for service from all the members of its pool of ninety thousand potential consumers, the Harris County Center defined a set of priority access criteria that is narrower than the state definition of "priority population" in order to triage service requests. While this is the first step toward operationalizing a benefits management system, defining access criteria alone is to benefits management what billing rate computation alone is to cost management. In other words, access criteria do not spell out what a consumer is entitled to receive. It only serves to identify whether a resident who presents for service qualifies, in terms of their presenting problems, as a consumer.

Because access criteria do not provide clear a priori guidance as to what is individually available and appropriate for each consumer or condition, a center must also have some methodology for determining the necessary level of service provision and setting guidelines concerning appropriate service expectations. Without clear service expectations, efficient benefits management cannot occur. The best a center can do in this instance is to fall back on cost management in order to ensure that in the aggregate the expenses associated with services that are provided do not exceed the projected revenue.

At the Harris County Center, the intake process is further refined by defining more explicit "portals of entry" and by streamlining and integrating the sequence of activities associated with intake, eligibility determination, and treatment planning. It is hoped that well-timed execution of these critical activities will lead to the most cost-effective service planning.

Service Planning Guidelines

Given that service determination and planning are critical steps in the benefits management process, the current trial-and-error method of planning for services in most CMHCs must be replaced. In other words, the determination of who does what for the consumer must "get it right" the first time in order to avoid cost overrun, inappropriate care, and ineffective treatment. But this is not possible without clear and standardized service planning guidelines, whether derived from internal historical experience or, preferably, based on industrywide standards. Such guidelines are being aggressively developed at both of our example centers, although their existence and execution are still exclusively manual, relying as they are on paper forms and paper documentation.

Updating Client Benefits Status

In addition to being able to ascertain eligibility and benefits entitlements, a center operating in a managed care environment must also be able to update the benefit status of every consumer, preferably via a dynamic (online) linkage with the funder or payer. In recent years, with increasing emphasis on maximizing Medicaid reimbursement for services provided to Medicaid eligibles, most centers have developed the capacity to update their consumers' Medicaid eligibility status on a routine basis. In most CMHCs, billing coordinators also obtain eligibility and benefits information on privately insured clients when they first enter treatment or when an adjustment is made to their charges.

Our two example centers have automated linkage with their state Medicaid offices to facilitate the laborious process of determining Medicaid certification. Each month, the centers obtain a file containing all the enrollees for the counties they serve. Computer programs then use the transmitted data to perform the following:

- When a consumer is already identified as Medicaid eligible in the center's data base, his status is updated with the transmitted data to reflect his current as well as retroactive certification. Retroactive certification and retroactive changes in certification have presented some of the most frustrating challenges to the information systems, although they are not insurmountable.
- When a consumer has not been identified as Medicaid eligible in the center's data base, his record is matched against the transmitted file of Medicaid enrollees. Matching criteria include first and last names, birth date, and social security number. At Valley Mental Health the list of "new" enrollees is used by the billing staff and the consumer's clinician to initiate the enrollment process. At the Harris County Center, the list of new enrollees is used to convert their services into claims for submission to the Medicaid intermediary.

As a means to increase its pool of Medicaid certified consumers, the Harris County Center has developed a computerized process to identify consumers who meet Medicaid eligibility criteria but are not Medicaid-certified. This process relies on the indexing of each non-Medicaid consumer's family income against the federal poverty guideline and her diagnosis against the diagnostic criteria that define Social Security Supplemental Income (SSI) eligibility. This information is distributed to primary clinicians to encourage the identified consumers to enroll in the Medicaid program. A small grant from the Social Security Administration actually funds some benefits coordinator positions to assist the agency's potential eligibles in obtaining Medicaid certification.

Planned Versus Used Benefits Patterns and Exhaustion Rates

As a CMHC develops the capacity for benefits management, it should also combine benefits data with other data to increase its management capacity. With valid and reliable information from the cost and benefits management phases, for example, a center can begin to analyze and project service liability in terms of planned (allowed) versus actual cost, or in terms of actual versus available service utilization. Such analyses should be available by consumer, consumer group, payer or health plan, and staff or provider type. These analyses should highlight the variances between available versus used benefits by individual consumer, consumer category, provider type, and payer category. Valley Mental Health is experimenting with this analytic capacity, but its application is limited to the Medicaid capitation population.

In the long run, a benefits management system must also expand the above analytic ability to include the capacity to identify actuarial profiles of benefit exhaustion rates. These rates show how fast the benefits are used up over a given time period, although annual rates will probably be most useful since most contracts are specified for one year's duration. The profiles must, of course, be differentiated to account for variations across problem types, illness categories, consumer types, and provider types.

Training of Staff About Benefits Management

The close relationship that exists for cost management between information system capacity and human resource development is also relevant with respect to benefits management. That is, as benefits management modules are developed, staff must also be trained in the concepts and operational features of benefits management and capitation. Without full understanding and continuous practice by staff regarding benefits management, there is little hope for any CMHC to achieve and maintain a competitive stance and financial viability.

Our example centers have not developed formal training for clinical or support staff in the concepts of benefits management or capitation. Both centers, however, have begun training programs regarding access criteria and portals of entry and have expended significant effort to train staff in the treatment planning process. Valley Mental Health also conducted intensive program-by-program in-service sessions when it first entered into its capitated contract with Medicaid.

Access to Benefits Management Information

A significant information technology challenge remains: the ability to make all of the aforementioned information and analytic capabilities available at the desktops and fingertips of every intake worker, care planner, clinician, and utilization reviewer. This capacity clearly must be implemented in all CMHCs that hope to operate successfully as providers and managers of care in the managed care arena. Furthermore, as with the cost phase, there is a clear need to integrate business data with patient data, service data, and other pertinent clinical data (such as medication) to be able to manage benefits and benefits exhaustion efficiently.

While most CMHCs have some of the aforementioned integrative capacity, as a rule this has not been the focus of prioritized efforts. This state of affairs is not surprising, considering the fact that CMHCs have been so strongly influenced and driven by the fee-for-service rather than capitation paradigm.

Information Features in the Managed Care Phase

For purposes of this discussion, managed care is defined as a center's ability to guide, monitor, and control each consumer's regimen of services in terms of amount, duration, utilization, cost, and quality.

Standard Guidelines for Planning Care

As noted above, a center must first have the capability to document and monitor what is planned before any kind of actual versus planned analysis can be done. Only then can information comparing planned versus actual care, planned versus actual cost, and benefits exhaustion be made available to clinical and management staff so as to refine the service delivery process. The planned regimen of services or treatment must be developed or at least coordinated in some central or otherwise controlled manner.

In the traditional, fee-for-service environment, there is little or no incentive to do this since each program component is encouraged to draw down as much reimbursement as it can by providing as many services as possible. Usually, there is also no established limit on service provision. Consequently, a treatment plan is often a fuzzy statement of service intent that does not specify in advance the reasons for and the amount and type of services. Treatment plans are changed when the service pattern does not seem to "work." But an agency in the managed care atmosphere can ill afford to continue this trial-and-error approach to care management. Without a careful benefit exhaustion plan, both the consumer and the agency will surely encounter unpleasant surprises, the most serious of which is the inability to continue to treat the problem or illness effectively.

Utilization Management

A common mechanism for managing care is utilization management. This mechanism consists of prior approval of each consumer's service package on the basis of the consumer's benefit coverage, membership, and problem type, and then subsequent monitoring of service delivery to ensure that the actual provision and use of services do not exceed preapproved limits. Limits can, of course, be extended when more services are deemed necessary in order to reach effective outcomes.

The Harris County Center's clinical application software has a utilization review module that marks off visits (or days) from the count of preapproved visits (or days). It then alerts key monitors regarding the level of service use. Although not yet activated, these features can easily be modified to support formal utilization review in the center. The center's use of individualized service coordinators, who are responsible for planning and monitoring the care of their consumers across the full spectrum of the center's services, also ensures maximum coordination and control of service use.

Coordinating Care Across the Service Delivery Network

One of the clinical benefits of operating in a managed care environment is the realization that treatment responsibility has rarely, if at all, been the domain of a single staff member. Most consumers involved with a CMHC that has a significant continuum of care probably receive services from a number of staff in different programs.

The majority of CMHC consumers also suffer from illnesses and conditions that are long-term and chronic rather than acute. Thus, when a center provides a wide array of services over a large number of sites, it is often difficult to pinpoint the focus of care for its chronic consumers, who can access services at many points in the service delivery system.

These two critical variables—chronic illness conditions and a multiplicity of service sites—often make it difficult to coordinate plans of care across the array of service programs. Care planning, as a consequence, can easily remain piecemeal and at best be coordinated only within departmental boundaries (clinics, case management program, psychosocial program, etc.). For example, at the Harris County Center, prior to its intensive training program on integrated treatment plan development a year ago, 80 percent of consumers served in the psychosocial programs did not have a plan of care signed off by a psychiatrist or psychologist. Some consumers even entered these programs directly without going through formal portals of the system.

Further exacerbating this lack of care coordination is the fact that in almost all CMHCs the treatment plans, to the extent that they do exist, can only be found in the physical clinical record or chart. The lack of computer-assisted treatment planing makes it difficult to share the plans in a timely fashion horizontally across programs that serve the same consumer and vertically for providers to seek authorization from care managers or for case managers to monitor an individual consumer's benefit exhaustion rate.

Both of our example centers are aggressively examining these deficiencies with the intent to fast track all necessary systemic changes and implement them. Valley Mental Health is meeting this challenge functionally by reorganizing its entire performance evaluation criteria in terms of teams rather than individual providers. The Harris County Center has successfully reorganized two of its outpatient clinics into a multiservice center where teams, rather than individuals, work with each consumer to plan the services, provide or "commission" for them, and monitor them against the plan. This model is being replicated in other outpatient sites and subsequently at the interdepartmental and interagency levels of the center.

Electronic Integration of Access, Quality, and Cost Information

Any reengineering of a CMHC to address managed care issues must incorporate the trilogy of access, quality, and cost. Performance indicators pertinent to each area must play an integral role in monitoring how successful the center is in adapting and evolving to the full managed care environment. These indicators must be used by management and staff to continuously improve service delivery. One of the primary sources of data for constructing such indicators is the consumer treatment plan or plan of care, which heretofore has been primarily manual. When the rich data contained in the planned service goals for consumers are captured electronically and integrated with other information system components, the center's care monitoring capacity increases significantly.

But how does one capture and systematize the myriad of empirical treatment expectations that clinical staff have often proliferated idiosyncratically? Conceptually, it is possible to devise methods to extract, organize, and systematize these treatment expectations from the clinical service delivery process. But so far, no single method has proved empirically definitive in terms of user-friendliness, efficiency, and relevance. Two alternatives are being considered at Valley Mental Health:

1. Provide a mechanism to record the primary service coordinator's estimate of expected service utilization (augmented by other center providers involved in treatment). Service expectations are to be specified in terms of type and duration (for example, outpatient therapy once a week for eight weeks). The computerized system would then help staff monitor actual service provision in terms of these individualized goals by providing feedback, either online or in some report format.
2. Establish centerwide expectations by some consumer characteristic (most probably diagnosis). Actual services can then be monitored against these more

global expectations or guidelines. This latter approach emulates the diagnostic related grouping (DRG) method used by Medicare to control reimbursement for medical care.

There are advantages and disadvantages to adopting either of these approaches. Relying on the service coordinator's estimates, which are usually negotiated with the consumer at the time the service plan is developed, gives the clinician more latitude to prescribe services. However, this approach tends to create a much narrower "window" for the agency to assess its total treatment liability. That is, it is difficult for the agency to monitor how much remains for each consumer in terms of dollar resources or service benefits. Consequently, the center is put in a constantly reactive rather than proactive position in terms of care and resource management. On the other hand, a more global, agencywide method of estimating service liability creates a broader scope of action for management but restricts the latitude of the service coordinator. The drawback here is that the guidelines, being of the "one size fits all" nature, do not allow for appropriate adjustment to individual consumer situations. As with most organizational changes, only time will tell which approach is more viable for implementation. The information system dilemma, however, remains in that no concrete implementation can happen until a choice is made between the two alternatives.

Effective Practice Guidelines

Quality evaluation is based on the premise that some standard of quality exists against which to plan services in order to maximize treatment efficacy and to assess the outcomes of actual services. Put differently, evaluation is based upon the capacity to plan services according to sound practice guidelines, and to then monitor and assess whether or not treatment follows the agreed-to plan of action. Because practice guidelines for chronic illness conditions among CMHC consumers are sorely lacking, it is extremely difficult to implement this quality evaluation process.

In its effort to systematize and establish the best practice guidelines, Valley Mental Health has assigned to a multidisciplinary committee the task of researching the field in order to ascertain which CMHCs may have already accomplished this task and whose work could be adapted or augmented for adoption by the center. At the time of this writing, the committee had identified the following salient issues in terms of challenges for the center to overcome:

- Dependency on the subjective judgment of the primary service coordinator, which leads to frequent changes in service expectations or plans, particularly as multiple providers (staff or program) become involved at different stages of care or as consumers are seen in many components of the continuum of care.

- The lack of agencywide consensus regarding clinical expectations, which is due to the difficulty in getting clinicians to agree on what is appropriate care under a variety of situations. Alternative solutions are being investigated, particularly by examining what others have done (for example, Oregon, Joint Commission on Accreditation of Healthcare Organizations (JCAHO), American Psychiatric Association [APA], etc.) and by examining the center's historical service data to derive trends and patterns of care.

- Methodological problems that are inherent in special managed care contracts. For example, when dealing with its capitation contract to serve persons with severe and persistent mental illness, should the center establish expectations on a per clinical episode or an annual basis?

The Harris County Center, on the other hand, plans to address the issue of practice guidelines by defining a series of "service arrays" in the next phase of its system of care reorganization. This was started with the definition of priority access criteria (discussed above under eligibility criteria). Conceptually, these service arrays resemble practice standards or guidelines generally found in other healthcare sectors. The information system challenge is to facilitate the electronic storage, dissemination, and access to information about service array by intake workers, care planners, clinicians, and utilization reviewers.

Other Information System Development Challenges

At both centers, four major information system implementation challenges remain in terms of care management. Most of these have so far been broached only conceptually rather than empirically:

1. Arrive at clear operational definitions of practice standards or guidelines that take into account significant consumer and care characteristics (for example, diagnosis, presenting problems, ethnocultural imperatives, etc.).
2. Define the data array underpinning the objective measurement of factors that determine the appropriateness of the service package.
3. Provide historical trends of service provision patterns (such as drug prescription, modal visits planned, etc.) by provider, provider category, consumer type, or problem category.
4. Offer information regarding the provider's performance in terms of rates of adverse incidents, cost overruns, or significant deviations from practice standards.

Information systems will not reach their maximal contribution to managed care until these features are fully operationalized and made routinely and easily accessible to clinical and management staff.

Information Features in the Managed Outcome Phase

Outcome in the present context is defined as a measurement of change that can serve as an indicator of the impact of services on the consumer. From a societal viewpoint, the outcome focus should also be on programmatic impacts on society, the community, or the immediate environment in which the CMHC operates. While this broader outcome perspective is valuable within a managed care context, the primary starting point should be the concerns of clients, payers, and funders. The development of customer-focused indicators of mental health program performance has in fact been the objective of significant national effort in recent years.

Collecting Clinical Data

In each CMHC, much data actually exists that can be systematized and transformed into indicators of consumer-focused outcomes. These data are gathered during clinical service delivery when clinicians ascertain their client's status at various programmatic or temporal points in terms of symptomatology, clinical functioning, life circumstances, behavioral manifestations, and the like. Many CMHCs have actually been collecting client satisfaction data using their own instruments or standardized questionnaires.

The easiest task in developing an outcomes management system may be to first systematize the natural clinical data collection process to render it usable for consistent and reliable measurement and reporting. One can then turn to other, more esoteric outcome assessment approaches that approximate formal research.

Regardless of the data source and collection methods, outcome measurement must be standardized for similar programs, illness conditions, patient populations, and the like. For ease of data collection and information generation, the process should also be automated with the goal of making data reporting timely and relevant for decision making at all CMHC organizational levels. Standardization addresses the set of basic questions, "Which instrument is used to measure outcome, for which consumer population, at which stage in the care process, how frequently, and by whom?"

For example, it might be decided that a symptom checklist is to be self-administered by outpatient adult consumers at intake and the third visit, administered by staff to all inpatient adults at admission and the fifth day of hospitalization, but not used with children. In this example, outcome (that is, the effect of service on symptom reduction) would be operationalized as a change score on the symptom checklist.

Examples of Outcome Measurement Approaches and Instruments

Turning to our example centers, we find that the Harris County Center has identified four outcome subprojects. First is a project to define outcome measures in terms of the center's overall achievement of the impacts intended by its mission statement. This measurement process addresses the more global—that is, less focused on the individual consumer—outcome issues but still uses client-specific data as the basis for computing the indicators. Because mission statement objectives are global, the outcome indicators—such as ratio of jail days encountered by our consumers in relation to total number of consumers served—will not be directly applicable for each consumer. More consumer-relevant measures are to be defined in the other three outcome subprojects. Each of these outcome subprojects focuses on a circumscribed service arena: the adult mental health division, the children and adolescent division, and the mental retardation division. Staff from each of the divisions are to select their own sets of outcome measures. The role of the information system is to provide technological support to develop and maintain these outcome management subsystems.

While many decisions remain, the following preliminary measures are good candidates at the Harris County Center:

- The CSQ-8, which is a general consumer satisfaction scale with eight items. Added to the eight-item scale will be items that solicit input from consumers regarding specific aspects of the programs where they receive services.
- The CBCL (Child Behavior Checklist), which was already adopted by the Texas Department of Mental Health/Mental Retardation. This scale will be used locally in the child and adolescent programs.
- Some as yet to be determined symptomatology measurements will be used for adults.
- A goal attainment scaling approach in the mental retardation division that will track a consumer's progress against standardized plans of care, much like what is adopted at Valley Mental Health (discussed next).

Valley Mental Health plans to address consumer outcome by adopting a measure for each of the following areas: functionality, symptomatology, client satisfaction, and goal attainment. Currently, the center participates with other Utah CMHCs to pilot and evaluate several outcome instruments in order to determine a set of measures for statewide adoption. As part of this effort, the center is piloting the General Well Being Scale for adults, the CBCL for children and adolescents, the Multinomath Community Ability Scale for use with consumers with serious and persistent mental illness, and a modified goal attainment scaling methodology for use in measuring consumer's achievement of the goals of treatment or care (to be discussed next). Consumer satisfaction will be measured using the instrument developed by the Mental Health Corporation of America.

Example of Modified Goal Attainment Scaling

In order to measure outcome in terms of the extent to which planned clinical or behavioral changes match the intended treatment plan objectives, centers can modify the goal attainment scaling method initially developed by Thomas Kiresuk. Modifications would consist of customizing the instrument to fit their particular data collection and processing situations and deriving data from the treatment plans.

The following example from Valley Mental Health illustrates how modifications to simplify Kiresuk's methodology do not sacrifice the utility of the goal attainment approach to outcome measurement. For each problem or goal that is the focus of treatment, three measurements are taken, on a one-to-ten scale. The first measure ascertains "where the consumer would like to be" regarding the desired change; the second concerns where the "consumer" feels she is at the time of the measurement; and the third focuses on where the "therapist provider" thinks the consumer is.

Data collection occurs (1) at the time the managed care plan is originally developed, (2) on scheduled review dates individually determined with the consumer, and (3) when the consumer completes or terminates treatment.

Because these measures are consumer identifiable, changes in the scores obtained at different data collection points, as well as the differences between the three scales at each measurement, can be computed to indicate the level of attainment of each consumer's problems and goals. These change scores can then be examined and aggregated to provide global indicators of outcome or impact by consumer, program, or provider (staff) types.

Parameters of a Sound Outcomes Management System

The following are some basic requisites to ensure valid, reasonable, and reliable outcome measurement systems:

- The measures are practical for use (that is, easy for staff and consumers to understand and accept) and are not intrusive to the clinical care process.

- The measures possess sound psychometric properties of high internal consistency, high reliability, and sound face and construct validity.
- The measures include benchmarks for the center to gauge its own performance or improvement in comparison with similar agencies, providers, or programs.
- The measurement process safeguards consumer and staff confidentiality.
- The ultimate purpose of the outcome management process is to ensure continuous improvement in internal management, service delivery, and quality of care instead of providing data for punitive actions.

Collaborative Development, Data Integration, Performance History

Because formal and consistent outcomes management is really in its infancy in most CMHCs, its development must be multidisciplinary and underwritten by consistent cooperation between clinical personnel, technical staff, management, and researchers. Each group has responsibilities for and significant stakes in the process, and its interests and concerns cannot be easily presumed by the other groups. For example, while researchers pay close attention to the reliability and validity issues, clinical staff must heed practical considerations such as synchronization with the treatment process and acceptability to consumers; at the same time, information system staff must ensure the technical feasibility of data capture, data processing, and information dissemination.

As discussed above, an outcomes management system includes a multiplicity of data sets originating from many sources. These data sets must be carefully integrated among themselves and with other data in order to provide meaningful information for decision making.

Many salient issues remain, and their resolution requires an examination of outcome information from many perspectives and vantage points. For example, how does one compare the effectiveness of a youth program relative to the effectiveness of an adult program, when different outcome measures are used in each? What are the consumer characteristics that influence treatment expectations and thus must be considered when extrapolating from the outcome data to a judgment concerning the relative impact of treatment? How does one relate outcomes expectations to the severity of illness conditions?

Because most CMHCs have only recently begun the process of implementing a comprehensive approach to outcomes measurement, tracking, and management, historical and longitudinal data are not yet available and comparisons against baselines are not possible. Since firm and reliable baselines are unavailable, whether for groups of programs, groups of consumers, illness types, or provider types, outcome results cannot be expected to be immediately useful for programmatic decision making. Thus managers and policy makers should carefully avoid inappropriate judgments until such time as sufficient baseline data exist to provide reasonable confidence in the conclusions drawn from outcome data. In particular, utmost caution should be exercised when voicing negative pronouncements against programs, staff, or treatment processes based on such data since the state of the art of outcome measurement is still far from being reliably and empirically grounded.

In concluding this chapter, we ask the bottom line question: "Can CMHCs reengineer their information system capacity to help them meet the challenges of managed care?" From the examples presented above, we think that the answer is a qualified yes. That is, while CMHCs and related agencies serving publicly funded clients can meet such challenges, they must first be ready to make significant technological investments and, more importantly, commitments by management at the highest levels. These organizations must also retrain their staff regarding new roles and functions that are dictated by the managed care environment.

The delivery of integrated and well-managed behavioral healthcare requires sound clinical and management decisions that take into account cost, benefits, quality of care, and outcome information. These decisions must be fully supported by well-integrated, useful, and decision-relevant information rather than fragmentary data. As in other industries, accurate, up-to-date information is absolutely essential to excellence in performance. Well-honed information technology and capability are therefore the key ingredients that provide the competitive edge to ensure an organization's service quality, positive impact on consumers, and financial viability. Without information system reengineering and total organizational reengineering, it will be difficult for CMHCs to survive the impending shift away from autonomous fee-for-service care delivery and financing methods.

Notes

P. 124, *Medicaid portion of their health care system:* Oss, M. E. (1995, July). Market place perspective. *National Council,* p. 10.

P. 125, *Integrate Care at the Clinical Level:* Gorski, T. (1995, Spring). Trend watch: The evolution of managed care practices. *Treatment Today,* p. 10–12.

P. 125, *move toward greater cost-effectiveness:* Carbine, M. E., & Zablocki, E. (1995, April 21). Moving hospitals into capitation game means staff cuts, IS upgrade, education. *Physician Manager, 6*(8), 1–2.

P. 128, *Data Standards for Mental Health Decision Support Systems:* Leginski, W. A., Crose, C., Driggers, J., Dumpman, S., Geertsen, D., Kamis-Gould, E., Namerow, M. J., Paton, R. E., Wilson, N. Z., & Wurster, C. R. (1989). *Data standards for mental health decision support systems.* National Institute of Mental Health. Series FN No. 10. DHHS Publication No. (ADM)89–1589. Washington, DC: U.S. Government Printing Office.

P. 133, *nitty-gritty cost computation process:* Newman, F. L., & Sorensen, J. E. (1987). *Integrated clinical and fiscal management in mental health.* Norwood, NJ: Ablex.

P. 145, *significant national effort in recent years:* Mulkern, V., Leff, H. S, Green, R. S., & Newman, F. (1995). Performance indicators for a consumer-oriented mental health report card: Literature review and analysis. In *The Evaluation Center at HSRI: A compilation of the literature on what consumers want from mental health services* (pp. 1–217). Cambridge, MA: The Evaluation Center at HSRI.

P. 146, *the CSQ-8:* Larsen, D. L., Attkisson, C. C., Hargreaves, W. A., & Nguyen, T. D. (1979). Assessment of client/patient satisfaction: Development of a general scale. *Evaluation and Program Planning, 2,* 197–207; Nguyen, T. D., Attkisson, C. C., & Stegner, B. L. (1983). Assessment of patient satisfaction: Development and refinement of a service evaluation questionnaire. *Evaluation and Program Planning, 6*(3–4), 299–313.

For Further Reading

Leginski, W. A., Crose, C., Driggers, J., Dumpman, S., Geertsen, D., Kamis-Gould, E., Namerow, M. J., Paton, R. E., Wilson, N. Z., & Wurster, C. R. (1989). *Data standards for mental health decision support systems.* National Institute of Mental Health. Series FN No. 10. DHHS Publication No. (ADM)89–1589. Washington, DC: U.S. Government Printing Office.

Newman, F. L., & Sorensen, J. E. (1987). Integrated clinical and fiscal management in mental health. Norwood, NJ: Ablex.

Nguyen, T. D., Attkisson, C. C., & Stegner, B. L. (1983). Assessment of patient satisfaction: Development and refinement of a service evaluation questionnaire. *Evaluation and Program Planning, 6*(3–4), 299–313.

Oss, M. E. (1995, July). Market place perspective. *National Council News, 10,* p. 4.

CHAPTER EIGHT

COMPUTERIZATION IN HOSPITAL-BASED DELIVERY SYSTEMS

Warner V. Slack, Charles Safran, and Howard L. Bleich

The increasing availability of digital computers in the early 1960s had many physicians concerned about the potential encroachment of this new technology on the profession of medicine and on the traditional rapport between doctor and patient. Would these machines result in the dehumanizing processes that had been associated with the Industrial Revolution? Would modern times destroy the art of medicine? The debate was frequently lively, and a rejoinder that we found useful in those days, one borrowed from experimental psychologists, was that any doctor who could be replaced by a computer deserved to be.

Coupled with these concerns were excessively high expectations. It is often true that the less direct experience people have with a machine, the more they tend to react to it with both fear and unreasonable admiration. The electronic digital computer, with its capacity to hold large amounts of data and to execute

Note: We are indebted to our many colleagues at the Center for Clinical Computing and at Beth Israel and Brigham and Women's hospitals, who worked together with us to design, develop, implement, and maintain the computing systems described herein.

The following articles referenced in this chapter have been adapted with the permission of the publishers: *New England Journal of Medicine* (1985), and *M.D. Computing* (1989, vol. 6, pp. 133–135), (1989, vol. 6, pp. 141–149), (1989, vol. 6, pp. 183–185), (1992, vol. 9, pp. 6–10), (1992, vol. 9, pp. 278–280), and (1993, vol. 10, pp. 357–360).

multiple, complex instructions with great speed and accuracy, is indeed an awe-inspiring device—one that stimulates comparisons with the brain itself and fosters remarkable prophecies.

In medicine, as fear of the computer waned, expectations increased, and with expectations high, prophecy became a substitute for accomplishment. Computer manufacturers, in turn, moved to capitalize on these great expectations. Some advertised their machines as panaceas for the medical community; they sold what they called "total hospital information systems," which were partial at best and contained little information. When the dust settled—much of it on expensive, unused computer terminals—hospitals that had purchased these systems found that they had spent a great deal of money and received little in return, perhaps a partially working billing system. From the patient's perspective, the principal difference was that bills were higher because of the computing costs; in addition, the bills arrived, if at all, somewhat later than before.

Digital computers in hospitals and clinics in the United States are still used primarily for fiscal purposes, just as when they were introduced thirty years ago. Typically, financial data have been recorded throughout the hospital on pieces of paper, aggregated in a data-processing area, keypunched onto Hollerith cards or magnetic media, and fed to the computer. From these data, the computer produced bills for patients or third-party payers, payment checks for the hospital's creditors and employees, and a large number of printed reports. These computers, which are programmed to handle batches of financial transactions, are poorly suited to interactive clinical applications and have had little influence on the practice of medicine.

In keeping with the times, trends in the vernacular of fiscal computing now have a managerial flavor. The management information system (MIS) is in vogue. Not to be confused with a clinical computing system (some bemused clinicians think the M in MIS stands for medical), an MIS is typically designed and implemented primarily for financial purposes. What few clinical needs are served by MIS are for the most part a by-product of accounts receivable.

In recent years, however, investigators have demonstrated that the needs of individual clinical departments, such as the laboratories, the admitting office, the medical records department, the pharmacy, the pathology department, and the radiology department, could successfully be served by computers. With few exceptions, these programs were electronically isolated from one another, or interfaced in such a manner that they could not readily share information.

An Integrated Clinical Computing System

In 1976, Howard Bleich and Warner Slack approached the administration of Boston's Beth Israel Hospital with a plan to develop not isolated computer applications for individual departments but a single, hospitalwide clinical computing system. Our primary purpose was to use the computer to help doctors, nurses, and other clinicians provide better care for their patients. We were convinced, however, that the finances of the hospital would also benefit from the clinical computing system.

We had several goals. First, information should be captured not on pieces of paper but directly at computer terminals located at the point of each transaction. The computer in turn should provide immediate benefit to the person who enters this information.

Second, information captured at a terminal or automated device anywhere in the hospital should be immediately available, if needed, at any other terminal. Rather than printed reports, which become progressively out of date from the moment they are produced, terminals providing immediate access to the most up-to-date information should be the principal means of retrieval.

Third, the response time of the computer should be rapid. For the busy physician, nurse, or medical technologist, delays that can be measured in seconds are often unacceptable.

Fourth, the computer should be reliable; in the event of a failure, the defect should be corrected within minutes, and users should never lose data.

Fifth, confidentiality should be protected; only authorized persons should have access to the data.

Sixth, the computer programs should be friendly to the user and reinforce the user's behavior. There should be no need for users' manuals. It should be easier for the physician to obtain a laboratory result from a computer terminal than from a telephone call.

Finally, there should be a common registry for all patients. For each patient there should be one and only one set of identifying information in the computer, available at all times to authorized users, and preserved if possible in perpetuity. Whenever an error in the common data base is detected and corrected at any terminal, that correction should be immediately available at all terminals. The common registry should be shared throughout the hospital by all programs that involve identification of a patient.

In collaboration with our colleagues throughout Beth Israel Hospital, we developed and instituted such a hospitalwide clinical computing system. In the fall of 1982, on the basis of experience gained at Beth Israel, we were asked to assume responsibility for developing a similar computing system at Boston's Brigham and Women's Hospital. The development of the systems for the two hospitals was under the direction of the Center for Clinical Computing (CCC), an affiliate of the Harvard Medical School.

Salient features of these systems are their widespread use and popularity among clinicians and other hospital workers, the accurate data that they provide for the hospitals' financial needs, and their low cost. During the developmental years, the total cost at Beth Israel Hospital was approximately 1.5 percent of the operating budget, and at Brigham and Women's Hospital, where financial programs were also included, the cost was approximately 2 percent of the operating budget.

In 1989, upon completion of the CCC's project at Brigham and Women's, administrative responsibility for computing was transferred to the hospital; in 1995, the same transfer occurred at Beth Israel.

The clinical computing systems at Beth Israel and Brigham and Women's hospitals are in routine use in psychiatry and psychology as well as primary care medicine and all medical and surgical specialties. The principles of the clinical computing in these two hospitals would apply equally well to institutions devoted exclusively to psychiatric and psychological services.

Departmental and Laboratory Computing

Beth Israel and Brigham and Women's hospitals are both major teaching hospitals of the Harvard Medical School. Beth Israel has 478 beds and 60 bassinets, an active inpatient psychiatric service (with a closed ward), and active outpatient psychiatric and psychological services. Each year there are approximately thirty thousand admissions and two hundred thousand outpatient visits. Brigham and Women's has 739 beds, 96 bassinets, and an active ambulatory psychiatric service. Each year there are approximately forty thousand admissions and three hundred thousand outpatient visits.

The Computers

The programs that provide clinical computing were written initially in the MIIS dialect of MUMPS (marketed by Medical Information Technology, Inc.) and were run on separate networks of Data General minicomputers, one network at each hospital. The computing systems are now being transferred to new, more modern software platforms with the ability to handle an ever-increasing number of terminals and printers. The new platforms should provide more modern visual presentation to the user together with increased speed and efficiency.

Registration

At Beth Israel and Brigham and Women's hospitals, the first components of the clinical computing systems were implemented in the medical records, admitting, and outpatient departments. These registration programs make up the core of the systems. Although the computer programs were tailored to the individual needs of each hospital, the programs were similar in function. For each patient who has been cared for at Beth Israel since its system of medical record numbers was established in 1966, and for each such patient at Brigham and Women's, the name, address, telephone number, social security number, and names of parents and spouse are stored in the computers in common registries, a separate one for each hospital.

When a new patient arrives, whether as an inpatient or an outpatient, he or she is interviewed and the data are entered, in the patient's presence, at a computer terminal. The computer then assigns a medical record number. Once the patient's data are in the registry, they are preserved indefinitely; thereafter, initiation of a hospital admission, outpatient visit, or major clinical procedure requires only that data be checked and updated; data need not be reentered. The patient's identifying information can be corrected at any terminal by any authorized person who has access to the registry; however, an audit trail of the information entered previously is preserved and can be displayed if a question of accuracy arises.

Laboratories and Clinical Departments

Programs in the laboratories and clinical departments were then developed and integrated with the registration programs. Computer terminals in the hematology, chemistry, virology, endocrinology, immunology, and microbiology laboratories communicate with the common registry of patients. To register a specimen, the technologist identifies the patient in the registry and indicates which tests are to be performed. Automated devices in the laboratories are electronically connected to the computer networks. Results obtained with these devices, as well as those that are entered manually, are displayed on terminals in the laboratories, where they are checked by a technologist.

A markedly abnormal result or any result that has changed substantially since the previous determination is automatically flagged; such results are rechecked by a senior technologist and telephoned to the clinician at the number provided by the computer. Once verified, results are released for viewing by clinicians at terminals located throughout the hospitals.

In a similar manner, the computing systems have an important role in the clinical departments (blood bank, cardiology, cytology, pathology, pharmacy, psychological testing, pulmonary function, and radiology). At Beth Israel, technologists in the electroencephalography, electromyography, and evoked potential laboratories use the computer to identify each patient, indicate the study to be performed, and record the results of each study, which are then approved by a staff neurologist and made available for viewing on the hospital's terminals.

In virtually every laboratory and clinical department, the results of diagnostic studies are captured directly from the diagnostician (for example, psychologist, surgical pathologist, or radiologist), technologist, or automated device and made immediately available on terminals throughout the hospitals and clinics.

Financial Computing

Virtually every service provided to a patient—whether an outpatient visit, inpatient admission, diagnostic study, medication order, or blood transfusion—must be registered in the computer before it can be performed. Manual registration and identification procedures that were once used throughout the hospitals, procedures that were fraught with error and lost charges, have largely disappeared. After the service has been performed and its results have been recorded in the computer, the charge is automatically added to the patient's file. In this way, more than 90 percent of each patient's charges are obtained as a by-product of the clinical computing systems.

At Beth Israel, these charges are transferred by magnetic tape each day to the hospital's fiscal computing system (in a separate facility not in our network), which prints the bills and performs other financial operations. The time required to collect unpaid bills (calculated as the amount of money not yet collected divided by the mean amount of the charges added per day) dropped from 65 days in 1977, when the registration programs were first introduced, to 39 days in 1982. And now?

At Brigham and Women's Hospital, accounts receivable is part of the clinical computing network. The clinical computing system produces billing tapes, both for inpatients and outpatients, that are transferred to such third-party payers as Medicare, Medicaid, and Blue Cross. In turn, remittance tapes from third-party payers, which accompany the payment checks, are read by the computer and used to match the payment received with the accounts of the individual patients. When payment has not been received, the computer automatically generates additional bills.

At Brigham and Women's, the time required to collect unpaid bills was reduced from 100 days in 1983 to 59 days in 1988. Outstanding debts in the outpatient clinics were reduced by more than $6 million during a time when the cash collected from outpatient revenues increased by 45 percent.

At each hospital, the computer assigns a diagnosis-related group (DRG) to each patient and alerts the medical records department when additional coding may entitle the hospital to increased reimbursement. At Beth Israel, the computer prints reminders listing the abnormal laboratory results of patients on Medicare that may entitle the hospital to additional reimbursement.

Clinical Information in the Care of the Patient

Clinicians, medical students, and other authorized personnel gain access to the clinical information system by going to any terminal (or personal computer serving as a terminal in the network) in the hospital, pressing the ENTER key, and typing a confidential password.

Patient Lookup

Clinical data are retrieved through PATIENT LOOKUP, the most heavily used option in the system. To use PATIENT LOOKUP, the clinician must first identify the patient, which can be done by entering a name, medical record number, fiscal number, social security number, room number, or name of a nursing station. When a patient's name is typed in the form SMITH, JOHN, for example, the program searches the registry of patients (over one million, at Beth Israel Hospital) and responds with the names and identifying data of all patients with that name, followed by the names and identifying data of all patients whose names have a similar sound. Patients currently undergoing active care are presented first. To restrict a search to patients currently in the hospital, the user need type only the first few letters of the last name.

Once the patient has been identified, the computer displays a list of laboratories and departments from which authorized clinicians can view the results of laboratory tests and clinical procedures. If the clinician chooses the option ALL LABS—MOST RECENT RESULTS, the computer displays all results for inpatients for the previous two days and all results for outpatients since the most recent admission or visit to a clinic. Data from all laboratories and clinical departments are available as soon as the diagnostic studies have been performed.

If the user selects the DEMOGRAPHICS/DISCHARGE DIAGNOSES option, the computer displays the patient's demographic information from the common registry, as well as the dates of service and the initial problem; it lists the name of the attending physician for outpatient appointments, visits to the emergency unit, and hospital admissions; and it presents the final diagnoses for hospital admissions. Choosing CARDIOLOGY, CYTOLOGY, NEUROPHYSIOLOGY (EEG/EMG/EP), RADIOLOGY, or SURGICAL PATHOLOGY results in a display of examinations performed and a summary of the findings and their diagnostic interpretations. O.R. HISTORY/RECOVERY ROOM results in a display of the patient's surgical procedures, either scheduled or already performed. Choosing BLOOD BANK results in a display of the patient's blood type and associated antibodies, the patient's transfusion history (including adverse reactions), and an inventory of cross-matched blood (or autologous blood if the patient has previously donated) that is held in reserve and ready for use. And choosing PHARMACY results in a display of options to view a list of medications used during hospitalization (either current medications or a summary for the present or most recent admission). Adverse drug reactions can be recorded in the pharmacy system and will be displayed thereafter whenever the patient's medications are listed.

Most of the reports are available from the terminals for up to a year; after removal from the active disk files, this information is kept on magnetic tape for use in retrospective analysis.

Clinicians' Ancillary Options

These options help with the daily routines of patient care. The program maintains a PERSONAL PATIENT LIST, patients under the care of each physician and nurse. When a new patient is seen by a house officer or nurse practitioner in an ambulatory care clinic, the patient's name is automatically placed on the clinician's list. When a new patient is admitted to the hospital, the patient's name is automatically placed on the attending physician's list.

With EDIT PERSONAL PATIENT LIST, a house officer, attending physician, or nurse can add or delete names from her list. With VIEW HOSPITALIZED PATIENT LIST, clinicians can view the names of patients who are on their lists and are currently in the hospital or have been seen that day in the emergency unit. With PERSONAL PATIENT LOOKUP, clinicians can step through the clinical data of their hospitalized or ambulatory patients without having to enter the names. This option reminds clinicians about laboratory tests that have been ordered. A CROSS COVERAGE option permits a provider to authorize others to have access to his list of patients.

At Beth Israel, a UNIVERSAL PRECAUTIONS option offers physicians a teaching program on safety measures when handling blood and other fluids from patients, and a CONFIDENTIAL COUNSELING FOR HOUSE STAFF option gives the names, telephone numbers, and page numbers of clinicians in the Department of Psychiatry who are available to help interns and residents in distress. INCOMPLETE MEDICAL RECORD (the least popular of the ancillary options) informs the doctor about discharge summaries that need to be dictated and medical records that need to be signed.

Decision Support

Decision support options are designed to help the clinician take better care of the patient and to help the investigator conduct research.

At Beth Israel, an electrolyte and acid-base program automatically obtains laboratory data, such as the serum sodium concentration, serum creatinine concentration, and blood ph, from the hospital's computer network. It then directs a dialogue during which the clinician supplies clinical information, such as the patient's weight and evidence, if present, of congestive heart failure. On the basis of the abnormalities detected, the program then asks further questions as needed to characterize the electrolyte and acid-base disturbances. Upon completion of the interchange, the program produces an evaluation note that resembles a consultant's discussion of the problem. The note includes a list of diagnostic possibilities, an explanation of the pathophysiology, recommendations for therapy, suggestions for additional laboratory studies, precautionary measures indicated by the illness or its treatment, and references to the medical literature.

DRUG INFORMATION offers guidelines for the use of all medications in the hospital's formulary. To date, clinicians have requested information about fluoxetine more often than any other medication. These programs were written in Converse, a language for use in computer-based interviews, and then incorporated into the clinical information system.

ClinQuery, a program that retrieves clinical information, permits clinicians to search the computerized clinical data of the patients who were admitted (there have been more than 319,858 admissions to Beth Israel since 1984). To protect confidentiality, names and other personally identifying information are not displayed. Lists based on demographic information; on results from surgical pathology, cardiology, radiology, and the clinical laboratories; and on blood transfusions, medications, and discharge diagnoses (from psychiatry, medicine, surgery, and all other clinical services) can be used to identify patients with attributes of particular interest.

For example, a doctor who is deciding how best to care for a patient with an antidepressant medication could use ClinQuery to look for examples of successful therapy among patients with similar problems. An investigator with an interest in reasons for readmissions to the emergency room or to the inpatient psychiatric service can use ClinQuery to explore alternative hypotheses. An administrator with an interest in diagnosis-related groups among psychiatric patients can use ClinQuery to study demographic and clinical profiles.

PaperChase, a bibliographic retrieval program, permits users to search the National Library of Medicine's MEDLINE database of references to the medical literature. Users can perform a search and read abstracts; at a cost of $12 per article, they can order mailed photocopies of the full text. PaperChase provides access to close to nine million references to articles in four thousand journals dating back to 1966. Each month, twenty-five thousand new references are indexed and abstracted. PaperChase, the first program of its kind, is available in all of the Harvard teaching hospitals, as well as private offices and institutions throughout the United States and abroad.

At Brigham and Women's, in addition to PaperChase and ANTIBIOTIC IN-
FORMATION (a program written in Converse that provides consultation on the use
of antimicrobial agents), a number of programs that provide decision support have
been incorporated into the clinical computing system since 1989.

Access and Confidentiality

Each authorized user gains access to the clinical information system by means of
a unique computer-assigned confidential password, or key. The computers at
the two hospitals maintain a dictionary of keys and the names of their owners.
If an unauthorized person repeatedly tries to use an illegal key, the terminal springs
a "keytrap": it beeps the Morse code for SOS eighteen times and renders the terminal temporarily unusable until the computer center is called.

Clinicians can also gain access to the clinical information systems by telephone. A double password offers additional security for this extramural access.

Because any clinician may be called on to care for any patient, each clinician's
key permits access to the clinical data of all patients in the registry. Whenever a
clinician looks up a patient's data, however, this transaction is recorded in the computer and is, upon request, made available to the patient or the patient's physician.

If the patient is a hospital employee, a family member of a hospital employee,
a celebrity whose privacy may need special attention, or someone designated at
random, the computer displays a reminder:

> TO PROTECT EACH PATIENT'S CONFIDENTIALITY, ONLY THOSE WHO ARE
> RESPONSIBLE FOR A PATIENT'S CARE SHOULD USE THIS OPTION. WE RECORD
> THE IDENTITY OF EACH USER OF PATIENT LOOKUP AND WILL GIVE THIS
> INFORMATION TO THE PATIENT OR THE PATIENT'S PHYSICIAN UPON REQUEST.
> TYPE 'Y'ES TO PROCEED; OTHERWISE PRESS RETURN.

In the outpatient setting, and of particular use in psychiatry and psychology
where confidentiality is deemed particularly important, we have added a new feature whereby the author of any electronic note can designate it as a "monitored"
note. The author of a monitored note then receives feedback in the form of an
automatic message, which gives the name of the viewer, the date and time of
the viewing, and the reason offered for viewing the note.

Utility Programs

A set of utility programs is available to all authorized users of the clinical computing systems at the two hospitals. A KEY option allows a user to change her
key in case of a suspected breach in security. An option labeled HOW TO USE THE
COMPUTER TERMINAL offers instructions for the beginner and reminders for

the more experienced user. A TELEPHONE DIRECTORY provides the telephone number, beeper number, and room number of each member of the staff and of each department, as well as the weekly schedule of physicians in their specialty clinics. A DOCTOR'S OFFICE directory provides the address, telephone number, and specialty (at Brigham and Women's Hospital) of each staff physician. This program helps house officers contact attending physicians whose offices are outside the hospital.

ELECTRONIC MAIL, probably the first such communication system to be installed in a clinical facility (at Beth Israel in the mid 1970s) permits a person to send a message to an individual or a group. With this option, a clinical instructor in psychiatry can forward advice to a medical student or invite a group of students to a teaching session; a chief resident in psychiatry can notify the residents that an instructive, unscheduled conference is about to occur; and the blood bank can notify all who sign on at the computer that there is an urgent need for a particular type of blood.

Mail can be sent immediately, posted for future delivery, or retracted if it has not been read and the writer has had second thoughts. Users can also ask whether a message has been read, view messages previously sent, and reread their old mail. At the time of signing on, each user is informed about unread mail and offered the opportunity to read it then or later. Mail that has been read can be held in an arbitrary number of queues for future use, or it can be edited and forwarded to someone else.

In some cases the computer itself generates messages. When a patient is readmitted or seen in the emergency unit at Beth Israel, a message to that effect is automatically sent to all physicians on whose PERSONAL PATIENT LIST the patient's name appears. Physicians have told us that they very much appreciate this feature; it alerts them when one of their patients returns to the hospital, even if under the care of another physician, and it eliminates the need to telephone the emergency unit repeatedly to find out whether an expected patient has arrived.

At Beth Israel, a computer-administered health screening interview is available for all hospital employees. Conducted in private and with protection of confidentiality, the interview seeks information on medical problems and patterns of living for which behavioral change is considered desirable, and it offers advice and suggestions. An option labeled VIEW LOOKUPS OF YOUR OWN FILE enables any member of the staff of each of the two hospitals to determine who has had access to his clinical record in the computer.

Use of the Clinical Information Systems

The computer-assigned key that identifies each user provides an electronic signature for each transaction with the computer. We have used these signatures to determine the frequency with which the computer programs are used by staff doctors, house officers, clinical fellows, nurses, medical students, and health assistants in the two hospitals. It should be noted that these clinicians are voluntary users of the clinical information systems. They could, if they so desired, rely on printed reports or telephone calls to obtain their clinical information. The intensity of their use of the computer, therefore, can be taken as a measure of the system's helpfulness.

Use at Beth Israel Hospital

During the week of February 23–29, 1992, a total of 2,354 clinicians at Beth Israel—1,022 nurses, 523 health assistants, 305 house officers, 352 staff physicians, 103 clinical fellows, and 49 medical students—used one or more of the options in the clinical information system 69,784 times. The PATIENT LOOKUP option was the most heavily used. During that week, clinicians looked up data on hospitalized patients 34,614 times—a 172 percent increase over a comparable period in 1984. During the same week, clinicians looked up clinical data on ambulatory patients 21,497 times, an increase of 426 percent since 1984. As expected, clinicians in training were the heaviest users of PATIENT LOOKUP, with a mean of 45 inquiries per house officer and 25 lookups per medical student.

Among the decision support programs, PaperChase was used to perform 1,556 searches of the MEDLINE data base of references to the biomedical literature. Clinicians used the other decision support programs a total of 1,288 times, and they sent over 13,000 pieces of electronic mail.

Use at Brigham and Women's Hospital

During the week of October 3–9, 1988, 2,262 clinicians at Brigham and Women's—549 physicians and 1,713 nurses, health assistants, and students—used one or more of the options in the clinical information system 89,101 times. As at Beth Israel, PATIENT LOOKUP was used most often: clinicians made inquiries about 1,306 inpatients 40,998 times and about 5,402 outpatients 14,383 times, and physicians in training were the heaviest users. Among the 299 interns and residents who used the system during that week, the mean number of inquiries was 59.

During the same week in October 1988, clinicians used the consultation program on antibiotics 111 times, received 27,716 pieces of electronic mail, and used PaperChase to perform 947 searches of the medical literature.

At the time of this writing—seven years since the previously mentioned study was conducted—there have yet to be any reports of frequency of use elsewhere by clinicians comparable to this experience at Brigham and Women's Hospital.

And since 1988, in conjunction with an increasing number of terminals and their ready accessibility, use continues to rise.

Assessing the Clinician's Use of Computers

In discussions of the effects of new technology on the practice of medicine, an analogy is sometimes drawn between use of the digital computer and use of such instruments as the electrocardiograph, electroencephalograph, and X-ray machines. There is an important difference, however, pointed out by Alvan Feinstein years ago: when the electrocardiograph, electroencephalograph, and X-ray machines were introduced, they provided information not previously available in medicine. The introduction of the computer, by contrast, offered no new information. Everything the computer can do in medicine, with the possible exceptions of mathematical modeling, axial tomography, and magnetic resonance imaging, can at least in theory be done by the human brain and hand. On the other hand, X-ray vision is impossible for us, at least for the present.

What the introduction of the computer did offer to medicine was a new and rapid way to process existing information. The human brain has about 100 billion neurons, with a vast array of interconnecting fibers. The brain responds to hormones as well as electrical impulses, and it runs on about 10 watts of power. Each neuron can fire about one hundred impulses each second. The computer, by comparison, has perhaps ten million transistors with far fewer interconnections; it is unresponsive to hormones and consumes more energy than the brain. But each transistor can fire impulses about a million times faster than can the neurons in the brain.

Thus, the computer has a relatively small number of fast circuits; it is designed to perform many simple tasks, one or perhaps a few at a time. The brain, on the other hand, has a much larger number of relatively slow circuits; it is better equipped to cope with large amounts of information presented and processed simultaneously.

Great speed and reliability are the fortes of the "artificial automaton," as John von Neumann called the computer in the days of its inception. Learning how to make better use of new information is the goal in medical specialties such as radiology, electrocardiography, and electroencephalography; learning how to make better use of information already on hand is the goal in medical computing.

This difference is often overlooked in assessing the use of computers by doctors, nurses, medical students, and other clinicians. There is a tendency to assume that to introduce a computer is to introduce new, important clinical information that the clinician *should* acquire, and to assume that whether the clinician does so is a measure of her willingness and ability to master new technology. When terminals go unused, the explanation is sought in characteristics of the clinician, such as age, computer phobia, or computer literacy, rather than characteristics of the computer and its programs, such as how well they present information to the clinician.

There is no a priori reason for a clinician to use a computer when it offers no information that cannot be obtained somewhere else. The results of diagnostic studies are available in printed reports; educational information and consultation can be obtained from books, journals, and personal communication; and much bibliographic retrieval can be done with the *Index Medicus*. If a computer that has been programmed to perform these functions is seldom used, it probably offers no advantage over traditional methods of processing and presenting this available information. Attention should then be directed to the program rather than the clinician.

Age and Computer Phobia

Blaming the already beleaguered clinician for being too old or computer phobic is a handy approach for computer manufacturers, systems analysts, and program developers whose programs are disliked and little used. It is reminiscent of the way automobile manufacturers used to blame drivers rather than defects in their cars, until Ralph Nader set the record straight with *Unsafe at Any Speed*.

In our experience, age and computer phobia are unimportant as deterrents to the use of clinical computing. In a study conducted at Beth Israel in 1982, well before the widespread proliferation of personal computers, 94 staff physicians, 152 house officers, 19 medical students, and 487 nurses, each of whom was a user of our clinical computing system, were asked (by a computer-conducted interview) to give their opinion of the system. The staff physicians, who were older (and thus, according to conventional wisdom, more prone to computer phobia) than the medical students and house staff, were nevertheless equally well disposed toward the clinical computing system and its helpfulness to them in patient care.

Computer Literacy

The person who invents a machine is likely to be its first user. The earliest automobiles—Nicholas Joseph Cugnot's steam vehicle of the 1760s and Karl Benz's gasoline-powered carriage of the 1880s—were first operated by those who designed and built them.

So it was with the computer. Almost certainly, Blaise Pascal was the first to use his mechanical adding machine (in the 1640s), Gottfried Leibniz the first to use his four-function mechanical calculator (in the 1670s), and William Burroughs the first to use his business machine (in the 1890s). Had Charles Babbage ever completed his difference engine (developed in the 1820s), he would for sure have been the only person who knew how to use it. And so it has been with the more modern vacuum-tube and solid-state machines, with programming languages, and with computer programs themselves. Once a machine is in general use, however, it is no longer necessary for the user to understand its inner workings. Most of us drive our automobiles without knowing the theoretical foundations of the internal combustion engine; most of us use our telephones without understanding information theory, and turn on our electric lights without Ohm's law in mind.

During the first two decades of the use of computers in medicine (the 1950s and 1960s), doctors who wanted to use a computer typically had to program it themselves, often in machine language. Programming in machine language (with instructions that are executed directly by the computer, one by one, without first being interpreted or compiled into simpler units) entails some understanding of the machine's inner workings. In the 1970s, most doctors who used computers were still doing their own programming. They had higher-level languages (compilers and interpreters) and programming was easier for them, but they were still in close touch with the machine.

Now, of course, things have changed. Clinicians who know nothing about the inner workings of their computers can, to good advantage, use programs written by others. With a few simple keystrokes (though as yet in relatively few institutions), they can look up the results of diagnostic studies, get advice on patient care, search the biomedical literature, and communicate with each other by electronic mail. And microcomputers provide word processing, accounting, and statistical programs that require little more understanding of the machine than how to turn it on.

Still, the idea persists that the clinician must know the theoretical underpinnings of the computer—must be "computer literate"—to use it wisely and well. This notion is kept alive in part by well-meaning, influential medical school academics (typically nonusers themselves), who are unnecessarily embarrassed by their own computer illiteracy and who misguidedly believe that an in-depth knowledge of computational theory is a prerequisite for productive use of a computer.

Then there are those persistent professors, often erstwhile programmers themselves, who want a computer course to be a required part of the medical school curriculum. They want their students to be computer literate. (This is not unique to clinical computing, of course; there are those who argue that medical students should be required to know the mechanics of the continuous flow autoanalyzer before using serum electrolyte values in the care of patients.) They forget that most undergraduates were heavy users of word processors and spreadsheets before they got to medical school, and that doctors (particularly nonacademics) who never took a course in computing use personal computers to good advantage in their practices and at home.

If a medical student *wants* to know the theory behind a machine (be it a computer or an autoanalyzer), perhaps there should be facilities within the school to encourage this. But when curricula are already full, when important clinical courses such as pediatrics and obstetrics are themselves sometimes electives, the argument for a required course in computing is unconvincing.

A Behavioristic Paradigm

Years ago, John Watson, Edward Thorndike, and B. F. Skinner offered compelling evidence that behavior is shaped by its consequences. If the consequences are reinforcing, the behavior is strengthened; if not, the behavior tends to disappear.

Will physicians interact with computers? They will, if the interaction is helpful. If the consequences of using the computer (ready access to results of diagnostic studies, searches of the medical literature, and words of advice and consultation, for example) are rewarding, its use will be repeated. If, with successive entries at the keyboard, displays on the screen continue to be helpful, the clinician is likely to continue using the computer. And subjective assessment of the computer, as indicated by responses to survey interviews, will be positive. If, by contrast, useful information is cumbersome to obtain, the clinician is likely to lose interest.

This is not to say that if a clinician returns to use the computer again and again, this behavior is necessarily desirable; heavy use of the computer could reflect its ability to offer diversion from less enjoyable but more clinically important activities. The computer could conceivably encourage behavior that is unrelated, perhaps even detrimental, to patient care.

On the other hand, the overworked house officer with little time to spare and whose behavior is reinforced primarily by the approval of patients, peers, nurses, and attending physicians, is unlikely to use a computing system that does not, at least from the house officer's perspective, provide help in the practice of medicine.

We submit, therefore, that one of the best available criteria by which to judge the quality of a clinical computing system is the intensity with which clinicians such as house officers voluntarily use it. When extensive orientation programs, training programs, and user manuals are deemed necessary, the prognosis is not good. In our experience, there is an inverse relationship between the size of the manual next to the terminal and the quality of the programs on the screen.

Unfortunately, information about the routine use of computers by house officers and other clinicians is hard to obtain. Articles in academic journals tend to be long on description and short on data. Most companies that market commercial systems do not record their use. Some time ago we saw a press release claiming that one hospital was using a system with "more than 250 workstations, . . . making it one of the world's largest patient data management systems." A telephone call to the hospital revealed that most of the workstations had yet to be delivered, let alone installed.

When looking for a clinical computing system, it is important to ask where a proposed system is working best and then call the place that is named. (We have noticed that, not coincidentally, the site of installation tends to be geographically remote from the point at which the question is asked.) Speak with a user, rather than the person who made the decision to purchase; the latter may be more interested in defending the decision than in assessing the computing.

A Simple Experiment

On August 1, 1979, a computer terminal was installed in the library of Beth Israel Hospital. Patrons, most of whom had never used such a terminal before, were free to use it at any time, day or night. No instructions were provided, no user's manual was written, no announcements were made, and no publicity was given. On the screen was a message that read: "PAPERCHASE: A COMPUTER PROGRAM TO HELP YOU SEARCH THE MEDICAL LITERATURE. TO START THE PROGRAM, PRESS THE RETURN KEY."

Between 4:00 p.m. and midnight, 12 people signed on and performed searches; the next day, 39 people signed on and performed 75 searches. During the first year, 1,229 people performed 10,678 searches—more computerized searches of the Medline database than were performed at any other institution in the country. During the third year, 2,202 people performed 16,803 searches. House officers were among the heaviest users.

Data of this type, which were collected automatically, are essential in evaluating any clinical computing program.

Clinical Computing Today

A distinguishing feature of the clinical computing systems at Beth Israel and Brigham and Women's hospitals is the intensity of their use. As clinicians learned that the programs were reliable and that the computers were almost never down, they came to rely on terminals for help in the care of their patients, and they requested new features and suggested additional programs. When the laboratory programs were first made available at Beth Israel (before terminals were installed on nursing units), interns and residents discovered that results could be viewed on terminals in the laboratories as soon as the tests had been performed. They descended from the nursing stations and commandeered the laboratory terminals, sometimes to the consternation of the technologists. In response to the demands of the house staff, terminals were installed on the nursing stations and used with increasing frequency. As of 1995, clinicians at Beth Israel look up the results of diagnostic studies over fifty thousand times a week from over three thousand terminals located throughout the hospital, clinics, and private offices.

In hospitals where computers are primarily used for fiscal purposes, what computer to buy and what software to use are for the most part viewed as financial decisions. Typically, a chief financial officer (or, in accordance with a recent trend, a chief information officer) selects the hospital's computing system. But if he is not familiar with the principles and practice of medicine, the clinical needs of physicians and their patients may not be considered in the decision. If a hospital or clinic is seeking good clinical computing—where the *M* in MIS does in fact stand for medical—as well as good financial computing, the choice of a computing system should be regarded as a decision to be shared by clinicians and managers.

Notes

P. 151, *debate was frequently lively:* Weed, L. L. (1970). Technology is a link, not a barrier, for doctor and patient. *Modern Hospital, 114*(2), 80–83.

P. 151, *one borrowed from experimental psychologists:* Skinner, B. F. (1953). *Science and human behavior.* Toronto, Ontario: Collier-Macmillan.

P. 151, *excessively high expectations:* Schwartz, W. B. (1970). Medicine and the computer: The promise and problems of change. *New England Journal of Medicine, 283*(23), 1257–1264.

P. 152, *fosters remarkable prophecies:* Schwartz, W. B, Patil, R. S., & Szolovits, P. (1987). Artificial intelligence in medicine: Where do we stand? *New England Journal of Medicine, 316,* 685–688.

P. 152, *such as the laboratories:* Hicks, G. P., Gieschen, M. M., Slack, W. V., & Larson, F. C. (1966). Routine use of a small digital computer in the clinical laboratory. *Journal of the American Medical Association, 196,* 973–978; Collen, M. F. (1967). The multitest laboratory in health care of the future. *Hospitals, 41,* 119–125; Lindberg, D. A. (1967). Collection, evaluation, and transmission of hospital laboratory data. *Methods of Information in Medicine, 6,* 97–107; Kunz, L. J., Poitras, J. W., Kissling, J., Mercier, B. A., Cameron, M., Lazarus, C., Moellering, R. C., Barnett, G. O. (1974). The role of the computer in microbiology. In J. E. Prier, J. Bartola, & H. Friedman (Eds.), *Modern methods in medical microbiology: Systems and trends* (pp. 181–193). Baltimore: University Park Press.

P. 152, *the medical records department:* Weed, L. L. (1968). Medical records that guide and teach. *New England Journal of Medicine, 278,* 593–600, 652–657; Grossman, J. H., Barnett, G. O., Koepsell, T. D., Nesson, H. R., Dorsey, J. L., Phillips, R. R. (1973). An automated medical record system. *Journal of the American Medical Association, 224*(12), 1616–1621.

P. 152, *the pharmacy:* Gouveia, W. A., Diamantis, C., & Barnett, G. O. (1969). Computer applications in the hospital medication system. *American Journal of Hospital Pharmacy, 26,* 140–150.

P. 152, *the pathology department:* Aller, R. D., Robboy, S. J., Poitras, J. W., Altsuler, B. F., Cameron, M., Prior, M. C., Miao, S., Barnett, G. O. (1977). Computer-assisted pathology encoding and reporting system (CAPER). *American Journal of Clinical Pathology, 68,* 715–720.

P. 152, *the radiology department:* Lodwick, G. S., Turner, A. H., Lusted, L. B., & Templeton, A. W. (1966). Computer-aided analysis of radiographic images. *Journal of Chronic Disease, 19,* 485–496.

P. 152, *With few exceptions:* McDonald, C. J., Murray, R., Jeris, D., Bhargava, B., Seeger, J., Blevins, L. (1977). A computer-based record and clinical monitoring system for ambulatory care. *American Journal of Public Health, 67*(3), 240–245; Pryor, T. A., Gardner, R. M., Clayton, P. D., & Warner, H. R. (1983). The HELP system. *Journal of Medical Systems, 7,* 87–102; Simborg, D. W., Chadwick, M., Whiting-O'Keefe, Q. E., Tolchin, S. G., Kahn, S. A., & Bergan, E. S. (1983). Local area networks and the hospital. *Computers and Biomedical Research, 16,* 247–259; Stead, W. W., & Hammond, W. E. (1983). Computerized medical records: A new resource for clinical decision making. *Journal of Medical Systems, 7,* 213–220; Bakker, A. R. (1984). The development of an integrated and co-operative hospital information system. *Medical Informatics, 9,* 135–142; Barnett, G. O. (1984). The application of computer-based medical record systems in ambulatory practice. *New England Journal of Medicine, 9,* 135–142; Scherrer, J. R., Baud, R., Brisebarre, E., Messmer, E., & Assimacopoulos, A. (1986). A hospital information system in continuous operation and expansion: Concepts, tools and migration. In H. F. Othner (Ed.), *Proceedings of the tenth annual symposium on computer applications in medical care* (pp. 120–132). Washington, DC: Computer Society Press; Whiting-O'Keefe, Q. E., Whiting, A., & Henke, J. (1988). The STOR clinical information system. *M.D. Computing, 5,* 8–21; Hendrickson, G., Anderson, R. K., Clayton, P. D., Cimino, J., Hripsak, G. M., and Johnson, S. B. (1992). The integrated academic information management system at Columbia-Presbyterian Medical Center. *M.D. Computing, 9,* 35–42.

P. 152, *they could not readily share information:* Bleich, H. L., & Slack, W. V. (1992). Designing a hospital information system: A comparison of interfaced and integrated systems. *M.D. Computing, 9*(5), 293–296.

P. 153, *benefit from the clinical computing system:* Bleich, H. L., Beckley, R. F., Horowitz, G., Jackson, J., Moody, E., Franklin, C., Goodman, S. R., McKay, M. W., Pope, R. A., Walden, T., Bloom S. A., & Slack, W. V. (1985). Clinical computing in a teaching hospital. *New England Journal of Medicine, 312,* 756–764; Bleich, H. L., & Slack, W. V. (1989). Clinical Computing. *M.D. Computing, 6,* 133–135.

P. 153, *a similar computing system at Boston's Brigham and Women's Hospital:* Safran, C., Slack, W. V., & Bleich, H. L. (1989). Role of computing in patient care in two hospitals. *M.D. Computing, 6*(3), 141–148. Bleich, H. L., Safran, C., & Slack, W. V. (1989). Departmental and laboratory computing in two teaching hospitals. *M.D. Computing, 6,* 149–155.

P. 154, *MUMPS:* Greenes, R. A., Pappalardo, A. N., Marble, C. W., Barnett, G. O. (1969). Design and implementation of a clinical data management system. *Computers and Biomedical Research, 2,* 469–485.

P. 154, *one network at each hospital:* Bleich, H. L., Safran, C., & Slack, W. V. Departmental and laboratory computing in two teaching hospitals. *M.D. Computing, 6,* 149–155.

P. 154, *increased speed and efficiency:* Glaser, J. P., Beckley, R. F., III, Roberts, P., Mara, J. K., Hiltz, F. L., & Hurley, J. (1991). A very large PC LAN as the basis for a hospital information system. *Journal of Medical Systems, 15*(2), 133–137.

P. 156, *outpatient revenues increased by 45 percent:* Bleich, H. L., Safran, C., & Slack, W. V. (1989). Departmental and laboratory computing in two teaching hospitals. *M.D. Computing, 6,* 149–155.

P. 156, *entitle the hospital to additional reimbursement:* Safran, C., Porter, D., Slack, W. V., & Bleich, H. L. (1987). Diagnosis-related groups: A critical assessment of the provision for co-morbidity. *Medical Care, 25,* 1011–1014.

P. 158, *help the investigator conduct research:* Safran, C., Herrmann, F., Rind, D., Kowaloff, H., Bleich, H., & Slack, W. Computer-based support for clinical decision making. *M.D. Computing, 7*(5), 319–322.

P. 158, *electrolyte and acid-base program:* Bleich, H. L. (1971). The computer as a consultant. *New England Journal of Medicine, 284,* 141–147.

P. 158, *language for use in computer-based interviews:* Bloom, S., White, R., Beckley, R., & Slack, W. (1978). Converse: A means to write, edit, administer, and summarize computer-based dialogue. *Computers and Biomedical Research, 11,* 167–175.

P. 158, *program that retrieves clinical information:* Safran, C., Porter, D., Lightfoot, J., Rury, C. D., Underhill, L. H., Bleich, H. L., & Slack, W. V. (1989). ClinQuery: A system for online searching of data in a teaching hospital. *Annals of Internal Medicine, 9,* 751–756.

P. 158, *can use ClinQuery to study demographic and clinical profiles:* Safran, C., Porter, D., Slack, W. V., & Bleich, H. L. (1987). Diagnosis-related groups: A critical assessment of the provision for co-morbidity. *Medical Care, 25,* 1011–1014.

P. 158, *PaperChase:* Horowitz, G. L., & Bleich, H. L. (1981). PaperChase: A computer program to search the medical literature. *New England Journal of Medicine, 305,* 924–930.

P. 160, *computer-assigned confidential password, or key:* Safran, C., Rind, D., Citroen, M., Bakker, A. R., Slack, W. V., & Bleich, H. L. (1995). Protection of confidentiality in the computer-based patient record. *M.D. Computing, 12*(3), 187–192.

P. 160, *In the outpatient setting:* Safran, C., Rury, C., Rind, D. M., & Taylor, W. C. (1991). A computer-based outpatient medical record for a teaching hospital. *M.D. Computing, 8*(5), 291–299.

P. 160, *designate it as a "monitored" note:* Wald, J. S., Rind, D., & Safran, C. (1994). Protecting confidentiality in an electronic medical record: Feedback to the author when someone reads a clinical note. *American Medical Informatics Association Spring Proceedings, 42.*

P. 161, *it can be edited and forwarded to someone else:* Sands, D. Z., Safran, C., Slack, W. V., & Bleich, H. L. (1994). Use of electronic mail in a teaching hospital. *Seventeenth Annual Symposium on Computer Applications in Medical Care* (McGraw-Hill), 306–310.

P. 161, *available for all hospital employees:* Slack, W. V., Safran, C. S., Kowaloff, H. B., Pearce, J., & DelBanco, T. L. (1995). A computer-administered health screening interview for hospital personnel. *M.D. Computing, 12*(1), 25–30.

P. 162, *the mean number of inquiries was 59:* Safran, C., Slack, W. V., & Bleich, H. L. (1989). Role of computing in patient care in two hospitals. *M.D. Computing, 6*(3), 141–148.

P. 163, *the electrocardiograph, electroencephalograph, and X-ray machine:* Slack, W. V. (1993). Assessing the clinician's use of computers. *M.D. Computing, 106,* 357–360.

P. 164, *give their opinion of the system:* Bleich, H. L., Beckley, R. F., Horowitz, G., Jackson, J., Moody, E., Franklin, C., Goodman, S. R., McKay, M. W., Pope, R. A., Walden, T., Bloom, S. A., & Slack, W. V. (1985). Clinical computing in a teaching hospital. *New England Journal of Medicine, 312,* 756–764.

P. 164, *person who invents a machine is likely to be its first user:* Slack, W. V. (1992). When the machine stops. *M.D. Computing, 9,* 6–10.

P. 165, *the only person who knew how to use it:* Bleich, H. L. (1992). Charles Babbage and his steam-driven computer. *M.D. Computing, 9,* 6–10.

P. 166, *compelling evidence that behavior is shaped by its consequences:* Watson, J. B. (1924). *Behaviorism.* New York: W. W. Norton; Thorndike, E. L. (1932). *The fundamentals of learning.* New York: Teachers College, Columbia University; Skinner, B. F. (1938). *The behavior of organisms: An experimental analysis.* New York: Appleton-Century-Crofts.

P. 166, *if the interaction is helpful:* Slack, W. V., Van Cura, L. J., & Greist, J. H. (1970). Computers and doctors: Use and consequences. *Computers and Biomedical Research, 3,* 521–527; Slack, W. V. (1980). Use of computers. *MEDINFO 80: Proceedings of the Third World Conference on Medical Informatics* (pp. 1082–1083). Amsterdam: North-Holland; Slack, W. V., Boro, E. S., & Bleich, H. L. (1992). Barriers to clinical computing: What physicians can do. *M.D. Computing, 9,* 278–280.

P. 166, *responses to survey interviews, will be positive:* Bleich, H. L., Beckley, R. F., Horowitz, G., Jackson, J., Moody, E., Franklin, C., Goodman, S. R., McKay, M. W., Pope, R. A., Walden, T., Bloom, S. A., Slack, W. V. (1985). Clinical computing in a teaching hospital. *New England Journal of Medicine, 312,* 756–764; Slack, W. V. (1992). Democracy and the computer in America. *M.D. Computing, 9*(6), 341–342.

P. 166, *intensity with which clinicians such as house officers voluntarily use it:* Bleich, H. L., Beckley, R. F., Horowitz, G., Jackson, J., Moody, E., Franklin, C., Goodman, S. R., McKay, M. W., Pope, R. A., Walden, T., Bloom, S. A., & Slack, W. V. (1985). Clinical computing in a teaching hospital. *New England Journal of Medicine, 312,* 756–764; Safran, C., Slack, W. V., & Bleich, H. L. (1989). Role of computing in patient care in two hospitals. *M.D. Computing, 6*(3), 141–148; Slack, W. V. (1993). Assessing the clinician's use of computers. *M.D. Computing, 106,* 357–360.

P. 167, *PaperChase: a computer program:* Horowitz, G. L., & Bleich, H. L. (1981). PaperChase: A computer program to search the medical literature. *New England Journal of Medicine, 305,* 924–930.

P. 167, *performed at any other institution in the country:* Lyders, R. (1987). *Annual statistics of medical school libraries in the United States and Canada 1986–87.* 10th ed. Houston: Houston Academy of Medicine–Texas Medical Center Library.

P. 167, *2,202 people performed 16,803 searches:* Horowitz, G. L., Jackson, J. D., & Bleich, H. L. (1983). PaperChase: Self-service bibliographic retrieval. *Journal of the American Medical Association, 250,* 2494–2499.

CHAPTER NINE

COMPUTERIZATION IN MANAGED BEHAVIORAL HEALTHCARE COMPANIES

William R. Maloney and Eugene D. Hill III

This chapter examines the trends that have shaped information systems in managed behavioral healthcare companies in the past and how these same trends will continue to influence the industry in the future. It reviews the necessary components of state-of-the-art systems today and summarizes some of the more innovative applications that behavioral healthcare companies have implemented in recent years. The chapter concludes with a look at the future state of behavioral informatics in order to assess the level of development required by vendors in managed behavioral healthcare in the future.

This chapter has important implications for behavioral health providers and managed care companies as it describes the technological merging of the behavioral healthcare delivery system. Managed care functions are shifting from the behavioral health companies to the providers. This is most clearly demonstrated by the move from fee-for-service to capitation at the provider level. This merging of functions cannot occur without the necessary technological infrastructure supporting the providers of care and linking them to the management organizations.

Historical Roots of the Major Current Information Systems

Ever since the emergence of the first Blue Cross and Blue Shield plans early in this century, the financing of healthcare and the delivery of healthcare services have been divided into separate industries in the United States. The only exceptions to this rule before the 1970s were the small number of prepaid group health plans, which combined the financing and delivery of healthcare in a single organization. For the vast majority of Americans, however, the financing of healthcare was provided by health insurance companies, while the delivery of healthcare service was through independent hospitals, physicians, and ancillary providers.

The automation of these two industries did not occur in a coordinated manner. Systems were developed independently for the insurers and the providers of care. Much of the discussion later in this chapter on innovations in current systems and the future of behavioral health informatics focuses on integrating the tasks performed by these two separate industries.

The introduction of computer technology to the healthcare industry began in the late 1950s. For the first few decades it was largely limited to financial applications. Mechanical adding machines at the insurance companies and hospitals were replaced by computer systems running accounting software packages. Due to the expense and expertise required to run these early systems, many hospitals chose to purchase computer services through service bureaus rather than leasing or purchasing their own machines.

The insurance industry, on the other hand, had greater resources, greater processing needs, and greater competitive pressures. Sharing a service bureau with the competition was not a viable option for large insurers. This led to the development of proprietary in-house systems.

Hospital and Provider Information Systems

The healthcare informatics industry broadened significantly in the 1960s due to several important factors. The introduction of Medicare and Medicaid both increased the funding for healthcare services and made the financing of healthcare more stable and reliable. Hospitals could more readily commit the capital required to build internal information systems (IS) departments. At the same time, computer technology was becoming accessible and less expensive. Systems were becoming more reliable, better software was available, and the number of trained IS personnel was increasing.

An important legal development in the late 1960s contributed to the diversity and growth of the industry. The U.S. Department of Justice obtained a consent decree against International Business Machines Corp. for unfair competitive practices. Much of the evidence for the decision was compiled by Control Data Corp. As part of the terms of the agreement, IBM agreed to get out of the service bureau business. It divested itself of its own service bureau, selling it to Control Data. This accomplished the Justice Department's goal of increasing competition in the computer industry. Within the healthcare industry, IBM lost the advantage it had built in providing service bureau services through its Shared Hospital Accounting System (SHAS) package. Several former IBM executives recognized the opportunity created by IBM's exit from this market and created a new hospital service bureau with updated versions of the SHAS package. This new company, Shared Medical Systems (SMS), is still today the largest provider of hospital software in the country. Many other software companies owe their start to IBM's retrenchment. This expanded the number of information product options for healthcare providers.

The next major change in hospital computing came in the 1970s with the increasing use and popularity of minicomputers. These smaller, less expensive machines lowered the barrier for many hospitals, and later for group physician practices, to provide their own systems. The software industry expanded accordingly. Special applications were developed for departments within hospitals, further enlarging the market. In this manner, medical informatics moved beyond the accounting functions to administrative functions and simple clinical functions.

As software developers began to cater to the unique needs of hospital departments and large group practices, the number of unique and incompatible systems increased. This proliferation of systems was further encouraged by the growth of the microcomputer market in the 1980s. Eventually it was possible for even single-physician offices to have their own practice management systems. By the early 1990s, it was estimated that over seven hundred unique practice management applications existed for physician offices. Many of these were developed from scratch for mini or micro computers. However, even the largest commercially available applications still control less than 20 percent of the market today.

The provider side of the marketplace has been characterized by a plethora of provider and hospital systems. The hospital marketplace has several large vendors, most notably Shared Medical Systems (SMS) and Home Box Office (HBO), but it is fragmented among hospital departmental systems. The provider marketplace is somewhat less fragmented in behavioral healthcare than it is in physician office systems. A few vendors, such as CMHC Systems and Echo Systems, have emerged from behavioral health or social service backgrounds to develop systems specifically aimed at tracking behavioral healthcare services.

Additional Diversity in the Software Market

On the insurance side of healthcare, the large insurers continued to maintain their proprietary in-house systems. At times, commercially available packages would be purchased to add functionality; however, these packages were typically modified extensively. Over time this led to the development of enormous internal IS departments, which still exist today.

Changes in the legal framework supporting the insurance industry in the 1970s led to the growth of new branches of the industry. This, in turn, led to new areas of software development. The first major change came with the passage of the Early Retirement Insurance Security Act (ERISA) legislation. This improved the ability of large companies and coalitions of smaller employers to self-insure. This in turn led to the growth of a new branch of the health insurance industry, the third-party administrator (TPA), and new software applications to support the processing and paying of health insurance claims.

Many of the TPAs started out as very small companies. These companies, like the physician practices, were looking for smaller, less expensive solutions to their information needs. Many were willing to hire programming staff to build simple applications. Over time the best of these applications were enhanced and created a new commercial market for claims software.

Similar opportunities occurred for small software developers with the passage of the HMO Act in the early seventies. The act promoted enormous growth in the prepaid group health plan market, which had previously been limited to several well-defined areas of the country. These areas of early HMO development included Minneapolis, Seattle, Washington, D.C., and parts of California. After passage of the act, HMOs became available in most parts of the country. Today more than fifty million Americans are insured by HMOs. As with the TPAs, this led to the creation of new software applications and companies that have grown with this segment of the industry. Many of the managed care applications, for example, those developed by Computer Sciences Corporation, Amisys Managed Care Systems, and Health Systems Design, have been adapted by the larger behavioral health companies for the management of behavioral health plans.

A third type of company was developing alongside the TPAs and HMOs: the utilization review (UR) firm. They offered employers a middle ground between the restriction of a comprehensive HMO and the complete freedom of provider choice offered by the indemnity health insurers. The UR companies required case management applications to track the care a patient had received and track the authorization for care that a provider had been granted. However, they did not need to either pay for the care (as did the TPAs and insurers) or keep the medical records (as did the hospitals and providers). This led to another set of unique applications and the entrance of additional software vendors into the market. Many of the behavioral healthcare firms in existence today began as specialized utilization review firms (Table 9.1).

Thus medical informatics, and more specifically behavioral health informatics, is characterized on the insurance side of the market by large, antiquated, proprietary systems. These systems were originally developed to track benefits and pay claims in an indemnity, or fee-for-service, market. Due to their size and complexity and the sheer volume of claims they must pay daily, the insurers have been

TABLE 9.1. MANAGED CARE EVOLUTION

	1970s	1980s	1990s
Focus	Benefit administration	Risk selection Medical management	Risk management Vertical integration
Private sector	Indemnity Staff model HMOs	PPO U/R IPA and staff model HMOs Specialty U/R	Integrated healthcare Delivery systems HMO (risk) POS
Public sector	Indemnity UCR HMO (cost) Claims administration	U/R DRGs HMO (risk) Medical management	RBRVS HMO (risk) Risk contracting
Provider payment	Fee for service	Some capitation	Mainly capitation
Provider choice	Complete freedom of choice	Freedom of choice with financial incentives	Some choice within limited provider panel

slow to respond to changes in the marketplace. These systems impact behavioral healthcare, however, since many of the behavioral health claims must still be paid on these systems. This is especially true for those insurers that either developed a behavioral healthcare subsidiary or bought one of the existing behavioral healthcare vendors.

The HMO or managed care market has largely developed its own set of software applications, as we mentioned. These applications and the ones developed by the UR industry have a direct impact on the behavioral health marketplace since many of these applications have been adapted for behavioral health plans. The applications are more relevant to managed behavioral health firms than to indemnity companies with systems more narrowly focused on the payment of claims only, since managed care combines the authorization of care (the UR function) with the claims payment (the TPA/insurance function). Especially important in the current marketplace, the HMO applications have better systems for the management of risk under a capitated payment system. These applications allow utilization and cost to be tracked in a variety of ways which enable the plan manager to recognize, report, and predict cost trends against the capitation payments.

The Influence of Cost Containment

One of the most important agendas in the last fifteen years for healthcare generally, and behavioral healthcare specifically, is the reduction of cost. Most of the trends described in the previous paragraphs have had as their central focus reducing costs. In recent years it has become clear that the techniques are working.

Increases in healthcare costs, including behavioral healthcare costs, first slowed and for the past several years have declined in many regions of the country. The trends described above focused on changing the practices of the purchasers and providers of healthcare. A variety of techniques were used, including increasing monitoring of providers, increasing the cost to consumers, developing new non-indemnity insurance options, and altering provider incentive systems through capitation. With each new technique came a new set of software applications.

While it is clear that such techniques have reduced the overall cost of healthcare, they have done so at the price of greater administrative complication and expense. Today there are many more layers of administration, each with its own set of software applications that are often incompatible with each other and disconnected entirely from the other layers. A commonly seen example in behavioral healthcare is when a UR company aggressively monitors inpatient psychiatric care and decides not to authorize a specific number of days, yet the claim is paid anyway since there is no linkage between the UR firm's case management system and the TPA's claim payment system.

The administrative inefficiencies created by various cost containment efforts provide a target for future cost containment. Past cost reductions brought about by the methods described earlier in this chapter can be augmented in the future by streamlining healthcare administration. Cost efficiencies can be realized through better integration of information systems and reductions in the inefficiencies created by multiple administrative layers. Integration will reduce costs by eliminating problems such as the UR/claims interface issue. Better systems integration will allow applications to communicate and bridge the historic gap between the payment of healthcare (the health insurance industry) and the delivery of healthcare (providers and facilities). This gap has been at least partially crossed with the HMO systems, which is why they are the applications of choice for building managed behavioral health systems. However, much work still remains to be done to link providers and payers, thus eliminating the historic differentiation between these industries.

As the two healthcare industries merge into the integrated healthcare organization of the future, multiple levels of administration will decrease. A capitated group practice or physician/hospital organization (PHO) will monitor its own utilization, thus eliminating the need for the insurer to introduce a UR vendor into the payment process.

The Current State of Behavioral Health Systems

Behavioral healthcare vendors are a mixed lot. Some come from HMO backgrounds, having run captive clinics for health plans. Others come from employee assistance program (EAP) backgrounds. These vendors have been responsible for identifying and referring troubled employees to behavioral healthcare providers, but historically they did not provide that care themselves. Still other companies have come from the UR industry. Often, the UR-based companies had little contact with the employee, and instead worked behind the scene with the provider to ensure that care was appropriate and that all alternatives had been considered.

Today, as public-sector behavioral health entities explore managed care, new commercial vendors are emerging with backgrounds in public-sector and community mental health centers. Similarly, the provider community is actively developing alliances that are capable of managing capitation. These alliances can continue to work with the existing managed healthcare (HMO and insurance) and managed behavioral healthcare companies, or they can approach employers and other purchasers of healthcare directly. The fact that they have not managed clinics and hospitals for an HMO in the past (as is true with the first group) does not mean that they cannot do so in the future.

Integrated Healthcare Systems

Regardless of their background, managed behavioral healthcare companies are migrating towards the integrated healthcare organization model. As time passes, they have begun to look increasingly alike. This should continue in the future as they become further integrated into the healthcare system. Figure 9.1 demonstrates the progress of the various types of healthcare organizations towards the "integrated healthcare organization" of the future. These integrated organizations will provide medical/surgical as well as behavioral healthcare. They will perform all of the functions of the current insurance and healthcare delivery systems.

Of the current types of healthcare companies, the HMO most resembles the future integrated healthcare organization. This is because the HMO has traditionally performed both the insurance and service delivery roles. However, the integrated healthcare organization is envisioned as typically having a much larger presence in the communities it serves. It would probably include one or more of the dominant hospitals in the area and would connect a large percentage of the community's outpatient clinics through a community health information network (CHIN). Allina, which resulted from the merger of Minnesota's largest HMO and one of the area's largest hospital systems, provides a good example of this type of organization. In the first months of its existence, Allina purchased the organization that owns and supports DISC, the dominant practice management system in the region. Between the merger and the acquisition, Allina now has the major pieces of an integrated healthcare organization. Allina is not alone; a recent Dorenfest and Associates poll showed that 31.5 percent of hospitals responding

FIGURE 9.1. PROGRESS TOWARD THE INTEGRATED HEALTHCARE ORGANIZATION OF THE FUTURE

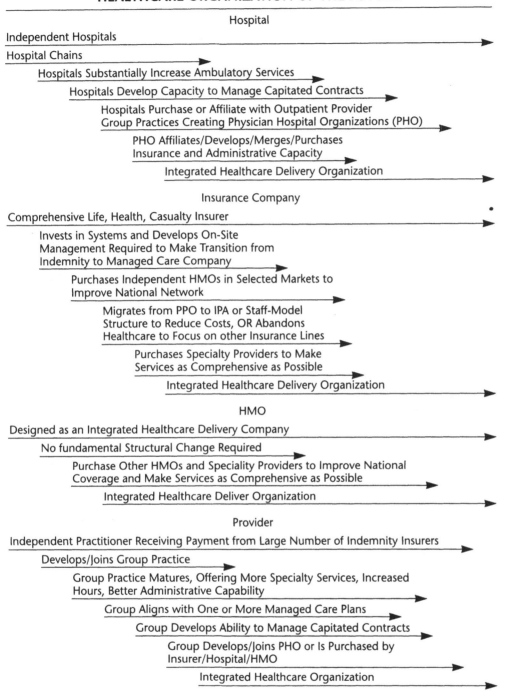

Hospital

Independent Hospitals

Hospital Chains

Hospitals Substantially Increase Ambulatory Services

Hospitals Develop Capacity to Manage Capitated Contracts

Hospitals Purchase or Affiliate with Outpatient Provider
Group Practices Creating Physician Hospital Organizations (PHO)

PHO Affiliates/Develops/Merges/Purchases
Insurance and Administrative Capacity

Integrated Healthcare Delivery Organization

Insurance Company

Comprehensive Life, Health, Casualty Insurer

Invests in Systems and Develops On-Site
Management Required to Make Transition from
Indemnity to Managed Care Company

Purchases Independent HMOs in Selected Markets to
Improve National Network

Migrates from PPO to IPA or Staff-Model
Structure to Reduce Costs, OR Abandons
Healthcare to Focus on other Insurance Lines

Purchases Specialty Providers to Make
Services as Comprehensive as Possible

Integrated Healthcare Delivery Organization

HMO

Designed as an Integrated Healthcare Delivery Company

No fundamental Structural Change Required

Purchase Other HMOs and Speciality Providers to Improve National
Coverage and Make Services as Comprehensive as Possible

Integrated Healthcare Deliver Organization

Provider

Independent Practitioner Receiving Payment from Large Number of Indemnity Insurers

Develops/Joins Group Practice

Group Practice Matures, Offering More Specialty Services, Increased
Hours, Better Administrative Capability

Group Aligns with One or More Managed Care Plans

Group Develops Ability to Manage Capitated Contracts

Group Develops/Joins PHO or Is Purchased by
Insurer/Hospital/HMO

Integrated Healthcare Organization

FIGURE 9.1. PROGRESS TOWARD THE INTEGRATED HEALTHCARE ORGANIZATION OF THE FUTURE, cont'd.

Behavioral Healthcare

Behavioral Healthcare Follows Trends Above as Independent
Behavioral Health Facilities, Providers, and Networks

Behavioral Healthcare Network Purchased by Insurer, HMO, Hospital System

Behavioral Healtcare Integrated into
Comprehensive Healthcare Delivery Sytem

Integrated Healthcare Organization

to a recent survey are already part of a CHIN, an alliance, or a joint venture. Another 40 percent plan to join one.

Within behavioral health the issues are similar. Allina includes the managed behavioral care division of the HMO and the inpatient and outpatient behavioral care delivery system of the hospital. The HMO has conducted utilization review of treatment services at the hospital in the past since it utilized the inpatient services of the hospital. However, the HMO's outpatient services were provided through its own behavioral health clinics.

The issue that remains for both behavioral health and the medical/surgical system is that of integration. In many ways the easy work is done and the hardest tasks lie ahead. Now that all of the pieces of the "integrated" healthcare organization are assembled, how do they become truly integrated? Significant integration will be required if the system is to deliver on its promise of cost reduction.

The HMO's utilization review of the hospital's inpatient psychiatric ward provides a good example. How can the cost of this work be reduced or eliminated now that the staff on either side of this review process are working for the same organization? The new company needs to integrate the systems of the HMO directly into its inpatient facility. The HMO has documented the preferred patterns of practice for inpatient psychiatry and the inpatient utilization review criteria. They have extensive records of inpatient utilization going back many years. This information needs to be shared, and it should be available online for the staff making the inpatient decisions.

Current Needs and Requirements

Given the mixed group of behavioral health vendors that are purchasing or developing software, it is not surprising that current software applications are diverse. It is possible to find many excellent applications and features across the industry.

However, since none of the existing behavioral health managed care vendors has completed the transition to the integrated healthcare organization, none of the vendors have systems that meet all of the requirements presented in Table 9.2.

Those vendors meeting some or most of the requirements are often lacking integration of the system elements. Typically, the various system components have been developed independently or were purchased from different vendors. It is the norm rather than the exception, for example, for behavioral health companies to have separate systems for provider maintenance/credentialing, case management, and claims payment. This creates difficulties at the interfaces between the systems, which must typically be resolved by increasing the number of administrative staff. It also makes adding advanced applications more difficult. Provider profiling, for example, is a difficult application to add to an existing system if the case management and claims records are not compatible with the provider files.

Only a few of the major behavioral healthcare vendors have had direct service as a major part of their business over the past five years. Consequently, integration of patient scheduling and other clinical and practice management functions will require the most development. Most of the vendors have left the practice management activities to their network providers in the past. As demonstrated in the Allina example above, this will not be possible in the future. Several of the major managed behavioral care vendors either have added or are in the process of adding the practice management component to their systems.

Table 9.2 lists the components of today's state-of-the-art behavioral health information system. Current vendors should have or at least be actively developing each of these components. For some of the components, the most integrated solution is to share the functionality with the sister medical/surgical organization. While this is an optimum solution, it is only positive if developed correctly.

For example, paying behavioral health claims on the claims system of the medical\surgical parent organization can be a good solution since it can result in a single integrated claims data base. Not having a single source for all claims data is a major flaw in many of the carve-out behavioral health plans. However, if paying the claims through the medical/surgical system means that behavioral health claims must be double entered or cannot be automatically adjudicated, then the solution is suboptimal. Obviously, having all the listed components is only part of the story. The components of the state-of-the-art system must be fully integrated with each other and with the medical/surgical systems.

While none of the managed behavioral health firms have all of the features listed above, most are working to add the options they are missing. Integration issues are a high priority for the majority of firms. As mentioned earlier, having case management and authorization systems that are not linked to the claims

TABLE 9.2. MANAGED BEHAVIORAL HEALTH SYSTEMS REQUIREMENTS

Finance	General ledger
	Accounts payable
	Billing/Accounts receivable
	Underwriting/Pricing
	Capitation management
	Contract management
Managed care	Case management
	Intake
	Authorization
	Referral
	Clinical protocols/Critical paths
	Rule-based (Expert system)
	Utilization reporting
Provider network	Credentialing
	Contract maintenance
	Profiling
Claim/Encounter procession	Automated adjudication
	Automated authorization matching
	Claim processing
Administration	Enrollment
	Eligibility
	Benefit plan maintenance
	Member relations support
Outcome	HEDIS reporting
	Client satisfaction
	Level of functioning
Practice management	Medical record/Treatment plans
	Scheduling (multiple clinics/facilities)
	Registration (enterprisewide)
	Billing/Accounts receivable (Patient level)
	Ancillary ordering
	Prescriptions
System requirements	Security
	Response time/Reliability
	User-accessible report writing features
	Access
	Sufficient, accessible PC locations
	User-friendly interface
	Mobile device option
	User-modifiable, Table-driven structure
	Imaging capability
	EDI
	Enterprisewide compatibility/Information interchange

payment system is a frequent problem being addressed by managed behavioral health companies.

Important Innovations Now Available

Despite the many issues that need addressing, there are also many new features which have been implemented by managed behavioral health firms in the recent past:

- Employee assistance systems allow the tracking of both problem type and diagnostic code to improve the referral process.
- Provider selection features at some of the managed care firms now provide instant information on provider specialty, availability, and distance from the client's residence.
- Initial provider profiling applications have been developed. While these are quite simple at this point, they show effort in the right direction. Importantly, the firms that have begun this development indicate that the profiles are as much for the providers as for managed care companies; many of these firms are sending the profiles to the providers.
- Optical scanning technology and scannable forms allow providers to receive authorization and prepare treatment plans in the most time-efficient manner. Treatment plans and claims are then fed directly into the computer system upon receipt, allowing claim turnaround times of less than a day for approved treatments.
- For providers that have (or are willing to purchase) a PC, electronic versions of this scanning system are available. These systems provide the therapist with "client" software for their machine, which includes electronic versions of the forms required by the managed care firms with which they are contracted. These systems are paperless, allowing the provider to receive authorizations, send treatment plans and claims, verify eligibility and benefits, and check payment status electronically.
- Telephone response systems have been developed which allow providers access to eligibility and claims information over the phone.
- Central scheduling functions allow the behavioral health company intake staff not only to find a provider but to schedule and confirm the initial session.
- Simple versions exist of online utilization review criteria and practice guidelines. These applications typically serve as reference guides to case managers. They allow the case manager access to "best practice" information to compare against the treatment options proposed by network providers.
- Simple artificial intelligence applications have been developed which match these "best practice" guidelines to treatment plans submitted electronically by

providers. These systems allow standard treatment plans to be approved automatically, while flagging outliers for clinician review.

- Systems are in rapid development for tracking client improvement or outcome. This type of system involves the automation of client and provider assessment scales. The client and provider fill out a scannable form or input information on a PC. Information is collected at the beginning and end of treatment and at prescribed intervals during treatment. Depending on the system, various analyses are provided of client improvement, treatment effectiveness, and client satisfaction with the treatment and the therapist.

◆ ◆ ◆

There is much work to be done for many present companies to reach the state of the art currently possible with today's technology and managed care know-how. This is especially true around the issue of integration. The legacy of healthcare information systems development described in the first section of this chapter has promoted an environment of specialized applications to the detriment of systemwide integration. Those behavioral health firms that have achieved a higher level of system integration have been rewarded with considerable administrative cost savings.

The features described in this section provide an overview of some of the progress being made currently toward reaching the optimal behavioral health system. The next section, however, demonstrates that the definition of state-of-the-art is moving at least as fast as the development efforts. The goal of integration within the behavioral health company's systems is being replaced by the goal of integration across the medical/surgical systems also. This in turn is expanded to include the entire "integrated healthcare organization," which requires communitywide integration. One of the main goals of future systems is an electronic or computerized patient record (CPR) that tracks client treatment regardless of where in the region that treatment was received. This will allow the system to develop a single comprehensive picture of the patient's history and each episode of care.

The Future of Behavioral Healthcare Informatics

The trends in behavioral healthcare informatics follow the trends in the healthcare industry. As healthcare migrates towards an integrated model, healthcare informatics must evolve to support this model. The future integrated healthcare organization will require information systems with each of the following components:

- An electronic medical record and central client registration, including the tracking of all patient services (within and external to behavioral healthcare). This allows creation of a single electronic patient history/medical record, which is augmented as services are delivered regardless of where within the integrated healthcare organization.
- Quick, online access to client eligibility information and treatment history by authorized personnel anywhere within the integrated system. At a minimum, information will be available throughout the enterprise. In most cases it will be available beyond the enterprise in community, regional, and national health information networks.
- Online practice guidelines, which are maintained and updated as new practice information is obtained. These guidelines serve as the core "expert" information in an expert system which provides clinicians with a range of appropriate treatment options during the assessment and treatment of clients. This expert system reviews the medical record as it is created; it provides feedback on drug interactions, nonstandard treatments, and outcomes that fall outside of acceptable ranges.
- A standard tool for measuring client progress and outcomes, updated regularly. Assessments are made by the therapist and client at pretreatment, posttreatment, and regular intervals throughout the treatment process. These measures are input into the system immediately following the treatment session; they serve as input to the client satisfaction assessment, the provider profile, and the outcome measurement applications. Over time, analyses of the measures are used to update the practice guidelines.
- Online provider matching, to automate matching of the client to the closest appropriate provider. This includes the capability to schedule the first visit and to generate automatic visit reminders for the client to help assure attendance at the session. Centralized scheduling and patient flow tracking are available for services provided throughout the enterprise and/or community to ensure that appropriate resources are available when needed, and to prevent over- and underutilization of resources.
- Greatly expanded healthcare service applications that are accessible to the membership through information systems without the face-to-face intervention of a therapist. This area includes member education applications and telemedicine. The goal of these applications is to provide the member with alternatives to seeing a therapist or otherwise accessing the medical system (telemedicine), and to help the member understand the therapeutic options if it is not necessary to access the healthcare system.
- A provider profiling system, including risk-adjusted utilization profiling, client satisfaction measures, outcome measures, and practice guideline compliance analyses.

- Menu-driven interfaces with voice recognition, touch screen, and point-and-click interface options to simplify data input and ensure that data (especially clinical data) are collected in a manner that aids analysis and trending.
- Mobile computing interfaces, to ensure that access to the system is available when required in the clinical process.
- Complete integration of all features. The system should be client-server or peer-to-peer, with consistent messaging standards across the network. This ensures most efficient use of processing power and compatibility of the functions. Maximally, all standards (communication, administration, clinical) will be national or international, for compatibility across the CHIN and other open systems. Minimally, standards must be at least enterprisewide.

The most important point to note about these features is that they span industries that were previously divided. The provider-matching software improves the productivity of the intake worker, which was typically an insurance and UR-industry function within the managed care systems of the recent past. In the description of the features of the future system presented above, provider matching is united with patient scheduling and resource allocation. These were previously functions of the healthcare delivery system. Uniting system features that belong to both industries better serves the integrated healthcare organization and lowers overall costs. It also greatly enhances customer service, in this case by scheduling without requiring the client to make another phone call to the provider.

Similar examples of crossing traditional industry boundaries exist with nearly all of the features in the list above. Healthcare information systems provide the enabling technology, allowing integration of the insurance and healthcare delivery functions. Integration of these functions in turn leads to lower cost, higher quality, and improved customer service by eliminating the gaps and redundancies inherent in the two-industry system.

Information Systems Infrastructure

The application features detailed above require the support of an information system infrastructure which is quite different from the systems of the past. Advances in microprocessing power and expense have brought the industry to a point where the cost and power of RAM and microprocessors is no longer the most significant constraining factor in determining the design of the system. Today's desktop workstation is faster and has more disk and memory than the file servers of just a few years back. Both are more powerful than the machines that ran entire hospitals in the 1970s. This trend will continue for many more years.

The power and flexibility of the development tools used by the programming staff have increased as well. Data bases have evolved from flat files to structured, hierarchical systems, and finally to flexible, relational systems. Application languages have also evolved, becoming more powerful, flexible, and object-oriented. All of this means that software developed today and in the future will be easier to create and easier to change. This is significant because developing and modifying software has become the most significant constraint to the advancement of health informatics. As the cost of microprocessors and RAM dropped, the cost and complexity of designing software and writing code emerged as the most expensive constraint to system development. While the full impact of object-oriented development has yet to be felt, it will have a very positive impact on the cost of software development in the future.

One of the most significant obstacles to adoption of object-oriented languages for development of behavioral healthcare software is the cost and effort already invested in "legacy" systems based on older and less flexible technologies. There are other issues, such as the development of healthcare-specific object classes and, of course, the standardization of healthcare protocols (for example, the American National Standards Institute or ANSI X12 standards); these represent significant hurdles to future development. However, the integration of new software within the existing software infrastructure will always remain one of the largest impediments to rapid deployment of new development languages and applications. Few companies are willing to start from the beginning rewriting their applications to utilize the latest object-oriented development environments. Rather, they will attempt to build their new systems around the old.

As an example, a common strategy employed as a temporary solution by many of the behavioral health firms is to build a Windows client (using Powerbuilder, Visual Basic, etc.) as the new front end to existing legacy systems. This gives the system an updated look and allows the user some simple multitasking capability that frequently was not available with the old systems. It does all this without requiring major modifications to the existing legacy systems.

The forces described above (increased processing power at the desk and the need to retain expensive legacy systems) combined with the expense of acquiring and using a communications bandwidth for networking will continue to fuel the trend towards client-server computing. Client-server development allows the healthcare company to take advantage of desktop processing power while retaining much of their investment in legacy systems. The vast majority of the overall computer processing power in all of the behavioral health firms is in desktop machines. These machines also represent the largest investment in computer hardware. Well-designed client-server systems take advantage of these desktop processors while maintaining the legacy systems as network servers. Client-server systems also offer IS departments the opportunity to develop individual parts of the system independently. The system can be migrated in a steady and orderly fashion toward the new technology.

Client-server architecture is especially helpful in uniting the insurance and healthcare delivery systems, since both sides can easily envision the other as a partner in a client-server relationship. A behavioral healthcare clinician checking the eligibility of a new client provides a simple example. The clinician has a client software application which registers the patient and requests eligibility verification from a server application at the insurance company. The server performs the necessary data base queries and returns the result to the client.

In time, as processing power continues to increase at the desktop, more of the server functions will migrate to the desktop as well. As this happens, it may be more useful to focus less on client-server relationships (especially to the extent that this implies remote procedure calls) and consider specialized objects that use standard messaging protocols to communicate across the network. This is the environment of the future integrated healthcare organization. Processing is performed wherever it can be accomplished most efficiently.

◆ ◆ ◆

Managed behavioral health companies are adding many new features to their systems. Some of these are quite innovative and provide a preview of future integrated health organization systems.

However, many of the current systems, while meeting minimum functionality requirements, are not well integrated. These systems require extensive human intervention at the interfaces in order to function correctly. This is especially evident in the reporting area and the interface between the case management and claims systems. To achieve the next level of healthcare cost savings, managed behavioral healthcare vendors must achieve the efficiencies inherent in well-integrated systems.

In order to serve the integrated healthcare organizations of the future, managed behavioral healthcare information systems must do more than simply integrate existing functions. The systems must also bridge the historic gap between healthcare insurance and the delivery of healthcare service. Uniting the functions of these two industries will improve healthcare quality, provide additional cost advantages, and enhance customer service.

PART THREE

COMMUNICATIONS

CHAPTER TEN

THE NEED TO KNOW
VERSUS THE RIGHT TO PRIVACY

Robert Gellman and Kathleen A. Frawley

O ne of the myths of modern medicine is that health records are confidential and highly privileged. The truth is that legal protections for health records are incomplete and inconsistent, that medical ethics are inadequate to address confidentiality problems in the modern health delivery system, and that new technology and changing administrative patterns are undermining whatever limited protections exist. Demands for nontreatment uses of identifiable healthcare information are escalating and weakening the ability of patients and providers to know how information is being used and disclosed.

Shortcomings of Existing Confidentiality Rules

Lack of adequate confidentiality rules is not unique to health records. In today's complex, computerized society, basic records about an individual's activities, transactions, and finances are maintained by such third parties as banks, employers, insurance companies, healthcare providers, credit card issuers, retailers, and others. In most cases, there are few formal protections for personal information maintained by third-party record keepers.

For example, the U.S. Supreme Court has held that an individual has no protectable legal interest when the government seeks account records about an individual from a bank. The same result is highly likely for other types of records.

Congress has enacted legislation that gives individuals a legal interest in some records maintained by third parties, but the protections are weak and scattered. Thus records of movies rented from a video store have limited legal privacy protection, as do cable television viewing records, bank records, and electronic communications such as electronic mail. Of these records, the video rental records have the strongest privacy protections. There are, however, no general federal laws regulating the use and disclosure of records about health, employment, insurance, consumer transactions, and many financial activities.

Legal and Ethical Principles

There are no clear constitutional protections for health records. The leading Supreme Court decision on health privacy is *Whalen v. Roe.* The case involved a constitutional challenge to a New York state law establishing a computer system for the reporting of the names and addresses of those who obtain certain prescription drugs. The Court declined to find a constitutional violation, relying in part on the protections against unauthorized use and disclosure in the reporting system. The Court noted that disclosures of private medical information are often an essential part of modern medical practice and could not find reporting to the state to be an impermissible invasion of privacy.

The case hints at a constitutional right of privacy for health records but does not hold that the right exists. The Court referred to the "vast amounts of personal information in computerized data banks or other massive government files" but went no further than the statement that the duty to avoid unwarranted disclosures "arguably has its roots in the Constitution." Had there been a greater possibility of public disclosure under the New York statute, the Court might have directly confronted the nature of the constitutional interest. Whatever constitutional interest may exist, the Court seemed to say that the statute did not pose a sufficiently grievous threat. In a concurring opinion, Justice Brennan would not rule out the possibility that there may be a need sometime for a curb on technology for central storage and easy accessibility of computerized data.

Some health records are subject to federal privacy laws. The fair information principles of the Privacy Act of 1974 apply to most personal information maintained by federal agencies. Health records maintained by federal agencies, such as facilities operated by the Veterans Administration or the Public Health Service, fall under the Privacy Act. There are also federal laws that apply to federal or federally funded facilities that offer treatment for alcohol or drug abuse. There is, however, no general federal law providing for the confidentiality of health records otherwise, and most health records have no federal statutory protection.

Whatever general confidentiality protections exist for health records must be found at the state level. State laws vary tremendously in scope and quality, and many are substantially out of date because they do not address computers, computer networks, or modern patterns of healthcare practice, finance, or administration. Communications between patients and physicians are privileged in most but not all states, but the protection of these laws is very narrow. The privilege only applies when a physician is testifying in court or in related proceedings, and many laws include significant restrictions that further limit the availability of the privilege. In any event, the privilege does nothing to protect patient information from being released to third-party payers, government healthcare agencies, peer review organizations, and other routine recipients. The physician-patient privilege offers no real protection to patients.

There are ethical rules and guidelines that require physicians to protect the confidentiality of patient communications. The most famous of these is the Hippocratic Oath, which instructs physicians to treat as confidential that which "should not be published abroad." Later ethical codes consistently recognized the importance of confidentiality, but they do not provide specific guidance on disclosure questions confronted in the modern practice of medicine. Ethics codes do not offer guidance on the disclosure of health records for health research, peer review, cost containment, third-party subpoenas, and other common uses.

Even if ethical codes adequately addressed all current issues, they could not provide uniform, comprehensive protections for the interests of patients. Ethics codes are typically applicable to healthcare professionals and not to others who have routine access to health information in the ordinary course of conduct. Thus there is no ethical code that applies to hospital orderlies, claims processors, billing offices, credit card companies, and others who see or maintain identifiable health information as they carry out their functions. This parallels a problem with health privacy statutes that also tend to apply to health professionals but not to most secondary users.

A 1993 review of health privacy and computers by the congressional Office of Technology Assessment reached these conclusions:

> The present system of protection for healthcare information offers a patchwork of codes; state laws of varying scope; and federal laws applicable to only limited kinds of information, or information maintained specifically by the federal government. . . . The present legal scheme does not provide consistent, comprehensive protection for privacy in healthcare information, whether it exists in a paper or computerized environment.

Another report by the Institute of Medicine reached a similar conclusion about the inadequacy of current rules. It found three weaknesses in legal confidentiality protections for health records. First, the degree to which confidentiality is required varies according to the holder of the information and the type of information held. Second, legal obligations often vary widely within a single state and from state to state. Third, current laws offer patients little real protection against redisclosure.

Increasing Use and Misuse of Health Records

The absence of legal and ethical protections for the confidentiality of health records is an increasing problem because the modern healthcare treatment and payment system entails greater routine use and disclosure of identifiable health records. Records are used intensively for treatment and payment, but these basic functions involve larger numbers of individuals and institutions than ever before. Secondary use of health records is another routine feature of the healthcare delivery system, and most patients and providers are not aware of the extent to which health information is used for purposes not directly related to the provision of healthcare.

Secondary users include

Public health agencies

Medical and social researchers

Rehabilitation and social welfare programs

Employers

Insurance companies

Federal, state, and local government agencies

Educational institutions

Courts

Law enforcement and investigation agencies

Credit investigation agencies

Accrediting, licensing, and certifying agencies

The media

Peer review organizations

Health data base organizations

Cost containment and outcomes researchers

For each of these classes of users, there may be several different types of activities that require the use of identifiable health records. There are, for example, many government agencies that use health records for purposes ranging from treatment to prosecution. For all users, records are available not only to those who carry out substantive functions but also to those who are engaged in administration, data processing, and transmission. Computers and networks increase the number of people who can access the information, the centralization of data, and the risks from breaches of security.

In addition, there is a thriving commercial market for identifiable patient information. Commercial marketing and mailing list companies maintain and sell lists of individuals with specific ailments. One data base maintained by a mailing list vendor includes fifteen million individuals, including those with hypertension, angina, diabetes, allergies, arthritis, osteoporosis, Alzheimer's disease, bladder control problems, and Parkinson's disease. This information is typically collected directly from patients. Other commercial ventures collect data from physicians in exchange for a fee and computer services, and aggregate data derived from patient records is used for commercial purposes.

There is also evidence of significant surreptitious trafficking in health information. An investigation in 1975 by a grand jury in Denver identified a private investigative reporting company that had for twenty-five years engaged in the business of collecting health information without the consent of the patient. Private investigators collected patient information directly from providers by telephone, by posing as doctors, by false pretenses, and through bribery of hospital employees. There was nothing in the finding of the grand jury that suggested that the conduct of this company was unique or even unusual. A similar investigation in Canada found a tremendous volume of trafficking in health information, and many subsidiaries of American companies were found to be providers or users of improperly obtained information. These investigations identified insurance companies as major customers for illicitly obtained health records.

The problem of the misuse of patient data cannot be treated as a symptom of computerization of records. Misuse of records clearly predated any significant computerization, and, in any event, the main threats cannot be presumed to come from computer hackers and others outside the healthcare process. Reviews of abuse of and illegal trafficking in other types of personal information have found that the principal problems are the result of actions by insiders misusing their ability to access records. This appears to be the case for health records as well.

A relatively new development for health data also has some significant privacy implications. Health data base organizations are being established to acquire and maintain identifiable patient information for large segments of the population. Information comes from many sources, and the resulting computerized data bases will be used for administrative, clinical, health status, and other purposes. A central repository of health data is a valuable asset with treatment, research, and commercial uses. A central repository also presents many privacy issues. How these data bases will be organized and controlled remains an open question. The failure of existing rules to provide adequate privacy protections for traditional health records only makes the privacy questions for health data base organizations even more pressing.

Overall, there are significant gaps in privacy protections for health records. The absence of clear legal and ethical rules is a major shortcoming that is constantly made worse by more intensive use, disclosure, and exploitation of health information.

New Legal Protections

In 1993, President Clinton placed health reform on the national and congressional agendas, and the issue was the subject of intense debate during the 103d Congress. The broad health reform legislation proposed by the President included an outline of a privacy policy for health records, with the promise that proposals for substantive privacy protections would follow within a few years. The President's privacy proposal was well received, but there was substantial support for the view that any major health reform legislation would have to address the privacy issue at the beginning. Most health reform proposals, from every point on the political spectrum, increased the use and transfer of patient data, and there was widespread recognition of the need for resolving privacy concerns comprehensively and in advance.

There was also strong public concern about confidentiality of health records. A 1993 poll conducted by Lou Harris found that an overwhelming majority (85 percent) of the public believe that protecting the confidentiality of health records is absolutely essential or very important in national healthcare reform. According to Dr. Alan Westin, the public put this priority even ahead of reform goals such as providing health insurance for those who do not have it, reducing paperwork burdens on patients and providers, and obtaining better data for medical research.

The leading health privacy bill considered during the 103d Congress in 1994 was the Fair Health Information Practices Act (H.R. 4077), introduced by Rep. Gary Condit (D-Calif.), chairman of the House Subcommittee on Information, Justice, Transportation, and Agriculture. The legislation was initially offered independently of other health reform efforts, but it was eventually linked to the broader Health Security Act (H.R. 3600) that was reported out of several committees in the House of Representatives. The entire health reform effort collapsed toward the end of the 103d Congress in late 1994, including the privacy part. While it did not become law, the Condit bill attracted considerable support from all sides. The bill is worthy of discussion because it is likely to provide a starting point for future legislative efforts and because it offers a comprehensive, coordinated, and current approach to the use, disclosure, and maintenance of health records.

Fair Information Practices

Congressman Condit called his bill the "Fair Health Information Practices Act" and deliberately avoided using the term "privacy." This was done in express recognition of the reality that health records are not completely confidential and that absolute privacy protections are not possible and cannot be assured. In contrast, a 1980 effort to pass a federal law on health records was called the Federal Privacy of Medical Information Act. The report accompanying the 1994 effort noted that the change in title "bears some significance."

Fair information practices originated with a 1973 report of an Advisory Committee in the federal Department of Health, Education, and Welfare. The principles of fair information practices then formed the basis for privacy (or data protection) laws in Europe and elsewhere around the world in the late 1970s and 1980s. In 1981, both the Council of Europe and the Organization for Economic Cooperation and Development adopted data protection standards based directly on a code of fair information practices.

While there is no universally agreed-upon formulation of a code of fair information practices, nearly all codes include the same eight basic principles:

1. The principle of *openness*, which provides that the existence of record-keeping systems and data banks containing data about individuals be publicly known, along with a description of the main purposes and uses of the data.
2. The principle of *individual participation*, which provides that each individual should have a right to see any data about himself or herself and to correct or remove any data that is not timely, accurate, relevant, or complete.
3. The principle of *collection limitation*, which provides that there should be limits to the collection of personal data, that data should be collected by lawful and fair means, and that data should be collected, where appropriate, with the knowledge or consent of the subject.
4. The principle of *data quality*, which provides that personal data should be relevant to the purposes for which they are to be used and should be accurate, complete, and timely.
5. The principle of *use limitation*, which provides that there must be limits to the internal uses of personal data and that the data should be used only for the purposes specified at the time of collection.

6. The principle of *disclosure limitation*, which provides that personal data should not be communicated externally without the consent of the data subject or other legal authority.
7. The principle of *security*, which provides that personal data should be protected by reasonable security safeguards against such risks as loss and unauthorized access, destruction, use, modification, or disclosure. Sufficient resources should be available to offer reasonable assurances that security goals will be accomplished.
8. The principle of *accountability*, which provides that record keepers should be accountable for complying with fair information practices.

These principles can be applied to address the privacy concerns for any records containing personal information. The federal Privacy Act of 1974 represents a legislative implementation of the principles for personal records maintained by federal agencies. Fair information practices formed the basis for the Condit bill.

Comprehensive Protection for Health Information

The Condit legislation defined as *protected health information* any identifiable health information created or used during the health treatment or payment process. In general, the legislation did not distinguish between treatment and payment as sources of health information that required formal protection. This reflects a recognition of the growing interrelationship between the provision of care and the payment for that care. There is likely to be a considerable overlap between the content of treatment records and payment records. Both types are likely to be used in ways that directly affect the rights, benefits, and privileges of patients.

Another recognition of the interrelationship between treatment and payment was the decision to allow disclosure of health records to third-party payers without the express consent of the patient. Past health privacy laws have tended to rely on the principle of informed consent as a prerequisite to disclosure of patient information. Thus, disclosure to an insurance company would normally require the written approval of the patient.

Under the Condit legislation, disclosures for payment would have been one of several types to be permitted without the express consent of the patient. The legislation rejected the "fiction of informed consent" as the basis for disclosures for payment. By authorizing payment disclosures under the statutory scheme, the bill would have offered patients better protection for their information than was available through signing of blanket disclosure authorizations that are a common feature of the healthcare payment process. The legislation would have allowed patients who objected to routine payment disclosures to provide an alternative payment method and avoid the unwanted disclosure.

One of the most notable features of the Condit legislation was the attempt to apply rules for maintenance, use, and disclosure of health information to everyone who obtained the information that originated in the health treatment and payment process. The bill accomplished this by defining as a *health information trustee* virtually everyone who received protected health information under the proposed statutory disclosure scheme. This included healthcare providers, insurers, public health authorities, health researchers, government health oversight agencies, and health data base organizations. Even those who are not normally a direct part of the health treatment process but who obtain protected health information only occasionally would qualify as health information trustees. Thus, those who receive protected health information in emergencies, pursuant to court rules, during law enforcement investigations, or because of subpoenas and search warrants would still be health information trustees and would have obligations under the bill.

The goal was to allow access to those who require health information to carry out a socially acceptable function while imposing a duty upon them to protect the information as a condition of access. The fair information practice standards would apply to physicians, orderlies, clerks, computer operators, auditors, prosecutors, judges, and others who obtain protected health information in order to carry out a specific activity. This would plug a significant gap in all existing laws and ethical rules governing health information by making the scope of the fair information practice rules nearly universal. Under the proposed legislation, there would be no institutional loophole through which health information could routinely pass and lose its legal protection.

In general, trustees would be required to

- Limit disclosure of protected health information to the minimum necessary to accomplish the purpose
- Use protected health information only for a purpose that is compatible with and directly related to the purpose for which the information was collected or obtained by the trustee
- Maintain appropriate administrative, technical, and physical safeguards to protect the integrity and privacy of health information
- Disclose protected health information only for an authorized purpose
- Maintain an accounting of the date, nature, and purpose of any disclosure of protected health information

These requirements implement the basic principles of the code of fair information practices. In addition, trustees would be accountable for complying with the law. The bill proposed criminal penalties, civil remedies, and administrative enforcement to implement the principle of accountability. Trafficking in protected health information for monetary gain would have been punishable by ten years in prison and a large fine.

Individual rights were to vary slightly depending on which trustee maintained protected health information. For health information used in treatment, payment, or oversight, individuals would have the right to:

- Inspect and have a copy of their health information
- Seek correction of health information that is not timely, accurate, relevant, or complete
- Receive a notice explaining their rights and how their information may be used

The specific application of the fair information practice principles to different types of trustees was adapted to balance the interests of patients and cost, need, and practicality. For example, the obligation to provide the subject of a record with access to the record and with the ability to seek amendment of the record did not apply equally to all trustees. It was only applicable to those who were providers, payers, public health authorities, health oversight agencies, or health data base organizations. These are the main parties who make decisions that directly affect the healthcare, rights, and privileges of individuals. It would not be appropriate or necessary for those who use health information for other, more incidental purposes, to provide access or make decisions about requests for amendment.

Uniformity

Another important feature of the Condit bill was uniform application to nearly all healthcare records throughout the United States. With the interstate transfer of health information becoming commonplace, it has been impossible to determine what law is applicable to a given record at any time. It is not uncommon for an individual to have a doctor in one state, a pharmacist in another (by mail order), an employer in a third state, and an insurer located in yet another state. As records are transferred back and forth during routine treatment and payment activities, state lines are crossed frequently. Even if all of the states have relevant health confidentiality laws, it is not apparent at any given time which law applies to which information.

Support for a uniform federal law for health records was absent in 1980. At that time, much of the medical establishment preferred state legislation and opposed federal health privacy laws. As computers and computer networks became more routine, and as more intense use of health records became institutionalized, the need for uniformity was recognized. By 1994, support for the principle of a preemptive federal law was nearly universal.

One of the strongest proponents of uniform federal legislation was the Workgroup for Electronic Data Interchange (WEDI). EDI is a technology that permits the exchange of computer-processable data in a standard format between organizational entities or trading partners. EDI has obvious applications in the healthcare business, where the transfer of patient information between providers, payers, and others is essential. Adoption and implementation of EDI was estimated to result in billions of dollars in savings. WEDI recognized that lack of uniform confidentiality legislation was an impediment to increased use of EDI, and it recommended the passage of preemptive federal legislation.

One area where complete uniformity was found to create troublesome policy conflicts involved records of alcohol and drug abuse treatment. Most of these records are subject to existing federal laws offering protections that, in some cases, exceed those under the proposed Fair Health Information Practices Act. To avoid reducing the level of protection for these records from its current level, the Fair Health Information Practices Act would have allowed the Secretary of Health and Human Services and the Secretary of Veterans Affairs to apply only those provisions of the new law that afford greater protection for alcohol and drug abuse treatment records.

The immediate prospects for federal legislation establishing rules for the maintenance, use, and disclosure of health records are uncertain. The legislation that was considered during the 103d Congress is likely to provide a starting point for future efforts. The Condit bill was reintroduced in the 104th Congress (H.R. 435), and other bills are sure to be added. It is likely that there will be federal legislation someday, but it is impossible to predict when or what it will contain.

Current Environment and Emerging Trends with Computer-Based Patient Records

In 1991, the Institute of Medicine published a report, *The Computer-Based Patient Record: An Essential Technology for Health Care.* This report recommended the development of computer-based patient records and the formation of a nationwide health information network. The IOM report clearly identified that the practice of healthcare in this country is seriously hampered by the lack of tools to efficiently access and manage clinical information.

As healthcare reform is addressed at the federal and state level, it becomes increasingly clear that more complete and accurate information is needed for:

- More effective delivery of healthcare
- Improving the quality of care
- Evaluating the cost of healthcare and the administrative costs associated with it

- Supporting public health and research activities
- Improving the ability of consumers to make informed choices
- Managing and containing the cost of healthcare

To meet these information requirements, the nation must move toward a health information infrastructure which will support computer-based patient record systems that capture clinical information, integrate it with clinical decision support and knowledge bases, and make it available for all legitimate users.

The development of community health information networks (CHINs) is currently ongoing in a number of states. The American Hospital Association's recent publication *Community Health Information Networks* defines a CHIN as "an integrated collection of computer and telecommunications capabilities that facilitate communications of patient, clinical, and payment information among multiple providers, payers, employers, and related healthcare entities within a community."

CHINs are generally either centralized (relying on a centralized data repository) or distributed (relying on separate data systems that may be linked to create composite records). Some CHINs are focusing on administrative and financial transactions, while others are planning to capture patient information for clinical decision support. Since computer-based patient records will be a key component of CHINs, privacy and confidentiality issues are arising with the increasing implementation of CHINs.

It is critical that providers, vendors, and CHIN sponsors and developers realize that the current guidelines for disclosure of individually identifiable health information for health records must be implemented when information is released from a provider's patient records to a CHIN. Written authorization from the patient or the patient's legal representative must be obtained unless the disclosure is permitted under federal or state statute or regulation, subpoena or court order.

Legal Issues

The legal obligation of healthcare providers to maintain the confidentiality of health information derives from state licensure laws and regulations, specific statutes and regulations on health record confidentiality, Medicare's Conditions of Participation, standards of the Joint Commission on Accreditation of Healthcare Organizations(JCAHO), and court decisions.

Unfortunately, there is little uniformity among state licensure laws and regulations on the requirements for health records, and much confusion remains over whether patient records may be created and stored in a computer-based format. One source of the many stumbling blocks on the road to computer-based patient records is the myriad of often conflicting statutes and regulations regarding who may access patient data and how data may be accessed. Many states have statutes and regulations specifically dealing with confidentiality of patient records and/or patient access to health records. Some states have special rules associated with records relating to diagnosis and treatment for AIDS, mental health, and substance abuse. However, most states do not have a comprehensive statute that protects the confidentiality of all healthcare information. The current legal standard governing the use and disclosure of health information generally depends on the type of information collected, the individual or entity collecting the information, and whether the information is required for payment or oversight purposes.

Security Issues

The legal requirements for confidentiality are the same for paper records and computer-based records. Providers must obtain authorization from the patient or the patient's legal representative for any disclosures of health information unless authorized by federal or state statute or regulation, or pursuant to a court order. Additionally, the challenge facing healthcare providers to protect computer-based clinical information from unauthorized use requires the development of adequate security mechanisms and procedures.

Three primary aspects must be considered in computer security: confidentiality, integrity (that is, accuracy and authenticity), and availability. Thus a secure computer system

1. Does not permit unauthorized users access to information
2. Maintains the continuing integrity of data by preventing alteration or loss, verifies the source of data to assure its authenticity, and retains a record of communications to and from the system
3. Is available to users, and recovers completely, rapidly, and effectively from unanticipated disruptions (disasters)

Data security measures must be implemented to protect computer-based records from accidental or intentional disclosure, loss, or unauthorized access. The American Health Information Management Association, in its position paper "Confidentiality of the Computer-Based Patient Record," indicated that such data security measures must include:

- Physical controls over access to the system inputs and outputs, such as unique passwords, key cards with access codes, fingerprints, voiceprints, or retinal patterns for user identification; audit trails and automatic monitoring of electronic transactions; automatic log-off; and the use of locks and badges

- A security system that controls access by defining authorized users and defining data access on a need-to-know basis (this allows for additional privacy controls for psychiatric and other treatments specified as involving sensitive information)
- Twenty-four-hour-a-day user support
- Strictly enforced policies prohibiting sharing of passwords, key cards, and access codes
- System ability to recognize access beyond the usual course of business, along with audit trails and ongoing monitoring of who is accessing what information
- Vendor contracts that identify specific protections and date of implementation
- Documented maintenance requirements, procedures, and maintenance logs
- Backup systems such as an alternate power source and off-line storage
- Documented instructions to users describing data access procedures during scheduled and unscheduled downtime
- Documented disaster recovery procedures

Since computer-based patient record systems have the capability to collect and store extensive information, unauthorized access could result in the disclosure of information on more than one individual. The potential for harm is therefore magnified. For that reason, safeguards must be developed to protect the patient's privacy and to ensure the confidentiality of clinical information. Data integrity and system security must be addressed in the provider's information security program.

To ensure the highest level of security, the network should be designed to permit authorized users to access only those portions of the data base that are relevant to their particular function or job. For example, a billing clerk may need access to encoded diagnostic and procedural information to process claims but should not have unlimited access to the clinical data base.

The network should be designed to monitor all attempts to access patient records. Any attempt to obtain information beyond a user's security clearance should result in some form of "lockout," rendering the user incapable of accessing the system until readmitted by the system's security coordinator. The system should track access, and audit trails should be monitored on a regular basis. The system should call back remote users who are requesting dial-in access to record and monitor access.

All users should be required to sign statements acknowledging that clinical information is strictly confidential, and that passwords and access codes are for their individual use only. Policies and procedures to address data integrity and system security must be developed, published, and strictly enforced. Formal information security education programs should be established by each organization that handles health information. All users should be required to participate in these programs at the time of employment and on a continuing basis. When a user's employment or medical staff membership ends, access to the system should be terminated immediately.

Hospital systems must struggle to balance the need to protect the privacy of patient records with the need to allow ready access to records for authorized medical personnel. They face this challenge whether their systems are on paper or in computer data bases. A few of the hospitals with computerized patient records have begun to set audit trails for authorized personnel who access patient records. The degree of audit information is increased if the records being accessed contain highly sensitive information, as is the case with psychiatric substance abuse or AIDS patients. Some hospitals have intensified the audit information trail for these types of records by an automatic set of prompts that precede access to the file. The first prompt states it is a record deemed to contain highly sensitive information. It then asks the person why he or she is attempting to access the information. The answer, along with the person's name, is on record and available to a supervisor and to the patient's physician.

Since networks permit access from multiple users and remote locations over public channels of communication, including telephone lines and radio waves, network security mechanisms should also include the use of encryption. Any patient information that is transmitted over networks must be encrypted to protect unauthorized access or alteration of data.

Recent reports in the media highlight concerns regarding computerization of psychiatric records. A health maintenance organization in New England was criticized for its policy of incorporating detailed psychiatric notes about patients into computerized medical records that are available to many physicians and staff members. The information included not only mental health diagnoses but also the notes of individual psychiatric sessions. As a result of public concern, the HMO is reconsidering how much personal information is placed in computerized records, and whether additional safeguards are needed to restrict computer access to sensitive medical data.

Concerns have also been raised regarding the practices of managed care companies that may breach confidentiality laws. Some plans require subscribers to call an 800 number and provide detailed personal information to an anonymous reviewer before receiving mental health benefits. While confidential information is required for treatment or payment and is protected under the law, it is not clear whether information to facilitate such initial referrals before treatment has formally begun is protected.

Organizational Issues

It is a generally accepted principle that the primary patient record is maintained and owned by the healthcare institution or practitioner providing care. This principle is established by statutes and licensing regulations in many states, which grant the provider control over the physical document but give the patient ownership-type rights to the information contained in the record. Therefore, the patient generally has control over the release of individually identifiable information, except in circumstances identified by case law, by federal or state statutes and regulations, and by provider policy. Once patient information has been released by a provider to an authorized requestor, the "ownership" of the information becomes less clear.

Policies and Procedures

A provider must develop policies and procedures regarding disclosure of health information. Employees responsible for information disclosure must be carefully trained and supervised to ensure their consistent compliance with the provider's policies and procedures for disclosure.

Any disclosure to external requesters should be accompanied by a statement prohibiting use of the information for other than the stated purpose and requiring destruction of the information after the stated need has been fulfilled.

In its 1993 position paper on disclosure, the American Health Information Management Association classified health information as

- *Nonconfidential information,* that which is generally common knowledge, and is unaccompanied by a specific request from the patient to restrict disclosure. As examples, nonconfidential information for medical services outside of behavioral healthcare may include

  Name of the patient
  Verification of hospitalization or outpatient services
  Dates patient received services

Each provider should develop policies and procedures about whether and under what circumstances to disclose this information, taking into consideration its patient population and state laws. For example, it is usually considered inappropriate and professionally unethical to disclose any information relating to patients undergoing psychiatric treatment, an abortion, or treatment for HIV/AIDS.

Healthcare providers have no obligation to disclose even nonconfidential information. If the treatment organization's policy permits, it may be disclosed to legitimate requesters on a "need to know" basis without the patient's authorization unless otherwise requested by the patient or the patient's legal representative, or prohibited by law.

- *Confidential information,* that which is made available during the course of a confidential relationship between the patient and healthcare professionals. Confidential information includes, but is not limited to, all clinical data and the patient's address on discharge.

This information may be disclosed only upon written authorization by the patient or the patient's legal representative, or where such disclosure is required by federal or state law, subpoena, or court order.

The American Health Information Management Association has made recommendations on the minimum requirements for an acceptable authorization for disclosure of health information.

An acceptable authorization must

- Be in writing or given via computer (facsimiles or copies may be accepted if allowed by the provider's policy).
- Be addressed to the healthcare provider.
- Specifically identify the patient (this generally includes the patient's full name, address, and date of birth).
- Identify the individual or entity authorized to receive the information.
- Identify the health information authorized for disclosure.
- Specify the reasons or purpose for the disclosure.
- Specify the date, event, or condition upon which authorization will expire unless revoked earlier.
- Indicate that the authorization is subject to revocation by the patient or the patient's legal representative.
- Be signed or authenticated by the patient or the patient's legal representative. (If authorization is given by someone other than the patient, that individual must indicate his or her relationship to the patient.)
- Be dated sometime following the patient's admission or outpatient encounter. Unless otherwise provided by state law, no more than six months should elapse between the date of signature on the authorization and the date the information is requested. (Note: Some states may require a shorter time period for which authorizations remain valid.)

The signed authorization from the patient or the patient's legal representative should be maintained with the patient's paper health record, along with a notation of the information disclosed and date of disclosure. If the record is computer-based, consideration must be given to other mechanisms for maintaining these authorizations.

The patient or the patient's legal representative has the right to revoke authorization to disclose information at any time. Revocation should be issued in the same manner in which authorization for disclosure was made. For written authorization, revocation of authorization should be submitted in writing to the healthcare provider and should be maintained with the patient's health record. If the patient or legal representative is unable to provide revocation in writing, an oral revocation may be accepted and should be documented by the person accepting the revocation. If authorization was given via computer, it may be revoked in the same manner. Revocation of authorization does not affect any health information disclosed prior to the provider's receipt of notice of revocation or any disclosure made for the purpose of obtaining payment for services provided in reliance on the authorization.

Most states allow a patient or the patient's legal representative to examine and obtain copies of the patient's hospital records, although some states grant patients the right to review their hospital records only after discharge. Rights of access to health records maintained by physicians and other individual healthcare providers are less clear.

Many states allow providers to refuse to grant patients access to psychiatric records, if the provider believes disclosure could be detrimental to the patient or if a third party could be endangered by the disclosure. However, in these states, the provider may be required to provide copies of the record to the patient's legal representative or attorney.

Unless otherwise prohibited by state law, the patient or the patient's legal representative should have access to health information. The provider should develop policies and procedures regarding inspection of records by patients and requests for correction and amendment.

If the patient or the patient's legal representative disputes information documented in the record, this should be discussed with the healthcare practitioner who made the entry in question. If the practitioner agrees that the entry contains an error, the practitioner should make the correcting entry in the patient's record. On paper records, the individual making the correction should draw a single line through the error, record the correct data, and then sign and date the corrected entry. The original entry must not be obliterated. When an error is corrected in a computer-based record, the system should preserve both the original entry and the amendment, as well as identify the person making the amendment. If the healthcare practitioner does not agree that a correction is warranted, this should be discussed with the patient or the patient's legal representative. The patient or the patient's legal representative may make a separate statement in writing or on computer disputing the information and offering an amendment. Such statement should be filed with or made part of the record and included with any future disclosure.

Employee Training

While issues related to the privacy, confidentiality, and security of health information are not new, organizations that handle health information are acknowledging the importance of formal training programs. Employees must understand the value of the health information that they handle. Programs should be designed to address these issues during orientation, at the time of employment, and on a continuing basis.

There are a number of issues that must be addressed in the organization's policies and procedures and training programs:

- What preemployment screening processes, if any, are used to screen potential employees who might have access to patient records or health information?
- What employee training programs are in place for raising the issues of confidentiality of health information?
- Do employees sign a confidentiality agreement at the time of employment? Is a confidentiality acknowledgement signed annually thereafter?
- Do employees understand their responsibilities for respecting patients' privacy and protecting the confidentiality of their health information?
- Does the facility have written policies and procedures outlining who may access patient information?
- What mechanisms are in place to control access to either paper or computer-based patient records?
- Is there a policy prohibiting the disclosure or sharing of passwords, access codes, key cards, or other user identifiers? Are these policies strictly enforced?
- Is the access of each employee restricted to the health information related to the employee's functions?
- When an employee or physician leaves the organization, are the password and access codes deactivated immediately?
- Is there a mechanism in place to track access to records by each employee so as to discourage unauthorized viewing?
- Are periodic audits performed to see if the organization's policies are being followed by employees and if they are still effective?

Contractual Issues

An organization must address access to health information by contractors and vendors. It is important to ascertain if the organization uses contractors or vendors to provide services that involve handling health information (such as correspondence management, transcription, storage and retrieval, microfilming, or information system support). These contractors or vendors must have policies and procedures regarding confidentiality and training programs for their employees and agents. Copies of these policies and procedures along with documentation of training should be provided to the organization.

Any contracts that are drafted should address the question of whether the organization has binding contracts with all third parties having access to its patient records, specifically, whether the contracts provide that the third party will:

- Keep the information in strict confidence
- Use the information only for the purpose of providing services under the contract
- Disclose the information only to those of the third party's employees who (1) need access to the information in order to provide services under the contract and (2) have signed a confidentiality agreement requiring the employees to hold the information in confidence
- Return the information in usable form upon request or at the end of the contract
- Indemnify the provider for all breaches of these obligations

Agreements between providers, vendors, and network developers and sponsors should be carefully drafted with the assistance of legal counsel and must include provisions to protect patient information against theft, loss, unauthorized destruction, or other unauthorized access.

◆ ◆ ◆

It has been recognized that there is a need for federal preemptive legislation to provide for more uniformity among the fifty states. The emergence of multistate providers and payers and the development of health information networks highlight the need for uniform national standards governing the use and disclosure of health information.

While it is unclear what approach Congress will take in addressing this issue, it is clear that the legal infrastructure is not keeping pace with information technology. In such an environment, the degree of privacy afforded individually iden-

tifiable health information depends especially on the practices of the individuals
and organizations who handle the information.

Notes

P. 191, *account records about an individual from a bank:* United States v. Miller, 425 U.S. 435 (1976).

P. 192, *limited legal privacy protection:* 18 U.S.C. §2710 (1988).

P. 192, *cable television viewing records:* 47 U.S.C. §551 (1988).

P. 192, *bank records:* 12 U.S.C. §3401–3421 (1988).

P. 192, *electronic mail:* 18 U.S.C. §§2701–2710 (1988).

P. 192, *Whalen v. Roe:* 429 U.S. 589 (1977).

P. 192, *Privacy Act of 1974:* 5 U.S.C. §552a (1988).

P. 192, *treatment for alcohol or drug abuse:* See 42 U.S.C. §§290dd-3; 38 U.S.C. §7332 (1988).

P. 193, *other routine recipients:* Gellman, R. (1984). Prescribing privacy: The uncertain role of the physician in the protection of patient privacy. *North Carolina Law Review, 62,* p. 261.

P. 193, *other common uses:* Gellman, R. (1984). Prescribing privacy: The uncertain role of the physician in the protection of patient privacy. *North Carolina Law Review, 62,* p. 261.

P. 193, *in a paper or computerized environment:* Office of Technology Assessment. (1993). *Protecting privacy in computerized medical information* (S/N 052–003–01345–2). Washington, DC: U.S. Government Printing Office.

P. 194, *little real protection against redisclosure:* Institute of Medicine. (1994). *Health data in the information age: Use, disclosure, and privacy.* Washington, DC: National Academy Press.

P. 195, *fifteen million individuals:* U.S. Congress. House. (1994). *Health Security Act:* Report 103–601, Part 5. 103d Congress, 2d Session.

P. 195, *users of improperly obtained information:* Canada. *Report of the Commission of Inquiry into the Confidentiality of Health Information in Ontario* (1980). Toronto, Ontario.

P. 196, *national healthcare reform:* Louis Harris & Associates. (1993). *Health information privacy survey.* New York: Author.

P. 196, *obtaining better data for medical research:* U.S. Congress. House. (1994). *Health reform, health records, computers, and confidentiality.* Hearings before the House Subcommittee on Information, Justice, Transportation, and Agriculture. Testimony of Dr. Alan Westin, Professor of Public Law and Government, Columbia University. 103d Congress, 1st Session.

P. 197, *Federal Privacy of Medical Information Act:* U.S. Congress. House. (1980). *H.R. 5935.* 96th Congress, 2d Session.

P. 197, *change in title "bears some significance":* U.S. Congress. House. (1994). *Health Security Act: Report no. 13–601, Part 5.* 103d Congress, 2d Session.

P. 197, *federal Department of Health, Education, and Welfare:* Department of Health, Education, & Welfare, Secretary's Advisory Committee. (1973). *Automated Personal Data Systems, Records, Computers, and the Rights of Citizens* (GPO 1700–00116). Washington, DC: Author.

P. 197, *the same eight basic principles:* Bennett, C. J. (1992). *Regulating privacy: Data protection and public policy in Europe and the United States.* (p. 99). Ithaca, NY: Cornell University Press.

P. 198, *complying with fair information practices:* U.S. Congress. House. (1994). *Health Security Act: Report no. 103–601, Part 5.* 103d Congress, 2d Session.

P. 198, *basis for disclosures for payment:* U.S. Congress. House. (1994). *Health Security Act: Report no. 103–601, Part 5.* 103d Congress, 2d Session.

P. 201, *passage of preemptive federal legislation:* Workgroup for Electronic Data Interchange. (1992, July). *Report to the Secretary of U.S. Department of Health and Human Services.* Published by author.

P. 201, *The Computer-Based Patient Record:* Dick, R. S., & Steen, E. B. (Eds.). (1991). *The Computer-based patient record: An essential technology for health care.* Institute of Medicine of the National Academy of Sciences. Washington, DC: National Academy Press.

P. 202, *"related healthcare entities within a community":* American Hospital Association. (1994). *Community health information networks: Creating the health care data highway.* Chicago: Author.

P. 203, *"Confidentiality of the Computer-Based Patient Record":* American Health Information Management Association. (1992, July). *Confidentiality of the computer-based patient record* (position statement). Chicago, IL: Author.

P. 206, *1993 position paper on disclosure:* American Health Information Management Association. (1993, December). *Disclosure of Health Information.* Chicago, IL: Author.

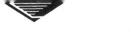

CHAPTER ELEVEN

THE RAPID GROWTH OF ELECTRONIC COMMUNICATION

Michael W. Hurst and William A. Roiter

For the behavioral healthcare industry in the 1990s and into the twenty-first century, technology and computerization will increasingly enable an enterprise that is fundamentally one human being helping another. Some readers may respond to this statement with a resounding (but, we think, ever decreasing) cry of "Heresy!" The authors, as practicing psychologists for fifteen years, managed care company executives, and behavioral healthcare communications advocates, would say that you may want to read on.

As of 1994, almost 60 percent of Americans with health insurance were covered by a managed behavioral healthcare program. Increasingly, states are applying for Health Care Financing Administration (HCFA) exemptions to allow their Medicaid programs to use managed care plan designs rather than strictly fee-for-service designs, and courts are allowing states to apply financial incentives to encourage Medicare participants to choose managed care programs. By the year 2000, it is extremely likely that over 90 percent of Americans covered by health insurance will have some form of managed behavioral healthcare.

The management of healthcare, including behavioral health, is predicated on the notion that "managed" care is as cost-effective as nonmanaged care or more so. A few studies have purported to confirm this belief. Even so, cost-effectiveness is a tricky notion in healthcare, for a multitude of reasons.

In the 1980s, when behavioral healthcare was maturing from a very rough beginning, the focus clearly was on managing costs, not care. But as the 1990s began to unfold, it was just as clear that the focus had become binocular; one had to simultaneously manage the cost as well as the quality of care.

The Increasing Role of Communications

Managing cost was originally a series of administrative steps. One of the first steps was contracting with providers (from practitioners up through hospital chains) for discounted rate structures in exchange for referrals. Another step was precertification, or making sure that a patient was eligible for treatment and that the intended treatment was approved. A third was utilization review, which is really a concurrent form of certification. In other words, a variety of steps evolved to administer the entire patient treatment cycle. These steps were designed to ensure that patients were eligible, that treatments were approved approaches rendered by approved providers, and that neither overtreatment nor undertreatment took place. Stated another way, a vast array of communications became necessary between providers, care managers, and payers.

The challenge for managing care has shifted emphasis from the "cost" to the "effectiveness" side of "cost-effectiveness." What is commonly meant by *effective* is that a process (for example, a treatment in healthcare) acts in the intended way with the intended results as a consequence of its application. The current term for the assessment of effectiveness is "outcomes."

Communications Increased by Outcomes Measurement Requirements

The assessment of outcomes can be systemic, as in the "report cards" of index statistics for large healthcare institutions, or it can be patient-centered, in terms of the patient's satisfaction with care. It can be disease-centered in terms of ameliorating a depression, eating disorder, psychosis, or whatever. It can be symptom-centered in terms of frequency, severity, and endurance of symptomatology. And so on.

The basic effectiveness question is, "What happened as a consequence of the treatment?" Corollary questions are: "Was what happened what we expected and wanted to happen for the resources that were used?" "Are there better outcomes that can be derived for the same expenditures of resources?"

The outcome question imposes further communications requirements between the manager/payers and the providers of care. As noted earlier in this chapter, years ago the managed care industry began simply, with such communications as a precertification call, a utilization review call or form, and a claim. It then evolved to include an eligibility inquiry and response; referral call and acceptance; evaluation report(s) and treatment authorization; clinical update and authorization; claim and claim remittance advice to the provider, reporting the status of the claim along with an explanation of benefits (EOB) to the provider and the patient; and finally an outcome report. In an effort to reduce the overwhelming overhead this sequence has imposed on all sides, there is an increasing movement toward capitating the provider.

The Effect of Capitation on Communications

Provider capitation means that the provider has taken the responsibility for the previously managed elements of treatment plan and authorization, update and reauthorization, and claims (none) with a patient-only EOB. The manager/payer provides some kind of host system for eligibility verification (typically telephonic but perhaps using a healthcare information network of some kind); most importantly, the manager/payer also takes on the role of auditor of outcomes. In other words, the provider takes the risk of providing cost-efficient care within the capitated fee for an entity (defined geographically or by business unit).

The behavioral healthcare industry may be moving away from more frequent, shorter communications required by the "inspection model" managed care systems to fewer but much longer communications that include much of the previously required information and probably more. The new communications require more analysis and are far more central to the viability of the provider's continued business as a capitated vendor. The manager/payer cannot tolerate the risk of accepting providers whose clinical practices jeopardize the manager/payer's business viability. Whether their providers are capitated or not, the managed care company is still answerable to their buyer of coverage: the employer, the healthcare buying group, or the government agency.

Hence as (not if, in our opinion) point-of-service network companies continue the march toward provider capitation with a mixed exclusive-and-contracted-provider network, and as (again, not if, in our opinion) the former brick-and-mortar staff model health maintenance organizations (HMOs) move toward point-of-service networks surrounding hospital or clinic or neighborhood delivery points, there is an ever-intensifying need for communications.

Ongoing Communications Required

As these structural delivery models change, the burgeoning communications requirements do not go away. The big questions will be "What kind of communications?" "What kind of information?" "Using what kind of media?" The questions really are not whether but how we communicate, what kind of communications we need, and the media in which we communicate to meet the binocular focus of the emerging managed behavioral healthcare system. Close communications between geographically dispersed providers and managers will be the key to cooperation in the service of better patient care.

The questions regarding communications are far less trivial than they may appear. Perhaps surprisingly to many in behavioral healthcare, they have been addressed and answered in many other industries. In addition, the healthcare industry as a whole, and behavioral healthcare as a specialty, imposes a number of special conditions on the variety of information, the confidentiality of information, and the basic type of information (numerical data versus character text) that is necessary to be shared among parties.

Cost Analysis of Communications in Managed Behavioral Healthcare

Table 11.1 presents the personnel data and communication transactions we used to evaluate the cost of behavioral healthcare communications using paper forms, telephone, and the U.S. Postal Service. We do not claim that all cases or all systems use each of these communication transaction sets; some require more and some require fewer. And some managed care organizations (MCOs) use the telephone (including fax) exclusively or the post office exclusively for communications. But at least we can look at the nonelectronic process and both the time and hidden costs that are involved.

The breakdown shown in Table 11.1 assumes that the practitioner is paid $60,000 per year, a conservative figure but perhaps a reasonable average given the mix of counselors, social workers, psychologists, and psychiatrists in various for-profit and nonprofit settings. We assume the use of a practice administrator (administrative assistant, secretary plus billing clerk, or otherwise) who is paid $30,000 per year. If the provider does not use an administrator, then the combined cost of the person(s) accomplishing the tasks can be substituted.

To estimate the fringe benefits, we used the common figure of 33 percent of salary (Social Security; federal unemployment; state unemployment, Massachusetts in this case, and Medicaid taxes).

Table 11.1 further displays the communication transaction sets that we use. The typical eight-session outpatient behavioral health case involves eight communications and one payment, with the total generally ranging from a minimum of three up to fourteen communications between the provider and the MCO. We assumed that the basic communications included the MCO making a treatment referral ("Tx Referral") to a provider; the provider requesting eligibility confirmation from the MCO; the provider sending a treatment plan ("Tx Plan") to

TABLE 11.1. COST OF FTES INVOLVED IN COMMUNICATIONS FOR ONE EIGHT-SESSION OUTPATIENT CASE

	Salary/year	33 percent benefits/year	Cost/minute
Provider	$60,000	$19,800	$0.67
Case manager	$48,000	$15,840	$0.53
Data entry	$22,000	$7,260	$0.24
Mail room	$15,000	$4,950	$0.17
Provider administrator	$30,000	$9,900	$0.33
MCO administration	$40,000	$13,200	$0.44

Example Communication Transactions to Support One Eight-Session Outpatient Case

Tx referral	Referral of a new patient to a provider from an MCO
Eligibility request	Provider requests patient's eligibility for claims payment prior to service delivery
Tx plan	Treatment plan produced by the provider and sent to the MCO for approval
Tx authorization	Approval of provider's treatment plan sent to the provider by the MCO
Tx questions	Case manager questions regarding the treatment plan
20 percent Tx returns	20 percent of treatment plans rejected, requiring an additional treatment plan
2 claims	2 claims sent by the provider to the managed care company
20 percent claims returned	At least 20 percent of claims returned for errors or omissions
Payment	1 check mailed to the provider for professional services

the MCO; the MCO sending a treatment authorization ("Tx Authorization") to the provider; the MCO case manager calling the provider ("Tx Questions") about some of the received treatment plans; the MCO returning 20 percent of the plans ("Tx Returns") to the provider because they are deemed insufficient, unreadable, or incomplete; the provider submitting two claims ("Two Claims") to the MCO/payer with 20 percent being rejected or pended with questions ("20 percent Claims Return") by the MCO/payer; and finally the MCO making a claim payment ("Payment") for all approved claims.

Table 11.1 provides the basic data and tasks for which we have calculated the time costs that are then used in Tables 11.2 and 11.3 for calculating the costs of communications in a typical eight-session outpatient case.

In Table 11.2 we made other assumptions based on our experience. It was assumed that the telephone charges totaled $1.00 per transaction type and were paid by the MCO. That is, all of the calls used to obtain an eligibility were assumed to total $1.00, even though we have found that it typically takes three chargeable calls

TABLE 11.2. CURRENT MCO AND PROVIDER COSTS

	$/minute	Minutes	Time Cost	Postage	Phone Charges	Materials	Total
TX referral							
Case manager	$0.53	3	$1.60	$	$	$0.20	$1.80
Mail room	$0.17	5	$0.83	$0.32	$	$0.05	$1.20
Provider administration	$0.33	5	$1.66	$	$	$0.05	$1.71
Eligibility request							
Provider administration	$0.33	15	$4.99	$	$	$	$4.99
MCO administration	$0.44	4	$1.77	$	$1.00	$	$2.77
Tx plan							
Provider	$0.67	15	$9.98	$	$	$	$9.98
Provider administration	$0.33	5	$1.66	$0.32	$	$0.15	$2.13
Mail room	$0.17	5	$0.83	$	$	$0.30	$1.13
Data entry	$0.24	7	$1.71	$	$	$	$1.71
Tx authorization							
Case manager	$0.53	5	$2.66	$	$	$0.10	$2.76
Mail room	$0.17	5	$0.83	$0.32	$	$0.05	$1.20
Provider administration	$0.33	10	$3.33	$	$	$0.05	$3.38
25 percent Tx questions							
Case manager	$0.53	10	$5.32	$	$1.00	$	$1.58
Provider	$0.67	20	$13.30	$	$	$	$3.33
20 percent Tx returns							
Case manager	$0.53	5	$2.66	$	$	$0.10	$0.55
Mail room	$0.17	8	$1.33	$0.32	$	$0.05	$0.34
Provider administration	$0.33	10	$3.33	$	$	$0.05	$0.68
2 claims							
Provider	$0.67	2	$1.33	$	$	$0.05	$1.38
Provider administration	$0.33	5	$1.66	$0.32	$	$	$1.98
Mail room	$0.17	5	$0.83	$	$	$	$0.83
Data entry	$0.24	5	$1.22	$	$	$	$1.22
20 percent claims return							
Provider administration	$0.33	15	$4.99	$0.32	$	$	$5.31
Mail room	$0.17	5	$0.83	$	$	$	$0.83
Data entry	$0.24	10	$2.44	$	$	$	$2.44
Payment							
Data entry	$0.24	5	$1.22	$	$	$	$1.22
Mail room	$0.17	5	$0.83	$0.32	$	$0.20	$1.35
Provider administration	$0.33	5	$1.66	$	$	$	$1.66
Totals		199		$2.24	$2.00	$1.40	$59.45
Total provider cost							$36.52
Total MCO cost							$22.93

to get through and actually make the eligibility request. On the other hand, we assumed the MCO provided a toll-free 800 number by which to make the telephone calls and for which we assumed they received a volume discount on their rates.

Table 11.2 provides the task, time, and cost breakdown for each element in the communications process between the provider and the MCO. The time estimates of the transaction elements are based on data gathered by the authors. Both of us are psychologists who were together in a group private practice for more than ten years and also were vice presidents of a large national managed care company; additionally, our current positions have provided us with the opportunity to analyze the work and communications flow of more than ten managed care companies and dozens of provider organizations.

The "Totals" line of Table 11.2 reveals that a typical eight-session course of outpatient treatment requires 199 minutes of communications time on the parts of the provider and MCO. After accounting for the percentage of cases requiring some but not all of the activities, the total cost of this time plus postage, telephone, and materials comes to $59.45.

At the bottom of Table 11.2 are two lines which break out the communications cost for the provider and the MCO. Remember here that we have assumed a group-practice type of provider with a practice administrator and all of the communications done by telephone or postal service. A solo provider might actually have at least the equivalent cost (a solo practitioner might average $90,000 net per year—the sum of practitioner and administrator salaries), and all the time would be added to the usual workday, making for fifty-hour workweeks, for example.

A provider's total cost for communications using paper forms, telephone, and postal service is estimated here as $36.52 for an eight-session outpatient treatment course. The MCO's total cost is about $22.93 for the same patient's treatment. If we use $80 as an average per-session reimbursement, then the provider received $640. Thus, for the provider, the communications costs represented $36.52 divided by $640, or 5.7 percent of the gross receipt.

Table 11.3 recomputes the cost of the exact same set of communication transactions, but now using an electronic messaging system. Such systems pass messages through a hub rather than providing a direct connection between provider and MCO. For example, a provider prepares messages off-line using electronic forms software. The communications software module then uploads messages to the hub for delivery to the MCO and both picks up and downloads messages from the MCO to the provider. We have used currently standard retail transaction rates in Table 11.3 in place of telephone costs. Some messaging systems provide a free 800 number for sending messages and charge according to the type or length of message. Other messaging systems have local access numbers but charge for the time connected. Inevitably, the sender pays, and that transaction fee is reflected in Table 11.3.

TABLE 11.3. MCO AND PROVIDER COSTS USING ELECTRONIC MESSAGING SYSTEM

	$/Minute	Minutes	Time Costs	Transaction Charge	Phone Charges	Materials	Total Cost
Tx Referral							
Case Manager	$0.53	3	$1.60	$0.59	$	$	$2.19
Mail Room	$0.17	0	$0.00	$	$	$	$0.00
Provider Administration	$0.33	2	$0.67	$	$	$	$0.67
Eligibility Request							
Provider Administration	$0.33	2	$0.67	$0.59	$	$	$1.26
MCO Administration	$0.44	0	$0.00	$0.89	$	$	$0.89
Tx Plan							
Provider	$0.67	10	$6.65	$0.89	$	$	$7.54
Provider Administration	$0.33	0	$0.00	$	$	$	$0.00
Mail Room	$0.17	0	$0.00	$	$	$	$0.00
Data Entry	$0.24	0	$0.00	$	$	$	$0.00
Tx Authorization							
Case Manager	$0.53	2	$1.06	$0.59	$	$	$1.65
Mail Room	$0.17	0	$0.00	$	$	$	$0.00
Provider Administration	$0.33	2	$0.67	$	$	$	$0.67
25 Percent Tx Questions							
Case Manager	$0.53	5	$2.66	$0.59	$	$	$0.81
Provider	$0.67	10	$6.65	$0.59		$	$1.81
20 Percent Tx Returns							
Case Manager	$0.53	0	$0.00	$	$	$	$0.00
Mail Room	$0.17	0	$0.00	$	$	$	$0.00
Provider Administration	$0.33	0	$0.00	$	$	$	$0.00
2 Claims							
Provider	$0.67	2	$1.33	$0.98	$	$	$2.31
Provider Administration	$0.33	2	$0.67	$	$	$	$0.67
Mail Room	$0.17	0	$0.00	$	$	$	$0.00
Data Entry	$0.24	0	$0.00	$	$	$	$0.00
20 Percent Claims Return							
Provider	$0.67	0	$0.00	$	$	$	$0.00
Provider Administration	$0.33	0	$0.00	$	$	$	$0.00
Mail Room	$0.17	0	$0.00	$	$	$	$0.00
Data Entry	$0.24	0	$0.00	$	$	$	$0.00
Payment							
Data Entry	$0.24	5	$1.22	$0.49	$	$	$1.71
Mail Room	$0.17	0	$0.00	$	$	$	$0.00
Provider Administration	$0.33	2	$0.67	$	$	$	$0.67
Totals		68		$5.32	$	$	$22.83
Total Provider Cost							$15.58
Total MCO Cost							$7.25

In Table 11.3 you can see that we did not project costs associated with treatment plans or claims being returned. Messaging systems that use "smart" electronic forms have internal logic for error detection, missing data, and inconsistent data, so that customers are extremely unlikely to have either treatment plans or claims returned for errors of these kinds.

You might also note that a number of the transactions take less personnel time electronically than manually, and therefore there is a reduced time cost. The difference stems from the fact that one never gets a busy signal nor is never put on hold, and the time required is purely the message preparation time since the software automatically handles the actual dial-up, transmission, and reception duties that a person literally has to do manually.

The impact of the time savings is seen in the "Totals" row near the bottom of Table 11.3. Here you can see a total time of 68 minutes, compared to 199 minutes using the telephone and postal service. Clearly one spends less time simply doing the task with the electronic methodology.

The bottom two lines of Table 11.3 show a provider cost of $15.58 and an MCO cost of $7.25 using an electronic messaging system in place of paper, telephones, and postal service. The provider's cost of communications now accounts for $15.58 divided by $640, or 2.4 percent of revenues.

Two conclusions are apparent. First, the cost of electronic communications for a typical eight-session outpatient treatment course is much lower at $22.83 compared to $59.45 (a total savings of 62 percent). Second, the biggest savings is attributable to the MCO (68 percent) rather than the provider (57 percent). In either case, however, the savings is substantial.

Because of the time and costs currently involved in such communications being done with standard manual systems, two trends have developed.

One trend has been to reduce the number of communications required to manage and treat a patient's behavioral health needs. Some MCOs have gone so far as to reduce the collection of clinical information by allowing a provider an "eight session pass-through," which refers to giving the provider up to eight sessions before clinical information must be reported and reviewed. The thinking behind this pass-through is based on the notion, but without carefully evaluated data, that most cases are either resolved within three sessions or require ten sessions or more.

While this pass-through can reduce the paperwork load, it also reduces the data available to evaluate treatment effectiveness. Providers and MCOs alike have no way of knowing what kind of treatment is effective or ineffective with various problems when there is no initial or continued evaluation. The initial evaluation data can be the basis for retrospective and concurrent outcomes analysis. These outcomes data are gaining importance in the minds of employers and their benefits consultants as the industry moves financial risk from the MCO to the provider.

The second trend has been to develop more cost-effective communications. Clearly, we would advocate reducing the cost of communications by going electronic rather than reducing the communication of clinically important information. It is clear that electronic communications have their time and cost advantages. But what does it mean to have "electronic communications," and what does it cost to put it in place?

Two Main Types of Electronic Communications

Currently, in mid 1995, there are two main types of electronic communications that you may have heard or read about. The most common is electronic data interchange.

Electronic Data Interchange (EDI)

EDI generally applies to completely standardized interchanges of data between all participating members of the same industry. That is, all senders and receivers participating in the standard setting agree on exactly the same set of data, data types and definitions, and file record layouts ("data sets"), to transmit from one side that will be received by the other side and vice versa.

The American National Standards Institute (ANSI), a nongovernmental organization, agreed to sponsor committees to establish the transmitter and receiver data sets to which participants would mutually adhere. In the general EDI scheme of things, the ANSI "X12.aaa" series of standards apply to the agreed-upon data sets. For example, ANSI X12.837 applies to medical claims and ANSI X12.835 applies to claims remittance advice.

Even with this standard-setting organization, however, there are several interesting drawbacks to notice. First, ANSI is *a nongovernmental organization;* that is, it has no statutory enforcement or promulgation powers. Second, the participants agree to mutually adhere to the standards if they claim to use them; that is, they do not have to and they might change particular requirements on their own.

Quasi-agreement between so many parties—six years to agree on claims in the medical arena—is extremely difficult, but possible, to achieve. It also took three years to agree on the much simpler eligibility request/response transactions set (ANSI X12.270/271). Quite simply, it would be a revolution for competitors in an information-based industry such as ours to say that certain data is no longer proprietary, nor provides any proprietary advantage.

Transaction partners adhering to the agreements could theoretically communicate data at extremely high speeds with virtually no transmission errors. Compared to handwriting, typing, or word processing followed by U.S. Postal Service conveyance, electronic transactions are incredibly more efficacious *once they are established*. Getting them established can be both expensive and time-consuming.

EDI offers extremely fast, robust, and documented transactions. There absolutely is no comparison to the speed and documentation with which transactions are accomplished: seconds instead of days, with everything documented and without the "return receipt requested" or "certified" postal service transactions that can be signed or acknowledged by any party at the receiving site. In "true" EDI, all transactions are fully documented for both the sender and the receiver.

Electronic Commerce (EC)

In contrast to EDI as it is usually defined, EC applies to standardized transaction sets (forms) agreed upon by business partners. That is, only the business partners, not everyone participating in an industry or standard-setting committee, need to agree on the standardization.

EC communications include EDI, facsimile, telex, electronic mail, electronic forms, and file transfers of virtually all types (graphic images, for example, or entire data bases). In contrast to traditional EDI per se, which is a subset of EC, electronic commerce operates under a variety of transmission protocols; the communicating business partners have to agree on what those are in order to actually communicate.

Also unlike EDI, there are a variety of EC value-added vendors who act as an integrated source of software, networks, applications, information data bases, and so forth, to be used by subscribers to the vendor's services. For example, CompuServe, Prodigy, America Online, Microsoft, and AT&T are all vendors of this type. Other companies serve specialty markets: Physician Computer Network (PCN) and Physician's On-Line (POL) specifically address medical doctors, whereas InStream Corp. has the InStream Provider Network (IPN) specialized for the behavioral healthcare market.

Table 11.4 compares EDI and EC features, while Table 11.5 evaluates the cost and ease of implementation of either type of electronic communication system.

The Cost-Benefit of Electronic Communications for Providers

It should be obvious that we would recommend an EC solution rather than a traditional EDI solution for putting electronic communications in the provider site. As of 1995, the cost of implementing electronic communications varies according to the flexibility, investment, and return on investment (ROI) that you are seeking.

TABLE 11.4. COMPARISON OF FEATURES OF ELECTRONIC DATA INTERCHANGE (EDI) AND ELECTRONIC COMMERCE (EC)

EDI	EC
Standardized industrywide forms	Standardized by business partner
Centralized solutions	Decentralized solutions
Predefined EDI-datafiles only	EDI files, facsimile files, electronic formfiles or multimedia files
Long-term, worldwide standards will be universally cheapest	Short and moderate term transition

TABLE 11.5. COST AND EASE OF IMPLEMENTATION OF ELECTRONIC DATA INTERCHANGE (EDI) AND ELECTRONIC COMMERCE (EC)

EDI	EC
Time to implement—long: 1–3 years	Time to implement—low: 1–3 months
Initial (1–3 year) cost—high	Initial cost (1–3 years)—low
Long-term (3+ years) cost—low	Long-term (3+ years) cost—moderate
Flexibility—low	Flexibility—high
Maintenance—low	Maintenance—moderate
Robustness—high	Robustness—unknown

Fax transmission of claims and clinical records is relatively common and reasonably cheap ($500 up front for a good-quality, low-volume fax machine, plus continuing, and largely hidden, telephone charges). Facsimile has a very limited future at the present time as a communications medium for behavioral healthcare. It is about the least confidential and secure method available at both ends of the pipe. In a practice management or clinical information system, it requires optical character recognition (OCR) at either end or a live data-entry person to convert the fax image to usable data. For practical purposes (that is, to achieve any administrative savings), OCR itself requires that the form be machine-written rather than handwritten to achieve sufficiently high recognition validity and reliability. However, there is a place for facsimile-based communications as a very low-volume, low-initial-cost methodology.

A more general EC solution requires a PC with a modem, hard drive, printer, and appropriate software. In mid 1995, a reasonably configured system with a laser printer and the necessary hardware and software could be assembled for $2,000 initial cost and perhaps $250–500 per year for a solid maintenance agreement. Additional software, such as a practice management system and an "office suite" including word processing, spreadsheets, presentation developers, and information managers, would cost another $1,000 up front but would not be necessary to function as an online provider using an EC system.

Recall from earlier in this chapter that a provider currently spends about $36.52 per average eight-session outpatient case; using an EC system such as described above, the cost would drop to about $15.58 per case. The savings is $20.94 per case.

Now we estimate the average full-time equivalent practitioner to see 30 cases per week; with an eight-week duration, this means approximately 180 cases per year. If half of these cases had insurance programs that were electronically enabled for the basic transactions we outlined previously, then 90 cases would provide $1,884.60 in savings from current methods in the first year. If we assume the total cost of the necessary hardware, software, and maintenance is $2,500, then the system has paid for itself in sixteen months. The continuing maintenance cost (say, $500 per year) and the transaction fees ($600 per year) would be cost-justified by the first 52 cases seen each year after the first year.

We have only analyzed the cost-effectiveness of the system for electronic communications of typical outpatient case scenarios. The impact of the investment made in hardware, software, and maintenance can be extended greatly by adding a practice management system, accounting, and word processing for a minimal increase in initial costs and maintenance fees.

How Electronic Communications Change Clinical Practice

We have implemented EC systems in practices of many different sizes and types. The changes that occur depend on how much efficiency the provider wishes to derive by considering the work flow surrounding a treatment course. In some practices, almost no change in work flow occurs from the practitioner's standpoint.

One picks up a patient in the waiting room, conducts a session, completes paperwork between sessions, and drops it off (or retains it) for data entry, and starts with a new case. In this scenario, the practice gains all the advantages of EC without disrupting the old work flow processes. On the other hand, the practice does not gain the advantage of examining and streamlining their traditional work flows.

One group with whom we worked realized that if each practitioner had a portable computer with electronic forms and communication software, the practitioners could complete the paperwork electronically rather than on paper and eliminate the overhead of the extra step of paper recording followed by data entry.

Furthermore, the practitioners could complete the electronic forms far more quickly than the handwritten versions used before, saving additional time of their own. Even more interesting was that the practitioners could take their portable computers anywhere and complete the electronic "paperwork" at nonproductive downtimes just as they could with paper forms, but they did not have to carry all the paper around! In addition, the nearest telephone line would allow them to send the forms and data onward without having to wait to bring it in to a data-entry clerk.

Additional value was derived from reducing accounts receivable turnaround from thirty business days to eight. Eligibility verifications were reduced from an average of three days to one day.

From the MCO perspective, tremendous work-flow gains can be had from EC. With the appropriate intelligent software on the senders' desktops, MCOs can receive "clean" and complete data, minimize data reentry, verification, call-backs, and so on. Expensive case managers can deal with more clinical care issues and fewer issues of administration, data correction, data validation, and data recognition. The corollary is that the case managers and practitioners are in less of an adversarial role and more of a clinically collaborative role. Both case managers and practitioners spend less time on the telephone or writing notes to one another.

Furthermore, the MCO can automate the incoming electronic data flow to pass directly into their clinical information system applications and can automate the response from the applications to the providers. The savings in the mail room, data entry, verification, provider relations, and customer relations can add up very quickly if the electronically based communications system is designed and implemented properly. At worst, the MCO gains a savings relative to manual, telephonic, and/or postal communications.

Future Developments

Thus far we have spoken only to the issue of going electronic with currently available and reasonably easy-to-use systems. Much more is going on technically that really promises to change the way our industry can make use of technology.

For example, the Internet is rapidly becoming a major force. Software is now available to make it easy to access information present on the subsection of the Internet known as the World Wide Web (WWW). A great deal of work is under way to make the access even easier so that the end user does not need to know the arcane and difficult instructions now necessary to find addresses of information on the WWW. The big commercial networks (CompuServe, Prodigy, America Online, and shortly MicroSoft Network and AT&T) are now providing more access to the Internet and promise much more for the future. (See Chapter Twelve in this book for more detailed information on the Internet.)

However, as much as we may hear and read about the Internet in mid 1995, there are very significant issues surrounding its use for highly sensitive, confidential information such as we have in healthcare. Some of the issues have been solved by credit card payers and other financial vendors. Many have not. And some of the solutions to provide security are well beyond the means of most providers in healthcare.

Other major technological developments that will accelerate widespread use of computers in behavioral healthcare communications include voice data input and pen-based input systems. Both currently exist but are relatively expensive with few, if any, applications relevant to behavioral healthcare. Voice-recognition transcription systems are the closest to practical reality. Many entrepreneurs are hot on the trail of making these into viable technologies for the healthcare industry.

More futuristic developments might include secure clinical data repositories that allow access only to data elements approved by the patient for specified inquirers. A similar concept is a centralized credentials data repository with access controlled by the practitioners whose credentials reside there. Such repositories exist in particular facilities and occasionally across enterprises to regional healthcare systems, but access is rarely controlled by providers.

The future is in having such data more widely accessible (within the limits of security, confidentiality, and so on) to appropriate parties on a real-time basis such that when a person is on vacation hundreds or thousands of miles away from their regular healthcare provider and healthcare is needed, a local provider can tap the distant data to get a full update without having to grill the patient or family members for hours.

The future is also in having technology become much more wedded to the notion of facilitating our human communications. By this we mean that the technology is continuing to change in ways that adapt to human communications styles and methods rather than having human styles and methods change to fit the technology.

As these near-future and future developments take hold, we will all be able to look back and perceive the enormous revolution that has been taking place as we move through our lives and careers. It is important to realize, however, that if we do not participate in these developments as they occur, we may face a rude awakening a few years later with the knowledge and adaptability of a cave man displaced to modern times!

Welcome aboard!

Notes

P. 213, *As of 1994, almost 60 percent of Americans:* Oss, M. (1995, March). More Americans enrolled in managed behavioral care. *Open Minds,* p. 12.

P. 213, *states are applying for Health Care Financing Administration:* Winslow, R. (1995, April 12). Medical upheaval. *Wall Street Journal,* p. 1.

P. 213, *courts are allowing states:* No author. (1995, April 27). *Wall Street Journal,* p. 1.

CHAPTER TWELVE

HOW TO USE THE INTERNET AND ELECTRONIC BULLETIN BOARDS

Dick Schoech and Katherine Kelley Smith

Most behavioral healthcare specialists have heard of the information super-highway. While they may want to cruise the information highways and by-ways, they typically do not have much time and do not know exactly what they want to find. They are similar to people who want to explore the world but do not know exactly what they want to see. Luckily, books on the information super-highway, the Internet, BBSs, and other telecommunications phenomena in cyber-space are as numerous as books on world travel. That's because cyberspace, like the world, is a big place. However, while world travel agents exist in almost every neighborhood, few travel agents exist for cyberspace. Often we must venture out alone, which is both fun and frustrating. The problem is that some profes-sionals do not have time to roam the streets of cyberspace. They need a tour guide who points out the major options and sites for business and pleasure.

This chapter presents the basics of networking hardware, software, capabil-ities, and tools. It also presents scenarios of how these can be used to support be-havioral healthcare practice. Finally, it provides advice on how individuals and agencies can get started networking. Throughout, we provide contact addresses

Note: This chapter is an expansion of an article by the authors that appeared in *Behavioral Healthcare Tomorrow,* January–February 1995 (Vol. 4, No. 1, pp. 23–29). Reprinted by permission.

and phone numbers. As with all road maps and tour guides, some information is outdated before it is printed.

Cyberspace and Access to Cyberspace

Cyberspace is the nonphysical place where people meet and share resources using telecommunications. Just as we have many ways to travel the world, many ways exist to travel cyberspace. Each access avenue described below has advantages and disadvantages that impact the resources available to the traveler. The access avenues are summarized in Table 12.1.

Bulletin Board System (BBS)

A Bulletin Board System (BBS) is usually an individually operated personal computer that offers e-mail, conferencing, and file transfer to hundreds of local callers. Most BBSs are nodes of a larger network of BBSs that share messages, conferences, and files. One network, named FidoNet after the developer's dog, connects more than thirty-seven thousand local computer BBSs. Another network available

TABLE 12.1. AVENUES FOR NETWORKING

Avenue	Advantages	Disadvantages
Local BBSs	Inexpensive, usually easy to use, good way to start networking.	Can be unreliable; may not carry relevant information; limited Internet access.
Commercial networks	Commercial networks can have substantial information on their own network and may supply their own easy to use software along with technical support.	Monthly cost; access to the Internet may only be an add on and may be limited.
Internet using shell accounts from commercial, corporate, or academic sites	Typically fast, high bandwidth access from the organization's local area network. Technical support is usually available.	May not be full Internet access. Some features may be locked out and others may cost, may not be available from home.
Internet using SLIP/PPP connection	Full Internet access available via standard telephone lines. Technical support varies by vendor.	Monthly cost; may be difficult to set up and use; requires more powerful local hardware and software, and SLIP/PPP access via modem is slow.

in many cities is Free-Net. Its BBSs are oriented around civic and community information and free Internet e-mail. To find local BBSs or learn if a Free-Net exists in your area, contact your local computer store or library.

Local BBSs vary by the type of user interface and by the topics of the conferences, data bases, and files they contain. Graphic-oriented user interfaces are becoming popular. BBSs offer the beginning traveler an easy and inexpensive way to learn some of the language and capacities of cyberspace. BBSs are beginning to be connected to the Internet via e-mail and conferences. Once comfortable with a BBS, you may find networking the Internet not so overwhelming. Once a user logs onto a BBS, other BBS resources can be found. Usually a BBS has a list of other relevant BBSs that may be called. Table 12.2 lists several behavioral health-care-oriented BBSs in the United States and their phone numbers.

Commercial Networks

Commercial networks are large private networks that offer many networking features, including access to the Internet ranging from limited to full access. Examples include Prodigy (info@prodigy.com), telephone 800/PRODIGY; America Online (info@aol.com), 800/827–6364; Delphi (info@delphi.com), 800/695–4005; and CompuServe (info@compuserve.com), 800/848–1899. Information on commercial networks can be easily obtained by contacting a sales representative.

Many specialty networks exist. The Institute for Global Communication (IGC) (support@igc.org) provides PeaceNet, EcoNet, ConflictNet, LaborNet, Homeo-Net, and HumanServe. HumanServe is somewhat unique in that it shares human service conferences with both FidoNet and the Internet. The Maternal and Child

TABLE 12.2. BBSs ORIENTED TO BEHAVIORAL HEALTHCARE

BBS Name	Location	BBS phone
National Association of Social Workers	Las Cruces, NM	505–646–2868
ABLE INFORM	Silver Springs, MD	301–589–3563
Black Bag BBS	Collegeville, PA	610–454–7396
C CAD Online	Dallas, TX	214–647–5739
Disabled Children's Computer Group	Berkeley, CA	510–841–5621
Dissociation Net	Albany, NY	518–462–6134
Shrink Tank	California	408–257–8131
Testing Station	Indiana	317–846–8917
Statistics BBS	Kansas	316–687–0578
Bureau of Health Professions	Silver Springs, MD	301–443–5913

Note: There are many more bulletin boards that deal with these issues. Any one of these boards may have more information for further exploration.

Health Network (MCHNet) is a human service–oriented commercial network that was developed by the Maternal and Child Health Bureau within the U.S. Public Health Service; its Internet address is gopher://mchnet.ichp.ufl.edu and its mailing address is Institute for Child Health Policy, MCH-NetLink Project, 5700 SW 34th St., Suite 323, Gainesville, FL 32607–5367. HandsNet also is a human service–oriented commercial network, addressing topics such as disabilities, housing, poverty, child abuse, nutrition, hunger, and community development; its Internet address is http://www.igc.apc.org/handsnet/ and its mailing address is 20195 Stevens Creek Blvd., #120, Cupertino, CA 95014. Other human service–oriented commercial networks include: SpecialNet (teachers in the field of special needs, 800/634–5644); SCAN (university-affiliated programs for people with disabilities); and NACHC (National Association of Community Health Centers). The monthly charge for commercial networks is comparable to the charge for a telephone line and may vary depending on features used and connect time.

The Internet

The Internet is a worldwide network of networks, connecting an estimated 35 million people. The Internet has been labeled the information superhighway. Individual Internet users have an address that looks like the following: schoech@uta.edu. The first part of the address contains the user's initials, name, or nickname. The name is followed by an @ sign that is followed in turn by the name of the organization. The final part of an address contains a period followed by the type of organization. It is easy to recognize some types of organizations: *.gov* stands for government, *.edu* for education, and *.com* stands for commercial. Sites on the Internet are identified by their URL (uniform resource locator) address. A typical URL is http://www.uta.edu/cussn/cussn.html. *Http* stands for "hypertext transport protocol." The *www.uta.edu* indicates it is a World Wide Web site at the University of Texas at Arlington (*uta*), an educational (*.edu*) institution. At *uta*, files are stored in a computer directory named *cussn*. The executable html (hypertext markup language) program is called *cussn.html*. URLs are case-sensitive; that is, the computer interprets capital and small letters differently.

While Internet resources are usually free, you typically must pay for Internet access. Commercial networks, corporations, government agencies, universities, and Free-Nets typically provide Internet access. Also, specialty commercial Internet access providers exist in major cities. Different types of access may use different protocols or standards for communicating via computers. Typically, commercial networks, corporations, and universities offer "shell accounts," where users connected to their system are provided Internet access. The features of shell accounts vary by the supplier. They can be a fast 10M bps (bits per second) for direct connections or much slower, for example 2400 bps for call-in via modem over standard telephone lines. A bit is the smallest piece of information communicated. Seven or eight bits are required to represent one number or character. Communications at speeds of less than 14.4K bps are more likely to be text-based than graphical.

Home access to the Internet is available using a modem and a standard telephone line. However, even fast modems result in slow internet access because a tremendous amount of data transfer is required in the form of text, graphics, pictures, audio, animation, and video. Consequently, cable television companies and others are beginning to offer fast Internet access from people's homes.

A popular home Internet access method supplied by commercial access providers is a SLIP/PPP connection using a fast 14.4+ bps modem and standard telephone lines. SLIP stands for "serial line internet protocol," and PPP stands for "point-to-point protocol." With SLIP/PPP access, you connect to the Internet directly with a connection provided by a commercial access provider, not through someone else's computer system. While SLIP/PPP gives full access, currently the fastest dial-in modems are 10–20 times slower than more high-speed connections where your PC is connected directly to the Internet via a local or wide-area network. Such high-speed connections typically require a special card to be installed in your computer to connect you directly via a high-speed line.

A SLIP/PPP connection requires different software from the standard terminal emulation software used for BBS access. Many times the commercial Internet access provider supplying the SLIP/PPP connection will provide the software necessary for accessing and using the Internet. Some Internet software packages, like Internet in a Box, contain their own SLIP/PPP access software along with other tools for using the Internet. For a SLIP/PPP provider available through an 800 number anywhere in the United States, contact Netcom (800/353–6600) (info@netcom.com).

Features of Networks

What we do in cyberspace is limited by the features of the network on which we are traveling. Electronic networks can have some or all of the following features:

- *E-mail,* or electronic mail, is the sending and receiving of private messages. E-mail is the primary use of most networks.
- *Browsing* is a common network activity, also called "surfing." Browsing is similar to casual shopping in a large mall. BBS browsing may involve calling one BBS after another, checking out the new games available. However, the best

place to browse is on the Internet, where you can jump from topic to topic anywhere in the world. On the Internet, you can go from viewing pictures of temples in Thailand to viewing the world of a child through a home page constructed as part of a grade school assignment. A home page is a series of Internet computer screens on one topic.

- *Conferencing* is the organized discussion of topics between like-minded participants using telecommunications. Conferences are called different names on different systems: "forums," "newsgroups," "listservs," or "echos." Some conferences are simply public e-mail areas. Other conferences offer the user sophisticated tools to locate, browse, and reply to one or several messages on a selected subtopic. Conferences may also make available previous discussions on a topic organized in one or several large files. An example of a worldwide conferencing network carrying more than 8,600 conferences is UseNet. Table 12.3 lists some BBS conferences. Table 12.4 lists some Internet conferences, how to access them, and how to find additional resources.

- *File transfer* is the sending (uploading) and receiving (downloading) of computer files from one computer to another. On the Internet, file transfer is called FTP, which stands for "file transfer protocol." Internet FTP is often from sites that offer "anonymous FTP"; that is, the user can log on with the name *anonymous* to gain access. Some FTP sites require that users have an account and their own password.

- *Data base searching* is the common networking activity where the user examines and searches repositories of information. Many data bases exist. Check out the U.S. Department of Health and Human Services data base, whose URL is http://www.os.dhhs.gov/0/aspe/prog_eval/evaluation.html.

- *Chat* is the simultaneous typing and viewing of all interactions by two or more persons connected electronically. For example, PysComNet has provided on-line, real-time chat on psychopathology and suicidal behavior. Contact PsyComNet at psydoc@netcom.com.

- *Electronic publishing* is the publishing of anything from articles to music in electronic form. Request the electronic journal *Psycoloquy* from http://www.princeton.edu/~harnad/psyc.html, or play music selections from independent artists at http://www.iuma.com/IUMA-2.0/olas/.

Networking Tools

Network travel is limited not only by the network features above but also by available tools. Below are some of the tools available to the cyberspace traveler. Some are part of an electronic network, while others are features of the software with which a user accesses the network. Sometimes these tools are integrated into one software package.

- *Browsers* are software programs that allow users to use a network. The speed of one's network connection determines what type of browser one can use. If you have slow access, for example through a 2400 bps modem, you will probably use a text-oriented browser, such as Lynx. Lynx allows one to browse the Internet using text commands and menus rather than a mouse. Faster modems (14.4K bps on up) support a graphical interface. With these faster modems, access is similar to the graphical interface of Windows or a Macintosh. Netscape is a popular shareware Internet browser for the Macintosh or PCs running Windows.
- Readers and mailers keep track of messages sent and received and those waiting to be examined. A popular Windows shareware reader for the Internet is Eudora. Easy to use readers are typically supplied by commercial networks upon subscribing.
- The *World Wide Web (WWW)* is a hypertext linking of the resources on the Internet. Through the WWW, you can click on "hotwords" or pictures and jump from topic to topic or from web site to web site. You can identify a WWW site by its URL typically beginning with *http://www*. Table 12.5 lists some behavioral healthcare WWW sites.
- *Telnet* is a tool that allows one to connect or log in to another computer remotely. Once connected, access is like being directly connected to that computer. Researchers might use telnet to link to another computer that contains the software or processing capabilities they need. To try telnet, connect to the National Museum of American Art at siris.si.edu. Or try swais.access.gpo.gov for testimony, evaluations, and other information from the U.S. General Accounting Office, the Congressional watchdog agency. Log in as *gao* (lower case).
- *Gopher* is a menu-based tool for searching the Internet. Gopher options allow the user to perform tasks such as displaying documents or automatically connecting to another Internet site. You can identify a gopher site as the URL contains the word *gopher*. Two search-related gopher tools are *veronica* and *archie*. *Veronica* provides keyword searches to find gopher and other types of information sites, such as WWW sites, UseNet archives, and telnet-accessible information services. The result of a veronica search is a gopher menu comprising information items whose titles contain the specified keywords. *Archie* provides keyword searches for Internet documents and software.
- *MUDs* (multiuser dimension) and *MOOs* (multiuser domain) offer unstructured meetings via chat in structured domains. For example, MUDs and MOOs exist for computer games or virtual places such as Diversity University, a dynamic

virtual learning environment accessible via telnet (telnet moo.du.org 8888 or e-mail moo@erau.db.erau.edu). Diversity University has a social work department.

- *Agents* are software programs that automate electronic networking based on the specifications of the user. Overnight, your agent could connect to a local newspaper on the network and search for information about a local issue of interest. It could then check various electronic networks for your e-mail, download an electronic journal, and accumulate a listing of files that have the word *disability* in their titles. When you awake in the morning, you could consult your agent for the personalized information it had accumulated. Most agents are in the development phase.

- Several tools are being developed for simultaneous interactivity of Internet users. The *undernet* is an Internet relay chat (IRC) system that allows users to simultaneously chat with people from all over the world. *CU-SeeMe* technology, being developed at Cornell University, provides a slow video connection between Internet users. The *Mbone* provides Internet users with continuous full-motion video, for example, video from a camera on the space shuttle. A high-capacity computer and high-bandwidth Internet connection are currently needed to display Mbone video.

- A *WAIS* (Wide-Area Information Server) is an Internet search tool. WAIS tools use keywords and strings of characters to search a data base over the Internet. Contact compsych@splava.cc.plattsburgh.edu for a searchable data base over the Internet.

Scenarios of Networking and Its Impacts

Networking is a difficult activity to comprehend by reading technical descriptions. Perhaps a better way to understand networking is by examining scenarios in which people use networking for work and pleasure.

Networking for Fun

Paul is a fourteen-year-old who spends a lot of time in cyberspace for fun and escape. Cyberspace is familiar territory to Paul and his friends, who have been using computers for years. About half of BBS users are under the age of eighteen. Paul especially likes the MUD (multiuser dimension) type of games, where he can assume any personality he wants in a make-believe world and interact with peers. Paul frequently uses real-time conferencing (chat) to relieve boredom and frustration. Chat offers him a chance to talk to peers he has never met. During chat,

TABLE 12.3. BEHAVIORAL HEALTHCARE BBS CONFERENCES

Conference Tag	Description
12_STEPS	Twelve-Step discussion echo
ABLED	Disabled users information exchange
ABLED_ATHLETE	Abled athletes
ABLENEWS	Disability/medical news, views, resources
ADHD	Attention deficit hyperactivity disorders
ADOPTEES	Adoptees information exchange
AIDS-HIV	AIDS and HIV
AIDS.DATA	AIDS data
AIDS/ARC	AIDS and ARC
AMPUTEE	Amputee support
ANXIETY	Anxiety disorders
BATTERED	Family violence
BIOMED	Biomedical and clinical engineering topics
BLINDTLK	Blindness-related topics and discussions
CARCINOMA	Cancer survivors
CARE_GIVER	Care giver
CFS	Chronic fatigue syndrome
CHILD_ABUSE	Child abuse information and recovery
CHILD_ABUSE_ISSUES	Open Forum—prevention, detection, legal aspects and more
CHRONIC_PAIN	Chronic pain discussion area
CPALSY	Cerebral palsy
CUSS	Computer user in the social services
DADS	Dads
EDUCATOR	Education
HELP_MANKIND	Humanitarian issues
GAYLINK	Gay topic discussion conference
GAYNEWS	Gays/lesbians news echo
GAYTEEN	Gay teenager forum for teenagers to discuss their sexuality
GRAND_ROUNDS	Medical information
ICGAL	Issues concerning gays and lesbians
INTERNET	The Internet from a user's perspective
MENTAL_HEALTH	Mental health
PARENTS	Parents echo
PLEASE	Stopping the cycle of child abuse
PROBLEM_CHILD	Problem children
PUBLIC_PSYCH	Public psychology support conference
RARE_CONDITION	Rare diseases
RECOVERY	Twelve-Step oriented recovery chatting
SILENTTALK	Conference for the deaf and hard of hearing
SIP_AA	Alcoholism and recovery
SIP_ACA	Adult children of alcoholics
SIP_INCEST	Incest survivor's conference
SIP_MPD	Singleness in purpose—multiple personality disorder
SIP_NA	Narcotics anonymous echo
SIP_SAA	Twelve-Step recovery from sexual addiction
SIP_SSAS	Spouses of sexual abuse survivors
SIP_SURVIVOR	Twelve-Step discussions for survivors of incest
STRESS_MGMT	Learn how to reduce or eliminate stress fast!
SURVIVOR	Cancer/leukemia/blood and immune system/coping with
THI_CVA	Brain injuries
WELFARE	Welfare conference

TABLE 12.4. CONFERENCES ON THE INTERNET

Conference Description	Address to Subscribe	Message to Subscribe*
Abuse-l: Child Abuse	listserv@ubvm.cc.buffalo.edu	subscribe abuse-l [FN] [LN]
Affective-disorders	listserv@netcom.com	subscribe affective-disorders
Anxiety-depression-youth	listserv@netcom.com	subscribe anxiety-depression-youth
Anxiety-disorders	listserv@netcom.com	subscribe anxiety-disorders
Assessment-psychometrics	listserv@netcom.com	subscribe assessment-psychometrics
Attachment-l	listserv@netcom.com	subscribe attachment-l
Baccalaureate Social Work Ed	listserv@rit.edu	subscribe bpd [FN] [LN]
Bone marrow transplant list	bmt-talk-request@ai.mit.edu	subscribe
Breast cancer list	listserv@morgan.ucs.mun.ca	subscribe breast-cancer [FN] [LN]
Canadian Social Work	listserv@pdomain.uwindsor.ca	subscribe csocwork [FN] [LN]
Child Abuse Research	listproc@cornell.edu	subscribe child-maltreatment-research-l [FN] [LN]
Child-adolescent-psych	listserv@netcom.com	subscribe child-adolescent-psych
Children: special health care needs	listserv@nervm.nerdc.ufl.edu	subscribe CSHCN-L [FN][LN])
Clinical-psychologists	listserv@netcom.com	subscribe clinical-psychologists
Clinical-psychophysiology	listserv@netcom.com	subscribe clinical-psychophysiology
Computer Use in Social Services	listserv@stat.com	subscribe cussnet [FN] [LN]
Computers in Social Work Ed	mailbase@mailbase.ac.uk	join cti-soc-work-uk [FN] [LN]
Computers-in-mental-health	listserv@netcom.com	subscribe computers-in-mental-health
Criminal Justice	listserv@cunyvm.cuny.edu	subscribe cjust-l [FN] [LN]
Current-issues-in-psych	listserv@netcom.com	subscribe current-issues-in-psych
Depression-l	listserv@netcom.com	subscribe depression-l
Dignity Net	majordomo@laplaza.taos.nm.us	subscribe dnet
Dissociative-disorders	listserv@netcom.com	subscribe dissociative-disorders
Ejintvio: Intimate Violence	listserv@uniacc.uri.edu	subscribe ejintvio [FN] [LN]
Emergency-psychiatry	listserv@netcom.com	subscribe emergency-psychiatry
Employee Assistance Programmes	majordomo@utopia.pinsight.com	subscribe eap
Evalten: Evaluation and Statistics	listserv@sjuvm.stjohns.edu	subscribe evalten [FN] [LN]
Feminist Social Work	listproc@moose.uvm.edu	subscribe femsw-l [FN] [LN]
Femisa: Feminism	listproc@csf.colorado.edu	subscribe femisa [FN] [LN]

TABLE 12.4. CONFERENCES ON THE INTERNET, cont'd.

Conference Description	Address to Subscribe	Message to Subscribe*
Field Education	listserv@nmsu.edu	subscribe sw-fieldwork [FN] [LN]
Folks with mood swings etc.	listserv@sjuvm.stjohns.edu	subscribe madness [FN] [LN]
Forensic-psych	listserv@netcom.com	subscribe forensic-psych
Geriatric-neuro	listserv@netcom.com	subscribe geriatric-neuro
Healthre: Healthcare Reform	listserv@ukcc.uky.edu	subscribe healthre [FN] [LN]
Helplessness-l	listserv@netcom.com	subscribe helplessness-l
Hiv-aids-psycho-social	listserv@netcom.com	subscribe hiv-aids-psycho-social
Homelessness	listproc@csf.colorado.edu	subscribe homeless [FN] [LN]
Human Services Info Tech Assn.	listserv@cornell.edu	subscribe husita-l [FN] [LN]
Hypnosis-l	listserv@netcom.com	subscribe hypnosis-l
International Social Work	listserv@nisw.org.uk	subscribe intsocwork [FN] [LN]
Issues: the Human Service Records	cwkgroup-request@umassd.edu	subscribe cwkgroup [FN] [LN]
Managed-behavioral-healthcare	listserv@netcom.com	subscribe managed-behavioral-healthcare
Mental-health-in-the-media	listserv@netcom.com	subscribe mental-health-in-the-media
Neuro-psych	listserv@netcom.com	subscribe neuro-psych
Obsessive Compulsive Disorder List	listserv@vm.marist.edu	subscribe ocd-l [FN] [LN]
Outcome of Intervention	listserv@sjuvm.stjohns.edu	subscribe outcometen [FN] [LN]
Ovarian cancer list	listserv@ist01.ferris.edu	subscribe ovarian-cancer
Parenting List	majordomo@listserv.cso.uiuc.edu	subscribe parenting [your e-mail address]
Personality-disorders	listserv@netcom.com	subscribe personality-disorders
Phil & Science of Social Work	listproc@lists.vcu.edu	subscribe sciofslw [FN] [LN]
Psy-lanuage	listserv@netcom.com	subscribe psy-lanuage
Psych-nurses	listserv@netcom.com	subscribe psych-nurses

List	Address	Command
Psychiatric-social-workers	listserv@netcom.com	subscribe psychiatric-social-workers
Psychiatry-l	listserv@netcom.com	subscribe psychiatry-l
Psychiatry-resources	listserv@netcom.com	subscribe psychiatry
Psycho-analysis	listserv@netcom.com	subscribe psycho-analysis
Psycho-pharm	listserv@netcom.com	subscribe psycho-pharm
Psychotherapy-practice	listserv@netcom.com	subscribe psychotherapy-practice**
Psychotherapy-research	listserv@netcom.com	subscribe psychotherapy-research
Psycoloquy	listserv@pucc.princeton.edu	subscribe psycoloquy
Research-psychologists	listserv@netcom.com	subscribe research-psychologists
Right-to-die list	majordomo@efn.org	subscribe right_to_die [your e-mail address]
Rural-care	listserv@netcom.com	subscribe rural-care
Sexual-variants-and-disorders	listserv@netcom.com	subscribe sexual-variants-and-disorders
Social Science Research Methods	listserv@unmvma.unm.edu	subscribe methods [FN] [LN]
Social Work	listserv@uafsysb.uark.edu	subscribe socwork [FN] [LN]
Social Work Measurment Group	listserv@stat.com	subscribe swmg-list [FN] [LN]
Student Social Work List	listserv@ist01.ferris.edu	subscribe scwk-l [FN] [LN]
Substance-related-disorders	listserv@netcom.com	subscribe substance-related-disorders
Thana-tology	listserv@netcom.com	subscribe thana-tology
Transcultural-psychology	listserv@netcom.com	subscribe transcultural-psychology
Traumatic-stress	listserv@netcom.com	subscribe traumatic-stress
Weekly magazine for the Deaf	listserv@listserv.deaf-magazine.org	subscribe deaf-magazine [FN] [LN]

*[FN] = first name, [LN] = last name

**Announcement: the staff lounge: an informal gathering place for Mental Health Professionals will be open this and every Thursday at 10:00 P.M. E.D.T. on the Internet's Undernet Channel/password:#interpsyc. Aphasia questions should be directed to Ivan Goldberg at kg1@columbia.edu.

Note: Most printed lists of conferences on the Internet are outdated. However, you can quickly search for conferences on any topic once you are on the Internet.

TABLE 12.5. BEHAVIORAL HEALTHCARE WORLD WIDE WEB SITES

Sponsoring Organization	WWW site address
A Brief Introduction to Skin Cancer	http://www.maui.net/~southsky/introto.html
Alternate views of cancer treatment	http://werple.mira.net.au/sumeria/cancer.html
American Psychological Assn's PsychNET	http://www.apa.org
Behavioral Informatics Tomorrow conference	http://www.ispot.com:80/CentraLink/
Breast Cancer Information Clearinghouse	http://nysernet.org/bcic/
Cancer Patient: emphasis on sarcomas	http://www.charm.net:80/~kkdk/
CancerNet Web Contents	http://biomed.nus.sg/Cancer/contents.html
Chemosensitivity Testing for Cancer Patients	http://www-med.stanford.edu/CBHP/Chemosensitivity_Testing.html
Children with cancer	http://mmp.dgsys.com:80/special/SpeciaLove
Computer Uses in Social Work	http://www.ed.uiuc.edu/EdPsy-387/Beena-Choksi/CSWfin.htmlz
Deathnet: Right to Die Web Site	http://www.IslandNet.com:80/~deathnet/
Doug's Internet Resources for Counselors	http://www.uark.edu/depts/cned/web/counsel.html
Emotional Support Resources	http://asa.ugl.lib.umich.edu/chdocs/support/emotion.html
European Network for Human Services	http://www.uia.ua.be/u/enith
Int J of General Practice & Primary Care	http://www.cityscape.co.uk/users/ad88/gp.htm
International Agency for Research on Cancer	http://www.iarc.fr/
International Agency for Research on Cancer	http://www.iarc.fr/
Madness Web Site	http://www.io.org/~madness

Medical Matrix-Guide to Medical Resources	http://kuhttp.cc.ukans.edu/cwis/units/medcntr/Lee/HOMEPAHE.HTML
Milton's Interpsych Page	http://www.med.umich.edu/psychiatry/interpsych.html
NIH WWW server	http://www.nih.gov/
Oncolink	http://cancer.med.upenn.edu/
OncoLink, from the U. of Pennsylvania	http://cancer.med.upenn.edu/
Organ and tissue donation and transplant	http://www.gblhorizon.com/mktplace/share.html
Patient Advocacy Numbers	http://infonet.welch.jhu.edu/advocacy.html
Psychopharmacology and Substance Abuse	http://Charlotte.med.nyu.edu/woodr/div28.html
Resources for Bipolar Affective Disorders	http://www.ucar.edu/pendulum/
Safety Net: Domestic Violence Resources	http://www.interport.net/~asherman/dv.html
Social Disadvantage Research Group	http://marx.apsoc.ox.uk/sdrgdocs/index.html
Social Workers Advocating Network Tech.	http://falcon.cc.ukans.edu/~pthomas/swan.html
Telescan: Telematics Services in Cancer	http://telescan.nki.nl/
The National Cancer Institute's WWW (USA)	http://www.nci.nih.gov/
Trauma Info Pages	http://gladstone.uoregon.edu/~dvb/trauma.htm
U. Michigan Quick Information for Patients	http://asa.ugl.lib.umich.edu/chdocs/cancer/CANCERGUIDE.HTML
Virtual CUSSN	http://www.uta.edu/cussn/cussn.html
Virtual Library	http://golgi.harvard.edu/biopages/medicine.html
Virtual New Mexico	http://128.123.3.18/~connealy/
Web Sites for Social Workers	http://lamar.colostate.edu/~mcmurray/webstuff.html
Yahoo Cancer Resources	http://www.yahoo.com/Health/Medicine/Cancer/

Paul can engage in group discussions unhindered by the insecurities and shyness of adolescence or the oversight of adults. Lately, Paul and a girl friend, whom he has never met in person, have been chatting privately. Networking offers Paul a chance to flirt and discuss intimate topics with the opposite sex, something he is too shy to do in person. He sees his travels on the information superhighway as preparation for the day he receives his driver's license and can travel the highways of the world.

Networking for Self-Help

Mark received substance-abuse treatment in the city where he once worked. Having lost his job because of his addiction, he moved to a small town over an hour away to find employment. His new job involves long hours and does not allow time to attend treatment meetings in the small town. Mark initially established network connections to communicate with his counselor about aftercare activities. By browsing, Mark has found several network conferences that operate like treatment meetings. Through these conferences, Mark has met two other people who live nearby and are working on similar substance-abuse problems. When times are very difficult, they provide in-person and telephone support to each other.

Networking and Disabilities

John was a university professor in electrical engineering before a sudden stroke ended his career and resulted in his using a wheelchair and becoming nonvocal. His only means of communication outside the home is through electronic networking. Using electronic networks, John is able to solicit programming jobs that he can perform at home and electronically transmit to his employers. More importantly, he is able to communicate with colleagues around the world and maintain his professional identity and interests. He uses local BBSs for meeting and communicating with friends. He volunteers his talents to a local disability organization by checking all the files uploaded to their BBS for viruses. Recently, John set up his own BBS to help himself, his business, and his friends. He is hoping he can soon afford a direct connection to the Internet.

Networking and Professional Work

Lisa provides counseling services in a rural mental health agency. Her specialty is working with persons with depression. She periodically connects to a local bulletin board where she sends and receives messages from clients who are too disabled or too far away to come into the office. Some clients upload logs documenting the results of the treatment tasks they agreed to perform. Lisa analyzes the logs and sends advice back to the client via e-mail. She also uses the BBS to download relevant mental health shareware and demos of commercial software (http://www.uta.edu/cussn/cussn.html). She keeps current professionally by taking courses that she finds on the World Lecture Hall (http://microlib.cc.utexas.edu/world/lecture). In addition, Lisa participates in conferences on her specialty interests of depression, the homeless, and victims abuse. On the victims abuse conference, she often gives basic advice and provides participants with local resources.

Another resource that Lisa finds valuable is a national lithium data base. When she has questions about whether a client is a good candidate for lithium or whether the current lithium prescription is appropriate, she connects to the appropriate data base, inputs client information, and reviews the advice. Another way she uses networking is to subscribe to the *Electronic Journal of Intimate Violence* (ejintvio@uriacc.bitnet), which provides insights into violent behavior. Lisa especially likes using networks on trips. In the evening, she uses her portable computer to connect to the agency computer and answers e-mail about client and agency problems. Electronic networking helps bring her office emergencies to her hotel room for quick solutions. This evens out her workload, makes her return to the office less hectic, and helps her relax knowing that important problems are handled.

Networking and Community Activism

Carina is a local community activist in an older neighborhood suffering from decline and neglect. She maintains a data base of neighborhood information that is available to residents via a BBS. Carina's agency uses many volunteers who are homebound due to limited mobility, speech, or vision. Each volunteer has become an expert on a particular neighborhood problem by connecting to local BBSs and statewide gopher sites and downloading information relevant to the neighborhood. Each volunteer stores this information in the agency BBS data base and maintains his or her section of the data base.

Using the data base and volunteer expertise, Carina has been able to develop crime prevention programs, mobilize a group of residents to force a company to quit polluting, and fight for a redistricting plan that benefits the neighborhood. Her data comparing city expenditures and private-sector investments by zip code were instrumental in getting the city and banks to acknowledge their neglect. Once the neglect was documented, they joined forces to develop a long-range plan for neighborhood redevelopment.

Networking a Group of Agencies

Ann is in charge of information resources at United Way. She and the United Way member agencies decided to join forces and network to optimize resources and services. A pilot project began where a group of the more computer-literate agencies obtained Internet access for e-mail and file transfer. The next project was to develop linked home pages for volunteer recruitment and fundraising (funding bulletins from the APA Research Psychology Network at APASD-L@VTVM1.CC.VT.EDU). Anyone browsing the Internet could see pictures of other volunteers in action along with audio narration of volunteer experiences. Potential contributors could see agency projects needing funds and monitor the impact of their contributions. The United Way promoted the home page through corporate e-mail systems.

A final project involves developing a data base of indicators on community well-being. The United Way made census data (http://www.census.gov/) and data on local services and needs available to citizens using searchable data bases and clickable zip code maps. Citizens viewing the needs and resources information can complete an online survey to record their opinions. This project is being extended, with United Way helping some neighborhoods to develop a home page with links to the home page of the United Way and member agencies.

Considerations When Networking

Several characteristics of electronic communications should be considered when using electronic networks.

- The learning curve is quite steep for networks like the Internet.
- People compose e-mail messages as they type and rarely edit. This process brings to mind a quote attributed to Mark Twain: "Forgive my lengthy letter. If I had had more time, I would have written a shorter one." Thus, networkers are bombarded with an overwhelming amount of poorly written information. To increase the likelihood of success in your electronic communications, construct messages with your needs clearly identified in the subject line or first line of the message. Format the remainder for easy skimming during the several seconds a reader typically devotes to a message.
- Using electronic communications, people construct mental pictures of others that are often inaccurate. Face-to-face meetings of networkers yield many surprises.
- Networking can be addictive. People often neglect face-to-face contact in favor of networking. It is debatable whether communications and relationships via the network are as socially beneficial as person-to-person communications.
- Fewer communication cues are provided during networking than in person-to-person interaction. Often glyphs such as :-) (a smiley face turned sideways)

are used to communicate emotions. Flaming, or the angry response to an unintended attack, often occurs. Flaming occurs when a reader misinterprets the intentions of the sender of a message because the reader has no visual or auditory cues and is reading nonedited text. "Netiquette," or network etiquette, exists and is often enforced by sending "flaming" e-mail messages to violators (Table 12.6).

- A few people with a lot of time on their hands can dominate conference conversation. Setting and observing ground rules and netiquette is important.
- Do not assume that just because you sent a message, it was received. Request a verification reply on important communications. *Forbes* magazine recently tested the reliability of the Internet by sending 240 properly addressed test messages. Nine percent failed to reach their destination, and many others took up to two days to arrive.
- Do not consider e-mail to be private. We often see humble apologies to thousands in a conference by those who assumed e-mail to be private, only to discover that the e-mail was public due to a user or technical error.
- Communicating electronically has some unexpected benefits. On one project, I communicated with someone for months, only to find during a face-to-face meeting that he was nonvocal. We could not communicate in person, but only over the electronic network. I had made a friend and colleague electronically that I could not have made in a normal work environment.
- Networks are still evolving; e-mail addresses change, WWW sites change, and resources change. Books are useful but are quickly outdated. Bookstores can advise on the most recent popular resource books. The Internet itself offers the best way to keep informed, but time is required. Use Internet resource sites with search engines (http://www.yahoo.com/search.html) or the Internet yellow pages (http://theyellowpages.com/) to find information.

Considerations on Setting Up Your Own Network

Hardware and software requirements in setting up a bulletin board system can range from minimal to substantial. One can start with an old 8088-based computer and a monochrome monitor if desired. Usually BBS operators purchase a dedicated phone line, but this is not necessary either. The cost of bulletin board software ranges from free to thousands of dollars. Packages varying from simple to complex can be found on most BBSs. As with many things, a great deal of time initially goes into the setup. Fortunately, maintenance can be less time-consuming depending on the complexity of the network. For organizations operating networks, there are important issues of liability and screening for pornography and hate information.

TABLE 12.6. NETIQUETTE

Advice	Rationale
DO NOT USE ALL CAPITAL LETTERS	Text in all capital letters is hard to read. Capital letters are used to simulate SHOUTING.
Check out conference FAQs and keep instructions	When you join a conference, see if a FAQ (Frequently Asked Questions) file exists so you do not ask questions that have been answered over and over by others. Keep instructions for quitting the conference so you don't have to send a message to all conference participants asking how to exit the conference.
Separate personal e-mail from conferences	Sending personal e-mail to someone via a conference is rude and may cost some conference members who pay for Internet access by the amount of mail they receive. Also, always get permission to forward a personal e-mail message to someone else or to a conference.
Keep lines to 60 characters or less	Some mailers do not handle lines longer than 70 characters. Long lines may cause formatting problems for some users. Often portions of the original message are quoted to make the reply more meaningful. Short line lengths helps avoid the line-wrapping of these quotes.
Make messages meaningful	Messages such as "me too" typically do not add anything to the conversation, are unnecessary, and require others to do extra work to read and delete them.
Warn of long messages	Readers should be warned if a post is over several paragraphs, e.g., "long message" or "20 pages follow." This allows users to download the message and read it later.
Warn of cross posting	If you post a message to several conferences, indicate at the beginning which conferences will receive the post so that readers will know to avoid the message on the other conferences once they read it.
Avoid flaming	E-mail carries few emotional cues. People can easily become offended by misinterpreting e-mail. Try to state positions without attacking positions different from yours. Be real clear if you are using sarcasm or irony.
Be careful if advertising	Special conferences exist for advertising. One advertiser sent an advertisement to 7,000 conferences. The volume of flame/hate replies crashed his local network.
Use formatting to enhance readability	Terminal screens read differently from the printed text. Help readability by formatting. For example, separate paragraphs with a blank line.
Always sign your e-mail with your e-mail address	Often it is difficult to identify the sender from the message header. Signing all e-mail with your e-mail address allows people to contact you, no matter where your message is forwarded.
Have only one subject per message and use subject titles on your messages	Subject titles on messages help users skim through the volume of mail they receive. To keep conference discussions on track, use the same subject title of the original message, unless you change the topic significantly. Also, limit each message to the subject specified in the title.
Download large files during off hours	Downloading takes away resources from those performing more interactive tasks. Downloading during evening or night hours is more courteous to others.

Setting up a WWW site is typically easier and more costly than setting up a BBS. Tools are available that help design home page screens and maintain the site. As with any system, maintenance and keeping the information current can require a lot of time and effort.

Most BBSs and WWW sites that do well have a theme or mission, for example, providing human service information to the general public or providing conferences for professionals. It is important to plan the purpose and mission of the system before selecting your software. Once the Board is running, consider becoming part of a larger network system like FidoNet, and watch your BBS expand worldwide.

Considerations on Multi-Agency Networking

Since networking is powerful and well accepted, it would seem to be a logical step to develop human service networks in agencies and communities. This simplistic logic has caused much unnecessary work and grief for those hoping to establish electronic networks among human service providers and consumers. Many previous human service networks have failed due to lack of use, support, and maintenance. Use is a major issue with most current commercial human service networks. In a three-year project to encourage local agencies to network electronically, we found that several problems existed that hindered electronic networking.

The first problem is that electronic networks must be distinguished from face-to-face communication networks. Face-to-face networks exist when a group of people share information and resources. Electronic networks build on face-to-face communication networks, but they cannot create them. Many associations or organizations mistakenly hope that electronic networks will cause their members to communicate. If face-to-face communication or the need to communicate does not exist before the electronic network is developed, the network will have a higher likelihood of failure. The slogan "build it and they will come" has not worked in electronically networking human service organizations.

Second, agencies often do not have desktop computers for all staff. Networking is a personal activity, hence one that is most successful when staff have personal computers at work and home.

Third, many human service agencies are currently developing management information systems and do not have knowledge about electronic networking or the experience of empowering workers through networking. Until agencies have their basic management information needs met, they will be reluctant to invest in electronic networking, which is seen as a luxury.

Fourth, using electronic networks to accumulate information resources can still be difficult. Until networking becomes easier for the computer novice, the number of agency networkers will grow slowly. Training is the key, even if it is often overlooked and not budgeted.

Fifth, even when electronic networking is easy, it requires a change in work habits. Changing work habits is very difficult, and employee networking to improve services must be rewarded formally by the organization. If electronic networking is not valued, then networking is seen as an addition to one's normal duties rather than an integral part of doing one's job well. An important part of integrating networking into an agency is having electronic networking become a criterion in formal performance evaluations. Our project concluded that clients' and newly trained workers' use of electronic networks eventually pressures experienced staff to network.

Given the above discussion, we feel electronic networking in an agency faces a slow evolutionary process. The agency can begin by establishing a LAN (local area network) for internal e-mail and file transfer. This local experience can create the impetus to network outside the agency. The agency can then set up an account or subnetwork on an existing network to see if workers and clients will actually network. Next, the agency can establish a mechanism such as peer training, where each trained user mentors and trains a new user. Finally, the agency can secure the resources to make networking a rewarding experience. Anyone taking the trouble to connect to a network needs to receive personal messages and useful information. If potential networkers take the trouble to connect several times and find nothing of value, they will probably not continue networking. Electronic networks are like gardens; they cannot be left alone for any length of time without dire consequences.

In essence, the steps involved in multi-agency networking are to

- Secure top level support
- See how information is viewed and used by the targeted users
- Define the need to network and specify the benefits of networking
- Specify how networking will be rewarded
- Determine whether time exists for people to receive the training necessary to change work habits
- Set up a pilot effort and demonstrate it to staff
- Incorporate network use into agency policies and reward mechanisms

Impact of Networking

Many ethical and confidentiality issues will be faced and resolved as we move into electronic communications. The issues of the haves and have-nots will be a problem until electronic skills and access become as common as the television and the telephone. The impact that networking has on various behavioral healthcare professional groups differs, as we discuss next.

Impact on Citizens and Clients

With networking, citizens and clients will be more connected to the human service delivery system. They will be able to prepare themselves for treatment by browsing local, national, and international resource sites. Those with specialized problems will be able to examine the latest statistics and research on their problem. They will also be able to examine the resources available and familiarize themselves with appropriate interventions before deciding which intervention to choose. Self-help and in-home treatment via networking will be an increasingly attractive option. Homebound clients, such as those with agoraphobia, disabilities, and similar problems, will find telecommunications to be a boon in receiving treatment and support for their problems.

Impact on Practitioners

While practitioners will have better access to information, their clients will have this same access. Often clients approaching intervention will be more informed about a particular problem than the practitioner. Consequently, intervention will become more of a partnership, with the practitioner providing the wisdom of experience and the client providing the specifics of the problem and details on client progress. Networking will also allow practitioners to easily share information electronically with clients, colleagues, and managers. Detailed monitoring of client progress can assume a more important role, allowing client treatment to be more short-term. Conferences will be held, papers presented, and workshops given online in order to save time and money. Over time, we will work out which practitioner activities require face-to-face contact and which tasks can be better completed online.

Impact on Managers

As with the business world, agencies will become less hierarchical, more networked in structure, and more short-term and team-oriented. Telecommuting will become much more common because it saves resources and time and allows freedom in the design and timing of tasks. Managers' jobs will include more monitoring and evaluating to ensure that goals and objectives are being met.

The Future

Predictions about the future of networking tend to be very optimistic. Perhaps that is because these predictions come from members of the upper middle class, who currently have the resources to acquire networking technology. Consequently, they also have the resources to make their lives optimistic. This overly optimistic attitude should be considered when viewing three trends that are important to the future of networking for behavioral healthcare professionals.

Rapid Advancement and Merging of Technologies

Hardware technical advances will outstrip our capacity to apply these technologies. Consequently, software and applications will continue to lag behind. The merging of digital technologies may be more important than the rapid advance in hardware. For example, integrating the telephone, television, stereo, and computers into a universal home telecommunications device will be as important as the development of the Ford model T. The model T was an integrated and inexpensive tool to allow the average person to travel the highways and byways, whereas this new device will be a universal tool for traveling the information superhighway.

The Changing Nature of Stored Information

What we define as stored information will continue to change. Once the world of stored information was dominated by numbers, words, and symbols. Today, we see information as pictures, numbers, text, graphics, animation, movies, and sound. As all information becomes digital, we will obtain more powerful and easier-to-use tools to work with stored information. In addition, we will integrate existing forms of information (as in interactive multimedia) and invent new forms, for example, virtual reality. The value of information will change from what is inherent in the information itself to what is associated with its connectivity. For example, a treatment plan or program evaluation that was once a periodic stand-alone report will become integrated into the agency information system, community human service resource system, etc. Consequently, the value of the treatment plan and evaluation will be due to connectivity as much as to its content.

Virtual Communities and Global Villages

Communities will continue to experience the changes of moving into a global village. Neighborhood home pages will allow people in suburbs to experience some of the connectedness of traditional neighborhoods. Neighborhood news and gossip can be exchanged via e-mail and conferences. Networking of neighbors will replace the face-to-face approach that was popular when neighbors had no backyard fences, worked the same hours, attended the same social institutions, and required only one breadwinner per family. While suburbs will become more connected, people can easily become part of online communities anywhere in the universe. Networking is creating virtual neighborhoods. To experience one of the oldest online communities, check out the Well in San Francisco (http://www.well.com/).

For behavioral healthcare practitioners, this will mean again using the neighborhood as part of the intervention strategy. For example, news and progress on physical illness and injury can be automatically posted on a neighborhood home page as it is recorded in the hospital record, and other information can be included if the patient requests. Networking provides the new tools, but again the push to involve the neighborhood in helping remedy problems stems from cost savings as well as the philosophy of helping one's neighbor.

◆ ◆ ◆

Tom Hanna, a pioneer in human-service networking, found that technical networking problems are behind us and that future problems involve the organization of knowledge for presentation through computer-facilitated communication technologies. He shared his summary of the state of networking: "Hypermedia, including text, movies, still images, and sound recordings shape the new data environment. All are created by individuals, seeking to share their information via the network. This is the heart of the networking concept. At one time, I am a consumer of information and expertise, at other times I am a resource to those seeking the knowledge I happen to have. This user-provider relationship is at the core of networking."

This electronic sharing will continue to grow, as the electronic resources in this chapter indicate. Just as the value of travel was only understood as more and more people had the ability to travel, the value of electronic networking will only be seen when most professionals and clients are connected electronically. Today, our electronic world is restricted by limited Internet access and control over information by several national TV networks and media producers. Networking will provide a much bigger world, where we become the producers and consumers of what we want to interactively explore and project. As we enter the information age, the adage to "think globally and act locally" is advice with a new meaning.

Notes

P. 235, *under the age of eighteen:* Grosse, G. (1994, October). No place in a virtual world: Are kids being shut out of cyberspace? *Texas Computing, 1*(6), 12–14.

P. 245, *took up to two days to arrive:* Noer, M. (1995, June 6). *Forbes, 155*(12), 162.

P. 247, *problems existed that hindered electronic networking:* Schoech, D., Cavalier, A., & Hoover, B. (1993). A model for integrating technology into a multi-agency community service delivery system. *Assistive Technology, 4*(1), 11–23; Schoech, D., Cavalier, A., & Hoover, B. (1993). Using technology to change the human service delivery system. *Administration in Social Work, 17*(2), 31–52.

P. 251, *Well in San Francisco:* Rheingold, H. (1993). The virtual community: Homesteading on the electronic frontier. Reading, MA: Addison-Wesley.

P. 251, *at the core of networking:* Hanna, T. (in press). Towards consensus in human services computer networking. *Computers in Human Services, 12.*

Additional Resources

COMPSYCH is a computerized software information service for psychologists managed by Peter Hornby at State University of New York at Plattsburgh and Margaret Anderson at SUNY Cortland. The system provides four major services: (1) a catalog of descriptive information about available software, (2) a directory of software users, (3) an archive for PC software described in the journal *Behavior Research Methods, Instruments, and Computers,* and (4) an announcement service for conferences, job openings, and other information. Contact COMPSYCH at gopher://baryon.hawk.plattsburgh.edu/1/.ftp/pub/compsych

InterPsych is a nonprofit, voluntary organization established on the Internet with the aim of promoting international scholarly collaboration on interdisciplinary research and intervention efforts in the field of psychopathology. The organization offers a variety of scholarly electronic conferences via e-mail, and real-time conferences. Plans are under way for an electronically distributed journal. InterPsych has over seven thousand members throughout the world, including many leading academics, research scientists, clinical practitioners, and students. The membership is drawn from disciplines as diverse as anthropology, computer science, neuroscience, pharmacology, philosophy, psychiatry, psychology, and sociology. Send an e-mail message to the executive director, Ben Goldhagen (roadman@panix.com), or its founder, Ian Pitchford (I.Pitchford@sheffield.ac.uk).

A list of Internet resources for not-for-profits in housing, health, and human services is available from Munn Heydorn (munn@interaccess.com) or http://www.ai.mit.edu/people/ellens/non/online.html

For a major conference on how to use information services, computers, and emerging technologies to advance behavioral healthcare, contact CentraLink and preview the Behavioral Informatics Tomorrow conference information: http://www.ispot.com:80/CentraLink/

A list of human services Internet resources is available from Michael S. McMurray (mcmurray@lamar.colostate.edu) or http://lamar.colostate.edu/~mcmurray/webstuff.html

Internet references books are readily available along with several versions of the Internet yellow pages. Several possible books are

Badget, T. (1995). *Welcome to the Internet.* (2nd ed.). New York: MIS Press. (a single-authored, simple introduction)

Pike, M. A. (1995). *Using the Internet.* (2nd ed.). Indianapolis: Que. (an extensive reference book with a CD-ROM included)

Ferguson, T. (in press). *Health Online.* Reading, MA: Addison-Wesley.

CHAPTER THIRTEEN

THE PAST, PRESENT, AND FUTURE OF DATA STANDARDS

Ronald W. Manderscheid and Marilyn J. Henderson

Change is obvious at every level of the mental health and substance-abuse enterprise. Currently, more than 107 million persons are covered by some form of managed behavioral healthcare, and seventeen states have received waivers for Medicaid managed care that include mental health and chemical dependency. This dramatic change demands a new look at the state of information development, particularly data standards.

In a managed care environment, consumers, providers, payers, and management services entities are all concerned with and affected by the quality, appropriateness, and coverage of the data standards that are employed. To look at examples, consumers want informative report cards with which to choose behavioral healthcare plans. Providers are concerned with the instruments used to measure the outcomes they achieve, with their relationships to the volume and type of clinical encounters, and with capitation rates paid for care. Payers seek accurate information on costs and the effectiveness of expenditures. And management services entities need to understand how well capitation systems are working. Thus, for different reasons, all participants in the mental health and substance-abuse enterprise are concerned with data standards.

Within each of the examples cited above, statistical information systems need to be based upon data sources that employ common data standards if they are to be successful. In other words, summary information is only meaningful if based upon a common metric and common definitions. Hence, data standards form the basis for the mental health and substance-abuse information enterprise.

This chapter examines the degree to which current mental health and substance-abuse data standards must be updated to be responsive to the dramatic evolution of mental health and substance-abuse services under managed care financial arrangements. This is accomplished by reviewing previous efforts at development of data standards and examining these from the perspective of managed care information requirements. The chapter concludes by discussing potential partnerships to facilitate needed changes and by presenting recommendations for specific courses of action.

Early Efforts at Standardization

More than a century ago, the U.S. Census Office worked collaboratively with the New England Psychological Association to define seven distinct forms of mental illness (mania, melancholia, monomania, paresis, dementia, dipsomania, and epilepsia) to be used in the 1880 census of the population. This collaborative undertaking set the tone for ensuing work in national census activities.

Later, these efforts were expanded to mental health providers. Starting with the 1923 Census of Patients in Mental Institutions, conducted by the U.S. Bureau of the Census, diagnosis was used as one of the descriptive variables in state mental hospitals. This resulted from the joint efforts of the National Committee for Mental Hygiene and the American Psychiatric Association to introduce a standard classification of mental diseases into most of the nation's state mental hospitals. Subsequently, this classification was adopted by the Surgeon General of the Army, the U.S. Public Health Service, and almost all public and private mental hospitals.

In 1949, federal mental health statistical operations were moved to the newly created National Institute of Mental Health (NIMH). Almost immediately, NIMH set up the Model Reporting Area for Mental Hospital Statistics, a joint endeavor with the state mental health agencies. The first step involved a study of the eleven states having central mental health statistical offices, to determine definitions used, types and frequency of data collections, types of reports generated, etc. A major finding was that only two of the eleven states used the same definition of *first admission,* and that wide variation existed in the definitions of *discharge* and *resident patient.*

To remedy the situation, NIMH invited the eleven states to a meeting in 1951 (the first National Conference on Mental Health Statistics) to agree on a course of action and to begin the process of developing and implementing comparable data standards. By 1965, thirty-four states were participating in this voluntary, collaborative project. In 1966, NIMH expanded the project to include ambulatory mental healthcare and designated the annual National Conference on Mental Health Statistics as the principal vehicle for consensus building and standards development. Generally, this endeavor was very successful and set the stage for subsequent progress. Dr. Morton Kramer, currently professor emeritus at Johns Hopkins University in Baltimore, was largely responsible for these developments and the progress achieved.

Mental Health Statistics Improvement Program (MHSIP)

By 1976, NIMH had effected a reorientation from data standards for state mental hospitals toward one focused on mental health statistical standards for all mental health organizations. A new program was initiated at this time, the Mental Health Statistics Improvement Program (MHSIP), to continue and expand the collaborative relationship with the states and to evolve data standards that reflected current developments in mental health services.

For the first decade of the MHSIP, all work involved contributions in-kind by participating states since federal grants were not available. To the present, the states continue to contribute in-kind by encouraging staff to participate in MHSIP committees and by participating in national, voluntary data collections operated by the Center for Mental Health Services' (CMHS) National Reporting Program (NRP) for Mental Health Statistics.

The initial set of data standards evolved by the MHSIP was published in 1983. These standards were based on the mental health organization as the principal reporting unit. Separate minimum data sets were proposed for organizations, the clients they served, and the human resources available to provide care (Table 13.1). By the middle of the decade, these data standards had been widely adopted by the states. The approach employed was viewed by the World Health Organization (WHO) as a model for emulation by other countries.

The 1983 MHSIP data standards were quickly accepted by the mental health field. However, the environment was changing rapidly. Block grants were being introduced; a new focus was emerging on the population having serious mental illness; and state mental health planning was mandated under federal legislation. Managed care was also beginning to emerge in the early part of the decade but was not a major force until 1990.

As experience developed with the MHSIP data standards and as changes occurred in the environment, the MHSIP community recognized the need to up-

TABLE 13.1. 1983 MHSIP MINIMUM DATA SET ELEMENTS

Organization	Human Resources	Client
Name	Organization ID	Organization ID
Address	Date of report	Type of report:
Location	Record identifier	Census/discontinuation
Service area	Employment status	Date of addition
Telephone number	Job title	Date of last service
Director's name	Discipline/training	Census:
Ownership/control	Education	Active program elements
University/college connection	License/certification	Sex
Type of organization	Participation in private	Date of birth
Operating expenditures	practice	Race/ethnicity
Income by source	Principal place of employ-	Marital status at addition
Accounting year	ment	Residence location at
Staff:	Date of birth	addition
Discipline/training by	Sex	Presenting problem
employment/contract status	Race/ethnicity	Handicaps/impairments
Vacancies	Activity hours/sample week:	Diagnosis
Clinical consultants by	by program element	Referral source
Discipline by FT/PT	by major activity/service	History of MH services
Reporting year	Consultation/prevention	Expected payment source
No. discontinuations	hours by recipient group	Living arrangement:
No. client/patients on rolls		at addition
Program element (PE) data:		at discontinuation
PE's within organization		Discontinuations:
PE's provided by affiliation by		Volume of program
no. of clients		contact
Affiliates name/address		Circumstances at
Discontinuations by primary		discontinuation
diagnostic groups		Discontinuation referral
Census by diagnostic groups		Date of report
Primary age groups		
Inpatient/residential PE's:		
Beds		
Patient days		
Outpatient/partial care PE's:		
Additions by diagnosis		
On rolls end of year		
Partial care PE:		
Half-day sessions/week		
visits (Year)		
Outpatient PE:		
Operating hours/week		
Visits by type (year)		

Source: Adapted from Patton and Leginski (1983).

date the standards. In 1989, two new minimum data sets were added, one for financial information and the other for events. The original minimum data sets—organizations, human resources, and clients—were updated. In addition, a conceptual framework was developed for the MHSIP, based upon hierarchical, relational concepts (Figure 13.1). The clinical event was viewed as the basic unit of the system, to which one could link client, provider, and financial information, within an organizational frame. The revised and expanded set of standards was published in 1989.

These standards were subsequently expanded with specific recommendations for performance measures and for data standards for child mental health programs. The Ad Hoc Advisory Group to the MHSIP, a set of state, local, and consumer representatives, has played a particularly important role in developing the data standards and providing leadership to the field. Dr. John Hornick, director of planning for the New York Office of Mental Health, was the chairperson for 1994–1995.

In this same period, the National Institute on Drug Abuse (NIDA) and the National Institute on Alcohol Abuse and Alcoholism (NIAAA) worked with the states and local providers to define a minimum data set for a client data system (CDS) to be reported on every substance-abuse client who received care from a public provider. Items included in the minimum data set were designed to be compatible with the MHSIP, and MHSIP representatives were invited to participate in the standards development process. The CDS is still in operation.

NIMH awarded the first grants to states to implement the MHSIP data standards in 1989. The original grants (type 1) were for $100,000 per year, for up to three years of support. By 1994, virtually all the states and territories had received one of these grants. Throughout this early period of MHSIP development, two persons were instrumental in its success: Cecil Wurster, formerly chief of the branch with responsibility for the MHSIP program, and Dr. Walter Leginski, currently chief of CMHS programs for persons with mental illness who are homeless.

In 1992, the NIMH grant announcement was expanded to include a second phase of implementation grants (type 2) and decision application grants (type 3) for the states. The second-phase grants were intended to facilitate more complete implementation of the MHSIP standards; the decision application grants were for the purpose of developing and demonstrating the capacity to apply actual data to administrative, policy, or research problems. Both types carried stipends of $125,000 per year, for up to three years of support. As of 1995, when the grant announcement was revised by CMHS (the current organizational location of federal mental health data collection activities), about three-fifths of the states and territories had received second-phase implementation grants, and about one-fifth, decision application grants.

FIGURE 13.1. CORE INFORMATION REQUIRED FOR DECISION SUPPORT SYSTEMS IN MENTAL HEALTH ORGANIZATIONS

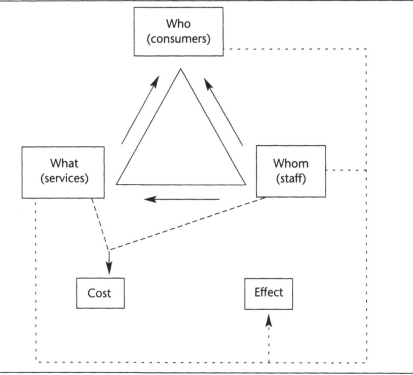

Source: Adapted from Leginski et al. (1989).

Current Efforts at Standardization

In 1995, CMHS adapted the grant announcement to the dramatic changes that were occurring in the environment. The new announcement focused attention on use of information for problem resolution; capacity development received less attention. The 1995 announcement was directed toward the facilitation of comprehensive state mental health planning and adaptation of the state mental health agency to healthcare reform initiatives being planned or implemented by the state. These topics are described in this chapter.

Historically, most state mental health agencies have employed statistical information to plan only for state-operated or state-funded programs. This planning typically has not included mental health organizations or practitioners from other not-for-profit or private-sector entities. Similarly, mental health services delivered through primary care organizations or practitioners, social service organizations, or self-help groups have not been encompassed in this planning.

As the states move toward managed care, it is essential that their planning be expanded to encompass the entire population with mental illness, as well as high-risk groups. This will permit each state to understand the dynamics of clients who move from private-sector plans to public-sector managed care programs or other safety net programs operated by the state. The new MHSIP grant announcement encourages the acquisition and analysis of quantitative data for such planning.

State healthcare reform initiatives are proceeding at a rapid pace. In most states, these initiatives center on application for a federal waiver to transform the state Medicaid program into a managed care plan operated by a private-sector management services organization. Frequently, these waivers are designed to develop separate managed care plans for populations with mental illness or substance-abuse problems, that is, carve-out programs.

To plan for managed care programs, the state needs to design a benefit package, develop homogeneous risk pools of consumers who will use different types and intensities of services, estimate the per-client per-year cost for each of the risk pools, develop a plan for how essential ancillary services will be provided and reimbursed, and prepare baseline service information prior to implementation of the managed care program so that performance can be assessed.

In the implementation phase for privatized managed care programs, state activities will change from planning to monitoring the performance of programs. In this phase, additional data are needed on population health status, enrollment, encounters, outcomes, and system performance indicators; the last-named need to be synopsized in report cards for payers or consumers. The new MHSIP grant announcement is designed to encourage states to use statistical information for these planning and implementation activities.

Key Consumer Input

Since 1990, NIMH and more recently CMHS have provided support for a Mental Health Consumer/Survivor Research and Policy Work Group, comprising consumer leaders from the field. The purpose of the group has been to provide advice to the government and to the MHSIP on the development and implementation of data standards for mental health. The Work Group has helped to define person-centered data systems that reflect a major shift in philosophy toward persons who use services. This has heightened awareness of consumer perspectives on service delivery, outcome, and recovery processes.

As a second major endeavor, the Consumer/Survivor Work Group has engaged in research through focus groups to define the cognitive maps that consumers use to think about service outcome. Currently, the work group is participating with CMHS and MHSIP in the development of a managed care report card for mental health and substance abuse. Development of this report card will create a method of providing feedback to consumers on plan performance. The final product will be made available to the states for use in their contracts with managed care organizations.

Data Standards for Behavioral Healthcare

The MHSIP data standards provide an excellent foundation for the information systems required by managed behavioral healthcare. However, the current system of standards requires expansion and modification to meet the full range of information needs in the future. We next identify essential developments in content, recording, and transmission standards.

Content Standards

Essential components of a good information system for managed care include, at the person level, data on the health status of the covered population, enrollment and encounter data for each covered person, and outcome data. In addition, the system will include information on disorder rates in the general population, descriptive information on the organization and operation of managed care entities and the providers that contract with them, and performance information on individual managed care plans (Figure 13.2).

Health Status Data. Health status data should be collected at the individual level in order to assess the individual's need for treatment. This would include information on the nature of the mental health or substance-abuse problem being experienced and the impact of that problem on the functioning of the person. The essential concept is to identify problem and functioning measures that are predictive of the need for mental health or substance-abuse services and that can be used in the development and assessment of clinical treatment plans.

Some work has been completed in this area. The National Co-morbidity Survey is based on the Composite International Diagnostic Instrument (CIDI). The CIDI is an instrument through which lay interviewers can assess psychiatric and substance-abuse diagnoses. Dr. Ron Kessler has completed methodological work on the CIDI to identify stem questions that are highly predictive of diagnosis. At present, the "CIDI stems" need to be codified into data standards, and a parallel

FIGURE 13.2. MODEL OF DATA FOR MANAGED CARE

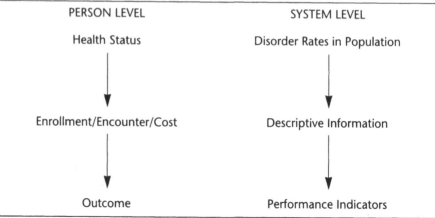

PERSON LEVEL	SYSTEM LEVEL
Health Status	Disorder Rates in Population
↓	↓
Enrollment/Encounter/Cost	Descriptive Information
↓	↓
Outcome	Performance Indicators

Source: Adapted from Leginski et al. (1989).

set of items on functioning needs to be added to these standards (see the following discussion of outcome measures).

Enrollment and Encounter Data. Enrollment and encounter data are required to monitor managed care plans. Enrollment data should be collected at the individual rather than the aggregate group level; they can provide an overview of the sociodemographic characteristics of an enrolled population. Together with health status data, enrollment information permits the construction of different risk pools when coupled with service use information. By contrast, encounter data are needed to provide a running account of services received *and* their costs for each client. Such information can be used by providers to determine whether they are exceeding agreed-upon capitation rates; it can also be used by states and other payers to monitor what types of persons are receiving what types of care and how this compares with the health status. MHSIP provides an excellent foundation for encounter data through the event data set developed as part of the 1989 standards.

Currently, the Subcommittee on Mental Health Statistics of the U.S. Department of Health and Human Services' National Committee on Vital and Health Statistics is debating what should be recommended for enrollment and encounter minimum data sets. The subcommittee will pay particular attention to what would differ in enrollment and encounter data standards for populations with mental health and substance-abuse problems, compared with other populations. The national committee is preparing to issue proposed enrollment and encounter minimum data sets to the entire health field; the work of the subcommittee will be incorporated into this product. In anticipation, the Ad Hoc Advisory Group to the MHSIP is preparing a report on enrollment and encounter data sets to submit to the subcommittee.

Outcome Data. Outcome data are a necessary component of an integrated managed care MIS. Yet, a major deficit of the mental health and substance-abuse fields is the lack of agreement among consumers, family members, clinicians, rehabilitation specialists, administrators, and researchers about how to measure the outcome of services. This deficit has hampered the development of improved clinical protocols, as well as the standing of these fields in the broader clinical community.

In recognition of the need for rapid developments in the area of outcome assessment, the National Alliance for the Mentally Ill (NAMI) has entered into a collaborative project with CMHS, NIMH, NIDA, NIAAA, and the Eli Lilly Co., to engage in three tasks: development of a set of principles for outcome measures and systems; implementation of a longitudinal demonstration to document an improved outcome measurement system; and evolution of a communication strategy that can highlight the progress being made in this area. Broad-based input will be sought from the mental health and substance-abuse fields on the products from this project.

Other projects are evolving to examine how current instruments, such as the Behavior and Symptom Identification Scale (BASIS-32), the Medical Outcomes Study Short Form (SF36), and the Global Assessment of Functioning (GAF) can be abbreviated and adapted for a managed care environment. Clearly, a need exists for the evolution of data standards for outcome measures.

Disorder Rates in the Population. Population data should be collected on a sample basis to allow for assessment of disorder rates and the overall health status of the general community population. These data comprise a necessary component for adequate services planning at the system level. The collection of these data over time can be used to provide information on overall system performance with respect to its effect on the general population.

The ability to obtain this type of data hinges on the efforts under way to develop and test good predictive health status measures that can be used within general population samples. The "CIDI stems" described earlier have already been incorporated into the 1994 National Household Survey of Drug Abuse, an annual household survey conducted by the Office of Applied Studies within SAMHSA. It is anticipated that they will also be included in the triennial periodic modules of the redesigned National Health Interview Survey, scheduled for initiation in 1996 by the National Center for Health Statistics.

Descriptive Information. Descriptive information is required on managed care entities and on the mental health organizations and providers that contract with them. Such characteristics as organizational structure and linkages, types of plans and services, types of payers and enrollees, types of organizational and individual providers, and sources of revenues and expenditures are relevant. This information is similar to that collected through the Inventory of Mental Health Organizations and General Hospital Mental Health Services (IMHO), currently conducted by CMHS.

The 1994 IMHO has already been modified to collect information on the participation of mental health organizations in managed care plans. In addition, a checklist was developed to collect information on the range of services available through these organizations. The evolution of the IMHO will continue to reflect the changes being made in managed care practices.

Plans are developed to collect information from managed care entities that operate or contract for networks of providers, as well as for health maintenance organizations (HMOs) that either provide directly or contract for mental health services. Initial work in this area is being undertaken in late 1995 through a CMHS meeting with managed care entities. Clearly, organizational data standards will require revision to accommodate these new requirements.

Performance Information. Performance information is required to evaluate managed care plans. *Report cards* are one specific form of performance information that will spark dialogue among key groups as they are developed. As noted above, CMHS is currently collaborating with the MHSIP and representatives of the consumer community to develop a mental health and substance-abuse report card, primarily from the consumer perspective. This report card will encompass the key dimensions of access, appropriateness, outcome, prevention, and satisfaction. It is anticipated that this report card will be available in prototype form for critical review by fall 1995.

Simultaneously, CMHS is working with other key groups in developing behavioral healthcare report cards to facilitate coordination among them. One meeting has already been held among these groups, and additional meetings are planned. These groups are the National Committee on Quality Assurance (NCQA), the Joint Commission on Accreditation of Healthcare Organizations (JCAHO), the American Managed Behavioral Healthcare Association (AMBHA), the Institute for Behavioral Healthcare (IBH), and NAMI. A collaborative endeavor among these entities can provide the framework for data standards in this area.

Recording and Transmission Standards

Equally of concern to the mental health and substance-abuse fields are recording standards for clinical data and transmission standards for sharing electronic versions of clinical and financial information. Recording standards are needed for the mental health and substance-abuse components of an electronic patient record, which is currently being developed. Transmission standards are concerned with the form in which information is sent and received electronically, as well as the format that is employed for such information. Both areas are intimately linked with privacy and confidentiality concerns.

Recording Standards. Recording standards are very important at present because they will ultimately define the clinical information that is captured about clients and the services they receive. In most instances, derivative statistical information will be limited by the nature and scope of this electronic information. CMHS is currently supporting an Ad Hoc Work Group for the Computerization of Behavioral Health and Human Service Records that will prepare recommendations for recording standards.

Transmission Standards. At present, most work on transmission standards is outside the fields of mental health and substance abuse. The National Institute on Standards and Technology (NIST) of the U.S. Department of Commerce is currently working in this area, and the European Common Union (ECU) has set up a project to identify appropriate transmission standards. At minimum, information representatives in the mental health and substance-abuse fields need to stay abreast of this work.

Partnerships for the Future

As we prepare for the twenty-first century, we need to envision how we will develop data standards for the future and the new partnerships and joint ventures that will be needed to make this possible. Clearly, task focus and partnership linkage are interdependent and synergistic. We suggest several major partnerships that could be very productive at the present time, together with a brief comment on the partners who can make these endeavors successful.

Partnerships to Revise Current MHSIP Data Standards. These partnerships must be a high priority in the short term. The areas that should be incorporated or revised have already been described above: health status, enrollment and encounter, outcome, and system description and performance. The key to future work in this area is to add new partners, such as managed care entities and HMOs, while continuing the excellent collaboration of CMHS with consumers, providers, and states initiated in the past. This work should be undertaken as soon as possible in order to maintain consistency of information collected on managed behavioral healthcare, as this field evolves rapidly.

Partnerships to Develop a Mental Health and Substance-Abuse Report Card for Managed Care. This is another high priority. Previous work has been described above. The critical issue at present is to achieve an appropriate level of consistency in report cards across public and private plans and different service settings. For example, report cards for private plans may not require the same range of information as those for public plans because the clients are vastly different and their service needs are not as extensive. However, when the same topic is covered on different report cards, then it is reasonable to expect that it be measured in comparable ways. All major entities developing report cards for managed behavioral healthcare—CMHS/MHSIP, the National Committee on Quality Assurance, the Institute for Behavioral Healthcare, the Joint Commission on Accreditation of Healthcare Organizations, the American Managed Behavioral Healthcare Association, and the National Alliance for the Mentally Ill—need to be partners in this endeavor. Private-sector managed behavioral healthcare entities that already have report cards should also be consulted.

Joint Activities with WHO. This holds promise for helping us learn from projects already carried out in other countries, as well as for developing a data base for comparative intercountry analyses. WHO also frequently serves as a conduit for the sharing of informal knowledge about regional projects being conducted in Europe, the Far East, etc. Within this context, joint projects with WHO on data standards can facilitate more rapid development of appropriate standards in the United States.

High priority needs to be given to the development of joint projects with WHO around data standards for health status and outcome, as well as data standards for a more discrete and operational array of mental health and substance-abuse services. WHO already has projects under way on the former topic, for example, revision of the International Classification of Impairment, Disability, and Handicap (ICIDH); and WHO has held several preliminary meetings with the United States and other countries on the latter topic.

Collaboration with AMBHA and the Group Health Association of America (GHAA). This collaboration is very important for establishing appropriate data standards for managed behavioral healthcare entities. AMBHA represents and understands managed behavioral healthcare entities that operate in a network environment; GHAA represents and understands HMOs and their mental health and substance-abuse components. An opportunity exists to work with AMBHA and GHAA in the development of future information projects within their organizations, as well as to elicit their participation in broader projects. CMHS needs to employ a federal leadership role to convene these entities with others in common data pursuits.

Recommendations for the Future

Here are several general recommendations for the future that ensue from the review previously outlined. Each reflects a different facet of the data standards enterprise for the mental health and substance-abuse fields. Some will be relatively easy to achieve; others, relatively difficult.

- *In the future, joint endeavors between government—federal, state, and local—and the private-sector mental health and substance-abuse industry will be the only feasible way to ensure essential consistency in data standards.* As all levels of government assume a smaller role in providing direct mental health and substance-abuse service with the growth of contracted managed behavioral healthcare, the focus of standards development will also need to shift to the private sector. Government will be able to make this shift and maintain accountability to the Congress and state legislatures through the types of partnerships and joint ventures described above. Such partnerships should be initiated in the near future.
- *Data standards development activities must reflect the views of all participants.* Partnerships between government and the private sector reflect part of the picture. Consumers, family members, and providers are essential to complete it. Although the MHSIP has done an excellent job in bringing these groups to key partnerships, more needs to be done to bring their points of view on data and information to the managed behavioral healthcare industry. Clearly, each of these groups is directly affected by any decisions reached by the industry; hence, they should have a voice in these decisions.
- *Adaptation to unanticipated future changes will be a necessary part of the data enterprise over the next decade.* Managed behavioral healthcare is now established. However, the future course is uncertain with respect to which structures and methods will predominate: separate managed behavioral healthcare plans, integrated general healthcare networks, HMOs that include behavioral healthcare, or other forms. Likewise, the development and adoption of computer technology is proceeding at a fast pace, but the future course is not completely clear. The data standards enterprise needs to anticipate and adapt to new developments when—if not before—they arise, rather than to lag behind those changes by several years. This can only occur if careful attention is given to developments in services and technologies as they occur, with reflection upon their data implications.

- *Data standards should adequately reflect "virtuality" in service delivery systems.* The most efficient, cost-effective way to achieve comprehensive, seamless service systems in the future is not likely to be through the development of a single service cafeteria in which all services are available, but rather through contractual and computer linkages among these services so that they are seamless from the perspective of consumers and providers. This approach represents a "virtual" organization. Such virtual organizations are likely to become very common as mental health and substance-abuse services are linked with general healthcare services, and social services, housing, and other services are brought under the managed care umbrella. Data standards should reflect these virtual organizations and be capable of permitting interface among their service components.

◆ ◆ ◆

The future holds considerable promise. We must be prepared to meet the challenges that it presents. Clearly, our past and present have positioned us to do this in an excellent manner.

Notes

P. 254, *that include mental health and chemical dependency:* Oss, M. (1995). More Americans enrolled in managed behavioral care. *Open Minds, 8*(12), 12. Gettysburg, PA: Behavioral Health Industry News, Inc.

P. 255, *the 1880 census of the population:* Manderscheid, R., Witkin, M., Rosenstein, M., & Bass, R. (1986). The national reporting program for mental health statistics: History and findings. *Public Health Reports, 101*(5), 532–539; Redick, R., Manderscheid, R., Witkin, M., & Rosenstein, M. (1983). *A history of the U.S. National Reporting Program for Mental Health Statistics 1840–1983.* (DHHS Pub. No. ADM 83–1296). Washington, DC: U.S. Government Printing Office.

P. 256, *The 1983 MHSIP data standards:* Patton, R., & Leginski, W. (1983). *The design and content of a national mental health statistics system.* (DHHS Pub. No. ADM 83–1095). Washington, DC: U.S. Government Printing Office.

P. 258, *set of standards published in 1989:* Leginski, W., Croze, C., Driggers, J., Dumpman, S., Geertsen, D., Kamis-Gould, E., Namerow, M., Patton, R., Wilson, N., & Wurster, C. (1989). *Data standards for mental health decision support systems.* (DHHS Pub. No. ADM 89–1589). Washington, DC: U.S. Government Printing Office.

P. 258, *care from a public provider:* Blanken, A. (1989, June). Evolution of a national data base for drug abuse treatment clients. In *Community Epidemiology Work Group: Epidemiologic Trends in Drug Abuse—Proceedings,* Rockville, MD, pp. 48–53; National Institute on Drug Abuse. (1990). *Client data system: Alcohol and drug abuse client minimum data set.* Unpublished manuscript. Rockville, MD: Author.

P. 260, *persons who use services:* Campbell, J., & Frey, E. (undated). *Humanizing decision support systems.* Unpublished manuscript, submitted to the MHSIP Ad Hoc Advisory Group. Rockville, MD: Center for Mental Health Services.

P. 261, *think about service outcome:* Trochim, W., Dumont, J., & Campbell, J. (1993). *A report for the state mental health agency profiling system: Mapping mental health outcomes from the perspective of consumers/survivors.* Alexandria, VA: National Association of State Mental Health Program Directors Research Institute, Inc.

P. 261, *report card for mental health and substance abuse:* MHSIP Task Force on Design of the Mental Health Component of a Health Plan Report Card under National Health Care Reform. (1994). *Mental health component of a health plan report card: Progress report.* Unpublished manuscript. Rockville, MD: Center for Mental Health Services.

P. 261, *The National Co-morbidity Survey:* Kessler, R., McGonagle, K., Zhao, S., Nelson, C., Hughes, M., Eshleman, S., Wittchen, H., & Kendler, K. (1994). Lifetime and twelve-month prevalence of DSM-III-R psychiatric disorders in the United States. *Archives of General Psychiatry, 51,* 8–19.

P. 262, *developed as part of the 1989 standards:* Leginski, W., Croze, C., Driggers, J., Dumpman, S., Geertsen, D., Kamis-Gould E., Namerow, M., Patton, R., Wilson, N., & Wurster, C. (1989). *Data standards for mental health decision support systems.* (DHHS Pub. No. ADM 89–1589). Washington, DC: U.S. Government Printing Office.

P. 263, *report on enrollment and encounter data sets:* Center for Mental Health Services. (1995). *Common core health data set project for enrollment and encounter: The preliminary results of a national survey of leading experts in mental health, substance abuse, chronic disabilities, long term care and managed care data collection.* Unpublished manuscript. Rockville, MD: Author.

P. 263, *adapted for a managed care environment:* Andrews, G., Peters, L., & Teesson, M. (1994). *The measurement of consumer outcome in mental health: A report to the National Mental Health Information Strategy Committee.* Sydney: Clinical Research Unit for Anxiety Disorders.

P. 264, *currently conducted by CMHS:* Redick, R., Witkin, M., Atay, J., & Manderscheid, R. (1994). Highlights of organized mental health services in 1990 and major national and state trends. In R. Manderscheid & M. Sonnenschein (Eds)., *Mental Health, United States, 1994.* (DHHS Pub. No. SMA 94–3000). Washington DC: U.S. Government Printing Office.

P. 265, *recommendations for recording standards:* Work Group for Computerization of Behavioral Health and Human Services Records. (1995). *National survey on the state of computerization among top managed behavioral healthcare companies in America.* Unpublished manuscript. Rockville, MD: Center for Mental Health Services.

EPILOGUE

Tom Trabin

Technology is advancing so rapidly, and computerization is transforming behavioral healthcare so dramatically, that any attempt to summarize the contents of this book would only be a series of still frames that capture a few moments in this high-speed cinema. So perhaps it's best to simply say, "Stay tuned for more news."

Nevertheless, we realize there is a constant and continuing need for the most up-to-date information on new technologies throughout the behavioral healthcare industry—among providers, administrators, and payers—for consumers, individual clinicians, small groups, and large organizations. That's why we at CentraLink and the Institute for Behavioral Healthcare have developed an ongoing series of informatics initiatives, including our annual national conference and exposition, "Behavioral Informatics Tomorrow," regular features and columns in our journal, *Behavioral Healthcare Tomorrow,* information found at CentraLink's Web Site, and more. We have created and want to support an ongoing community of professionals involved in the computerization of behavioral healthcare and hope to enrich your work as part of that community.

Through these services, reports, and dialogues, we intend to continue our commitment to providing you with the most important and useful information available on new information technologies and their creative applications. We think implementation of these technologies is one of the most vitally important challenges facing the behavioral healthcare field. If you would like more information about our forums, please contact us through our Web Site at http://centralink.com or call 415/435–9821.

ABOUT THE AUTHORS

Marion J. Ball, Ed.D., is a tireless advocate of health informatics who serves on the Board of Regents of the National Library of Medicine (NLM) and is a member of the College of Health Information Management Executives (CHIME). Through these and her many other activities, both at home and abroad, she works to effect the transformation of healthcare through information technology.

In July 1995, she completed a three-year term as president of the International Medical Informatics Association (IMIA). Within IMIA, she cochaired an international working conference on the health professional workstation and encouraged formation of a working group on the organizational impacts of health informatics. Earlier she was a member of the Institute of Medicine's Committee to Improve the Patient Record and cochaired the Information Technology Subcommittee, helping to shape recommendations for a computer-based patient record (CPR). Today she is active in telemedicine, telehealth, and associated topics, including the use of the Internet and World Wide Web for training and education.

Chief information officer at the University of Maryland at Baltimore, Ball holds a doctorate in continuing medical education from Temple University. She publishes and lectures widely.

Howard L. Bleich, M.D., is associate professor of medicine at Harvard Medical School and copresident of the Center for Clinical Computing. He was a founding fellow of the American College of Medical Informatics and is an associate editor of *M.D. Computing*. He received his bachelor's degrees from George Washington University and his medical degree from Emory University.

Bleich began work with computers in medicine in 1968, when he developed a computer-based consultation program to evaluate and suggest treatment for electrolyte and acid-base disorders. He was the principal investigator of the research that produced PaperChase, a self-service bibliographic retrieval program that permits physicians and scientists to search the National Library of Medicine's MEDLINE data base and other data bases for references to biomedical literature.

During the past fifteen years, Bleich and his colleagues at the Center for Clinical Computing have developed, implemented, and evaluated an integrated, hospitalwide clinical computing system in use for patient care at Boston's Beth Israel and Brigham and Women's hospitals.

Anthony Broskowski, Ph.D., is president of Managed Care Solutions, specializing in computer models for capitation, disease management, and integrated healthcare delivery systems. He previously served as director of healthcare information for Prudential Insurance Co. and senior vice president and senior analyst at Preferred Health Care, Ltd. (now Value Behavioral Health), a firm specializing in mental health "carve-outs." From 1977 to 1986 he served as the executive director of Northside Centers in Tampa, Florida, where he developed a comprehensive and innovative system of alternative mental health programs for adults and children.

Broskowski earned his Ph.D. in clinical psychology from Indiana University in 1967. Following three years as an assistant professor at the University of Pittsburgh, he completed a year of postdoctoral training at the Laboratory of Community Psychiatry, Harvard Medical School, and continued there for seven years as a member of the Harvard faculty. He has served as a consultant to major corporations, federal and state government agencies, and nonprofit human service agencies. He has published extensively on the topics of executive leadership, mental health program administration and systems of managed care, computer information systems, program evaluation, and management of risks; he has edited a book on the subject of organizational and clinical linkages between mental health and primary healthcare.

Peter Currie, Ph.D., received his doctorate in clinical psychology in 1983 from the California School of Professional Psychology in Los Angeles. After seven years in private practice, he cofounded Psychological Health Resources, Inc. (PHR), in 1990 and is currently president. PHR is a regional provider group that specializes in serving managed care organizations; since its inception, PHR has grown to provide behavioral health services to approximately three hundred thousand plan members. As PHR grew, Currie recognized the need to reengineer the group practice utilizing advanced information technology. He founded Psychological Health Technologies, a company focused on developing a computerized patient record called Psych Vision designed specifically for behavioral healthcare group practices.

Judith V. Douglas, M.H.S., holds master's degrees from Northwestern University and the Johns Hopkins University School of Hygiene and Public Health; she was a University Fellow at Yale.

Now a director of information services at the University of Maryland at Baltimore, Douglas previously worked at Blue Cross/Blue Shield of Maryland and the Kennedy Krieger Institute and taught at Towson State and Western Michigan Universities. She is a published author and editor in health informatics.

Kathleen A. Frawley, J.D., M.S., R.R.A., is director of the Washington, D.C., Office for the American Health Information Management Association (AHIMA). She received her bachelor's degree in English from the College of Mount St. Vincent in New York, her master of science in health services administration from Wagner College, and her law degree from New York Law School. She is certified as a registered record administrator by the AHIMA. She is a member of the New York Bar Association.

Frawley has written and lectured extensively. She was the recipient of the 1991 Distinguished Faculty Award for the Health Information Management Program at Touro College in New York. She has served as cochair for the Workgroup on Confidentiality, Privacy, and Security for the Computer-Based Patient Record Institute (CPRI) since 1992. She currently serves as secretary on the executive committee for CPRI.

Additionally, she represents AHIMA on the Workgroup on Electronic Data Interchange (WEDI) board of directors and Hospital Open Systems Team (HOST) board of directors. She is currently secretary on the Executive Committee for HOST.

Michael A. Freeman, M.D., is the chairman of the **Behavioral Healthcare Tomorrow** national dialogue conference, the editor-in-chief of the *Behavioral Healthcare* Tomorrow journal, and the general editor of the Jossey-Bass Managed Behavioral Healthcare Library. He also serves as the CEO of the Partnership for Behavioral Healthcare and the president of the Institute for Behavioral Healthcare; both organizations are dedicated to improving American and global mental health and addiction treatment benefits, management, services, and outcomes.

Dr. Freeman is a psychiatrist and a member of the clinical faculty at the Langley Porter Psychiatric Institute of the University of California, San Francisco,

Medical Center. He is a specialist and consultant in the managed behavioral healthcare purchasing, managed care, and services fields.

Robert Gellman, J.D., is a privacy and information policy consultant in Washington, D.C. He has served as chief counsel for subcommittees on information, justice, transportation, and agriculture in the U.S. House of Representatives. He has also held the chief counsel position for the House Committee on Government Operations. He received his bachelor of arts degree in 1970 from the University of Pennsylvania and earned his J.D. degree in 1973 at Yale Law School.

Wallace J. Gingerich, M.S.W., Ph.D., is professor of social work at the Mandel School of Applied Social Sciences, Case Western Reserve University, where he previously served as associate dean and interim dean. His current research is directed toward developing a computer-assisted record keeping system for case managers serving persons with chronic mental illness.

Gingerich publishes widely and has consulted with many public and private human service agencies on computer applications and brief therapy. His memberships include the National Association of Social Workers, the Council on Social Work Education, and the American Association for Marriage and Family Therapy. He received his M.S.W. and Ph.D. in social work from Washington University in St. Louis and was a postdoctoral fellow in mental health intervention design at the University of Michigan. Prior to coming to Cleveland, he practiced psychiatric social work in several community mental health settings in California and was a member of the faculty of the School of Social Welfare at the University of Wisconsin-Milwaukee.

Roger L. Gould, M.D., is a psychoanalyst and former head of the psychiatric outpatient department and community psychiatry at UCLA. His work in adult development was popularized by Gail Sheehy's book *Passages.* His many contributions to the psychiatric literature are summarized in his book *Transformations: Growth and Change in Adult Life* (1978). He founded Interactive Health Systems, a company devoted to developing psychoeducational and therapeutic programs in the field of adult development. He created the Therapeutic Learning Program (TLP), computer-assisted therapy designed to help adolescents and adults break through developmental blocks.

Marilyn J. Henderson, M.P.A., is currently the assistant chief of the Survey and Analysis Branch, Division of State and Community Systems Development, Center for Mental Health Services. Previously, she served as a survey statistician within the National Institute of Mental Health (NIMH) since 1976. At NIMH, she had primary responsibility for the development and implementation of national sample surveys of persons receiving services within mental health organizations. She has published widely on data collected through these surveys.

Eugene D. Hill III, M.B.A., is currently a venture partner at Accel Partners, a venture capital firm, where he focuses on healthcare service investments. His most recent position was president of behavioral health at United HealthCare Corp. He has been a managed healthcare consultant, venture capital advisor, and serves on the board of directors of Psychiatric Management Resources, CMG Healthcare, and Medintell Systems.

He served as president and chief executive officer of U.S. Behavioral Health from 1988 to 1992, a managed behavioral healthcare company he built from a start-up venture and sold to Travelers Corporation in 1990. Prior to his association with U.S. Behavioral Health, he was president and chairman of Sierra Health and Life Insurance, a company he founded. He also served as the administrator of Southern Nevada Memorial Hospital and Boston City Hospital. His early positions included responsibility for emergency medical services for the City of Boston and the City and County of Denver. He received his baccalaureate from Middlebury College and his M.B.A. in healthcare from Boston University; he completed Harvard University's Executive Program in Health Systems Management.

Michael W. Hurst, Ed.D., is a licensed psychologist who received his doctorate in counseling psychology from Boston University in 1974 and his baccalaureate from Massachusetts Institute of Technology in 1970. He is president of InStream Corp., where he has been the principal architect of the InStream Provider Network (IPN) along with enabling software for the behavioral healthcare industry. Previously he was corporate vice president, EAP and integrated care programs, of American PsychManagement (APM, now part of Value Behavioral Health) and chief operating officer of APM-Hurst after his own company was acquired by APM. He began his career at Boston University School of Medicine, where he remains associate professor of psychiatry (psychology).

William R. Maloney, M.B.A., M.P., has held a variety of positions on both the insurance and provider sides of healthcare delivery systems since he came to the field in 1986. During his career, he has been chief operating officer of a group practice; has developed a utilization review program for a managed care insurer; and has led HMO provider network development, provider and client contracting, provider credentialing, and managed care information systems. Prior to joining the national behavioral health consulting team at William M. Mercer, Inc., in 1994, Maloney was vice president of the Behavioral Health Strategic Business

Unit at United HealthCare Corp. in Minneapolis. He earned his bachelor's in psychology from the University of Illinois, his master's degree in management from the Kellogg School at Northwestern University, and his master's in planning from the Illinois Institute of Technology.

Ronald W. Manderscheid, Ph.D. serves as policy advisor on national healthcare reform in the Office of the Assistant Secretary for Health, U.S. Department of Health and Human Services, and as chief of the Survey and Analysis Branch, Division of State and Community Systems Development, Center for Mental Health Services. Previously, he was with the National Institute of Mental Health (NIMH) since 1973. He served as chief of the Statistical Research Branch, where he provided strong leadership in implementing the National Reporting System (NRP) and the Mental Health Statistics Improvement Program (MHSIP). He is noted for his publications on service delivery to persons with serious mental illness and the organization of the mental health service system. For the past three editions, he has served as editor of *Mental Health, United States.* In addition, he has served as the chairperson of the Sociological Practice Section of the American Sociological Association, and as president of the Washington Academy of Sciences and the District of Columbia Sociological Society. In 1993, he was a member of the Mental Health and Substance Abuse Work Group of the President's Task Force on Health Care Reform.

Kevin L. Moreland, Ph.D., obtained his doctoral degree in clinical psychology in 1981 from the University of North Carolina at Chapel Hill. After a postdoctoral fellowship in the Department of Psychiatry at Washington University's (St. Louis) School of Medicine, he worked at National Computer Systems (NCS) in Minneapolis, where he was involved in research and development on many psychological tests, including the Rorschach, MMPI-2, and Millon inventories, and their associated computer products and services. Moreland has published over fifty chapters and articles in professional journals. He coedited *Taming Technology: Issues, Strategies, and Resources for the Mental Health Practitioner* (1993, with B. Schlosser) and coauthored *Responsible Test Use: Case Studies in Human Behavior* (1993, with L. Eyde, G. Robertson, S. Kruge, et al.) and *The Rorschach Technique: Perceptual Basics, Content Interpretation, and Applications* (1994, with E. Aronow and M. Reznikoff). He is especially well known for his publications about computer-based psychological assessment. Currently on the faculty at Fordham University, Cornell University Medical College, and John Jay College of Criminal Justice, Moreland also presents workshops on psychological assessment throughout the country. He is on the editorial boards of *Assessment, Journal of Personality Assessment,* and *Psychological Assessment.*
Moreland's Internet address is moreland@murray.fordham.edu

Murray Naditch, Ph.D., M.B.A., is founder, president, and chief executive officer of Strategic Advantage, Inc. He holds a doctoral degree in psychology with honors, an M.B.A. in business strategy from the University of Chicago, an M.S. in operations research and marketing, and a B.S. in industrial administration from Carnegie–Mellon University. He is a graduate of the Executive Program in Business Strategy at the Harvard University School of Business.

Naditch designed and directed the Staywell Program, which originated at Control Data Corp. and became the largest heart-attack prevention program in American industry. He founded and was the former chief of the Department of Behavioral Medicine at the Bowman Gray School of Medicine at Wake Forest University and was a former faculty member in the Department of Psychology at Cornell University. He has been the principal investigator for five major federally funded and two privately funded research grants and has published more than forty papers in the scientific research literature. He is a licensed clinical psychologist and a Fellow of the Academy of Behavioral Medicine.

Tuan D. Nguyen, Ph.D., is the deputy director for decision support systems for the Mental Health/Mental Retardation Authority of Harris County, Texas. Since obtaining his doctorate in social psychology from Purdue University, he has been involved in numerous research, program evaluation, billing system, and statistical data system development projects in the fields of mental health, substance abuse, and forensic services. He has taught graduate-level courses and seminars at the University of California San Francisco, University of California at Berkeley, the California School of Professional Psychology, and the University of Texas Medical Center in Houston. He has made numerous professional presentations at local and national conferences on the topics of data system implementation and management, program evaluation, minority service utilization research, and minority mental health programs development. He serves on the Technology Leadership Group of the Texas Council of Community Mental Health/Mental Retardation Centers, the outcome subcommittee of the council's Managed Care Task Force, and the Management Practices Work Group of the council's Managed Care Readiness Task Force.

Gary Olsen, M.S.P.H., is the associate director for information systems and data processing at Valley Mental Health in Salt Lake City. For the past twenty-four years, he has assumed both clinical and information systems responsibilities in the field of mental health. He has presented numerous workshops and courses on management and use of data, on design and implementation of performance indicator methodology, and on graphical representation of data for managers. He has provided consultation on information systems design, request-for-proposal development, system implementation, and systems assessment. His most recent consultees include the states of Arkansas and West Virginia. He holds membership in the national Ad Hoc Advisory Group for the Mental Health Statistics Improvement Program (MHSIP) of the national Center for Mental Health Services, the MHSIP Advisory Group for the state of Utah, the national MHSIP task force on enrollment and encounter data design, and the American Management Association.

William A. Roiter, Ed.D., is a licensed psychologist who graduated from Boston University with a doctorate in counseling psychology in 1981 and a baccalaureate in education in 1973. He is a senior vice president of sales and marketing for In-Stream Corp. Previously he was vice president of sales for American PsychManagement (now part of Value Behavioral Health) after his and Michael Hurst's previous company was acquired by APM. He began his career at Elliot Community Mental Health Center, where he founded the first community health-center-based employee assistance programs for industry.

Larry D. Rosen, Ph.D., and *Michelle M. Weil, Ph.D.,* are coowners of Byte Back Technology Consultation Services in Orange, California. They are experts in the psychology of technology, with dozens of research publications and invited presentations over the past twelve years. Weil is a clinical psychologist with a private practice; she recently appeared on CNN, CNBC, and CBS's "48 Hours" to talk about technophobia. Rosen is a professor and past chair of psychology at California State University, Dominguez Hills, and recent winner of his university's Outstanding Professor Award. Their most recent work includes articles in the *Journal of Consumer Affairs* and *Computers in Human Behavior.* Internet address: lrosen@dhvx20.csudh.edu (or e-mail to:) 7420579@mcimail.com

Charles Safran, M.D., is currently director of clinical systems at Boston's Beth Israel Hospital and an assistant professor of medicine at Harvard Medical School. He was one of the founding members of the Medical Decision Making Group at Massachusetts Institute of Technology's Laboratory of Computer Science, where he began working in 1973. There he developed one of the first medical decision support systems to help oncologists choose cost-effective sequences of tests when staging patients with Hodgkin's disease.

In 1983, he joined Drs. Howard Bleich and Warner Slack at Beth Israel Hospital's Center for Clinical Computing in Boston. He began work on a data base combining, for the first time, clinical and administrative data that were routinely collected in the hospital's computer systems. The data base and its user interface, together called ClinQuery, have gained national and international attention.

Because of this work, Safran has been recognized as an expert on the storage, access, and use of integrated clinical and administrative data.

He is currently cochair of the National Library of Medicine/Agency for Health Care Policy and Research's national collaborative research project on the electronic patient record. He is a member of the board of directors of the American Medical Informatics Association and a respected colleague of medical informatics workers throughout Europe.

Dick Schoech, Ph.D., is a professor in administrative and community practice at the University of Texas at Arlington's School of Social Work. He has previously worked as the executive director of a comprehensive health planning council, as a regional mental health planner, and in several other human service agencies. He received an interdisciplinary Ph.D. in administration from the University of Texas at Arlington schools of business, social work, and urban studies. He is founder (1981) and coordinator of Computer Use in Social Services Network (CUSSN) and founder of CUSSNet, the electronic/BBS component of the CUSSN. He is also editor of *Computers in Human Services.*

He has written two books and numerous articles on human service computing and has been the principal investigator on grants to develop human service computing systems in the areas of child protective services, aging, mental health, and developmental disabilities. His Internet address is schoech@uta.edu

Warner V. Slack, M.D., completed his early work in computer-based medical interviewing at the University of Wisconsin. His efforts led to the development of the first computer-based medical history. Over the past twenty-five years he has done extensive research in the field of patient-computer dialogue. He has developed and studied programs that provide direct assistance to the patient in the management of common medical and psychological problems. He was an early advocate of the patient's right to participate in decisions about diagnosis and treatment.

During the past fifteen years, Slack and his colleagues at the Center for Clinical Computing (CCC), Harvard Medical School, have developed, implemented, and evaluated an integrated, hospitalwide clinical computing system (the CCC System), which is used in patient care at Boston's Beth Israel and Brigham and Women's hospitals. Pursuing his interest in the field of mental testing, he has also examined the use and misuse of the Scholastic Aptitude Test. The results of his studies, done in collaboration with Dr. Douglas Porter, have been influential in such reformative efforts as the "truth in testing" legislation passed in New York state. Slack is currently copresident of the Center for Clinical Computing, associate professor of medicine and psychiatry at Harvard Medical School, and editor-in-chief of *M.D. Computing.*

Katherine Kelley Smith, B.S.W., is a field consultant at the University of Texas at Arlington's School of Social Work. She operates Connect BBS, a human-service-oriented FidoNet bulletin board. She also develops data base applications for human service agencies. Her Internet address is ksmitty@uta.edu

Tom Trabin, Ph.D., M.Sc.M., serves as vice president for informatics and outcomes initiatives for CentraLink. In that capacity, he organizes and chairs national conferences and conventions on informatics and outcomes management for the behavioral healthcare industry, and also oversees those topic areas as associate editor of the *Behavioral Healthcare Tomorrow* journal. In addition, he consults with a wide range of organizations regarding behavioral healthcare issues and maintains a small clinical practice.

Trabin has significant executive experience in diverse behavioral healthcare settings. Formerly, he was director of managed care for U.S. Behavioral Health, a national managed care company, where his responsibilities included playing a central role in designing the company's case management information systems. He served in executive and strategic planning roles with Abbott Northwestern Hospital, a large not-for-profit hospital corporation. More recently, he was the organizing founder of Diablo Therapy Associates, a multidisciplinary clinical group practice. He also is active in governance of the California Psychological Association.

He is a licensed psychologist with a Ph.D. from the University of Minnesota. He also earned a master of science degree in management from the Sloan Program for Mid-Career Executives at Stanford Business School and was the recipient of a Bush Leadership Fellowship. He has authored several books and many journal articles for the behavioral healthcare field. His keynote presentations and workshops are well received at international, national, and regional conferences. He is well known for his work with behavioral healthcare policy, strategic planning, and operations issues, including how to meet the new challenges in information systems.

INDEX

Allina (community health information network), 178, 180

American Managed Behavioral Healthcare Association (AMBHA), 264, 266–267

American National Standards Institute (ANSI), data standardization, 222

Artifical intelligence, 16, 41

Ball, M. J., 3

Beck, A., 43–44, 48

Behavioral healthcare, industrialization of, 108–111

Behavioral healthcare computerization: and benefits management, 135–140; comparative cost analysis, 216–222; and cost management, 130–135; and managed outcome, 145–149. *See also* Community mental health centers; Computer-assisted therapy; Information systems; Managed behavioral healthcare computerization

Behavioral healthcare vendors, 177–184

Best practices: in county and community mental health centers, 143–144; and decision support technology, 35

Beth Israel Hospital, clinical computing system, 153–163

Bleich, H. L., 151

Brigham and Women's Hospital, clinical computing system, 153–163

Broskowski, Anthony, 11

Burlingame, G., 72

Bush, George, 95

Capitation management system, 112

Capitation-based financing: and electronic communications requirements, 215; versus fee-for-service, 126; in public healthcare, 125, 126, 132, 136–137

Case and claims managers, training for, 9

CASPER (Computerized Assessment System for Psychotherapy Evaluation and Research), 66–69

Center for Mental Health Services (CMHS), 256, 258, 259, 260, 263, 264, 265

Clarity Health Assessment System, 69

Client data system (CDS), 258

Clinical information systems, 152–163; access and confidentiality in, 160; clinicians' ancillary options, 158; computer use issues in, 163–167; computing systems in, 154; decision support options in, 158–160; financial computing in, 156; in laboratories and clinical departments, 155–156; patient lookup in, 157–158; registration programs, 155; utility programs, 160–161

Clinical/Management Information System (C/MIS), 69–70

ClinQuery, 159

CMHC. *See* Community mental health centers

Cognitive-behavioral programs, 43–44, 47–49

Colby, K., 40, 41

Community health information networks (CHINs), 178–180, 202

Community mental health centers (CMHCs), 124–149; access, quality, and cost information, 142–143; benefits management information access in, 139–140; best practice guidelines in, 143–144; and capacity expansions, 129; care coordination across service delivery network in, 141–142; client benefits status updates in, 137–138; clinical data collection in, 145–146; cost data versus billing rate data in, 130–131; cost variations and cost estimates in, 131–132; eligibility and benefits criteria in, 136–137; goal attainment scaling method in, 146, 147; and human resource development, 134–135; and multiple payer types, 132–133; outcome management system in, 147–149; outcome measurement approaches and instruments in, 146–147; planned versus used benefits patterns in, 138–139; service planning guidelines in, 137; standard guidelines for care planning in, 140; utilization management in, 140

COMPASS, 21, 22–24, 70–71

Composite International Diagnostic Instrument (CIDI), 261–262
COMPSYCH, 252
Computer phobia, 53, 95, 101–102, 164
Computer-assisted outcome measurement systems, 66, 67
Computer-assisted psychological measurement, 64–66
Computer-assisted therapy, 39–59; artificial intelligence approach, 41; cognitive-behavioral approach, 43–44, 47–49; as financial threat, 55–56; learning model approach, 42–43; in managed care setting, 55–56, 58–59; patient benefits, 59; professional benefits, 57–58; resistance to, 53–57; rigor and quality issues, 56; and sanctity of therapeutic relationship, 54–55; structured learning approach, 41–42. *See also* Therapeutic Learning Program (TLP)
Computer-based patient record (CPR), 3–4, 113–114; and data security, 117; and development of standards, 6; and health research, 118; human-machine interface in, 8; legal issues, 202–203; table-driven, 115, 119
Computerized clinical records, 14–15, 22–24, 27–28
Condit, G., 196–197
Confidentiality issues, 5, 191–210; absence of protection, 191–194; in clinical computing systems, 160; and employee training, 209; fair information practices codes, 197–198; health information trustee, 199; and the Internet, 226–227; legal requirements, 202–203; and managed care practices, 205; in payer-provider transmittals, 115–117; in payment disclosures, 198; privacy legislation, 196–200, 200–201; protected health information, 198; provider disclosure policies and procedures, 206–209; and secondary use of health records, 194–196; security measures, 203–205; in vendor and contractor agreements, 210
Continuous quality improvement, in virtual group, 122
County mental health centers. *See* Community mental health centers
Credentialing process, standardization of, 119
Currie, P. S., 108
Cyberspace: defined, 229; virtual group practices, 121–122. *See also* Internet; Networks/networking

Data security. *See* Confidentiality issues
Data standards. *See* Standardization
Decision support systems, 12–36; aid in DSM-IV diagnoses, 35; and alternative medicine, 80; and best practices, 35; for consumer use, 79–80; cost and benefits considerations, 33; and critical clinical pathways, 21; data collection and assessment systems, 19; decision-tree system (DTREE), 15–16; disease management protocols, 22; expert systems, 16–17, 28–30, 119; functions and characteristics, 13–14; and lack of standardization in clinical data, 34; legal liability concerns, 36; mathematical/algorithmic models, 15, 24–25; model base component, 14, 32; neural networks, 17–18; scenario-based, 74–78; screening and diagnosis systems, 19; selection criteria, 32–33; structural components, 14; structured computerized clinical records, 14–15, 22–24, 27–28; and treatment planning decisions, 20; triage or level-of-treatment decision systems, 19–20; use issues for, 35–36
Decision-tree system (DTREE), 15–16
Dilemma Counseling System, 42
Disease management protocols, 22
Distributed computer systems, 12
Douglas, J. V., 3

Electronic communications: comparative cost analysis, 216–222; cost-benefits to providers, 223–225; electronic commerce (EC), 223; electronic data interchange (EDI), 222–223; fax transmissions, 224; futuristic developments, 226–227; and outcome measures, 214–215; and provider capitation, 215; work-flow gains, 225–226
Employee assistance programs (EAPs), 177–178
ERISA (Early Retirement Insurance Security Act), 175
Expert decision support systems, 16–17, 28–30, 34, 114

Frawley, K. A., 191

Gellman, R., 191
Gingerich, Wallace J., 11
Gould, R. L., 39
Group Health Association of America (GHAA), 266–267
Group practice computerization, stages of, 111–115
Group thought function, 79

Hanna, T., 251
Harris County (Texas) Mental Health/ Mental Retardation Authority, 127–128, 131, 132, 133, 134, 135, 137, 138, 141, 142, 144, 146

Health Maintenance organizations (HMOs), 175, 176, 178–180
Healthcare information infrastructure, 4–5; and need for standards, 6
Healthcare networks. *See* Networks/ networking
Henderson, M. J., 254
Hill, E. D., III, 172
Hospital-based delivery systems. *See* Clinical information systems
Hurst, M. W., 213

IBM, Shared Hospital Accounting System (SHAS), 173–174
Information systems: capitation management systems, 112; client-server systems, 187–188; and data interchange security, 115–117; front- and back-office functions, 112–113; as group practice infrastructure, 110; incorporation of expert systems in, 114–115; legacy systems, 112, 187; reporting systems, 12; and standardization of data, 118–119. *See also* Clinical information systems; Practice management systems
Information technology, 3–10; in clinical functions, 113–146; in healthcare information infrastructure, 4–5; history of, 11–13; interface compatibility in interchange systems, 117–118; in managed behavioral healthcare, 7; and provider group-payer direct connections, 115–118; software infrastructure developments, 186–188. *See also* Computer-based patient record (CPR); Technological implementation
Institute of Medicine, Committee to Improve the Patient Record, 3
Integrated healthcare systems, 109–110, 178–180
Internet, 231–232; behavioral healthcare conferences, 237–239; confidentiality issues, 226–227; resources for not-for-profits, 252; World Wide Web (WWW), 226, 234, 240–241
InterPsych, 252

Jacobson, N., 65

Kessler, R., 261
Kiresuk, T., 147
Kramer, M., 256

L'abata, L., 41
Lambert, M., 72
Legacy system, 112
Level-of-care treatment, 8, 9–10; decision systems, 19–20

Maloney, W. R., 172

Managed behavioral healthcare computerization, 172–188; and cost containment, 55–56, 176–177; in county and community mental health centers, 140–145; current systems, history of, 172–177; hospital and provider systems, 173–174; and partnering with organized provider groups, 109–111; professional benefits of, 57–58; and provider network management, 7; resistance to, 55–56; therapy programs, 55–56, 58–59. *See also* Information technology

Managed care: and confidentiality laws, 205; increasing use of, 213; report cards, 264, 266; and standardization, 260

Manderscheid, R. W., 254

Marks, I., 43

Medicaid: cost determination and auditing process, 131; fee-for-service billing and reimbursement, 128; revenue goals, 132

Mental Health Consumer/Survivor Research and Policy Work Group, 260–261

Mental Health Statistics Improvement Program (MHSIP), 256–258, 262, 263, 267

Minnesota Multiphasic Personality Inventory (MMPI), 53, 64

Moreland, K. L., 63

MYCIN, 16

Naditch, M. P., 63

National Alliance for the Mentally Ill (NAMI), 263

National Institute of Mental Health (NIMH), data standardization, 255–258

Networks/networking, 228–251; activities and features, 232–233; behavioral healthcare conferences, 236; bulletin board systems, 229–230; client impact, 249; commercial/specialty networks, 230–231; E-mail, 232; electronic communication characteristics in, 244–248; futuristic developments, 249–251; hardware/software considerations, 245–247; impact on healthcare practice, 249; multi-agency use, 247–248; software tools, 233–235; user-friendly interfaces in, 6; work and pleasure uses, 235–244

Neural networks, 17–18, 34

Nguyen, T. D., 124

Olsen, G., 124

Organizational development (OD) consulting field, 9

Outcome information: computerization of, 145–149; marketing purposes of, 118; technology in, 8

Outcome measurement; computer-assisted systems, 66, 67; and electronic communications, 214–215

Outcome Questionnaire 45.1 (OQ-45.1), 71–72

PaperChase, 159

Pathware, 28–30

Patient-therapist assignment decisions, 20–21

Performance-based contracting, 109

Practice management systems, 178–179; cost/benefits, 119–121; selection of basic system, 119–121; as virtual group, 121–122

Problem Knowledge Couplers, 19, 30–31

Provider network management, 7–10

Provider profiles, 8–9, 23

PsychAccess system, 19, 27–28

PsychPro, 20, 24–25

Public healthcare: benefit packaging in, 136; capitation-based financing in, 125, 126, 132, 136–137; data system development federal guidelines, 128–129; high operational overhead, 125; need for information system redesign, 125–126; principal managed care capabilities, 125–126; privatization of, 125–126. *See also* Community mental health centers; Medicaid

QualityFIRST Behavioral Health Guidelines, 21, 25–27

RES Q (Reliable Electronic Survey Questionnaire), 72

Roiter, W. A., 213

Rosen, L. D., 87

Safran, C., 151, 152

Schoech, R., 228

Scientific knowledge development, 76–81

Security issues. *See* Confidentiality issues

Self-help programs, computer-based, 49

Selmi, P. M., 43

Shared Medical Systems (SMS), 174

Slack, W. V., 151, 152

Smith, K. K., 228

Standardization, 254–268; and client data system (CDS), 258; in community mental health center guidelines, 140; and consumer input, 260–261; and data standards content, 261–264; in decision support technology, 34; in electronic communications, 222–223; enrollment and encounter data, 262–263; and innovation, 118–119; and managed care, 260; MHSIP data standards, 256–258; and NIMH grants, 258; and outcome data, 263; by partnerships and joint ventures, 265–267; recording standards, 264–265; report cards for managed care, 264, 266; transmission standards, 265

Strategic Advantage, Inc. (SAI), 72, 73, 75

Strupp, H., 65

Technological implementation: attitudes and behaviors toward, 88–94; and computer phobia, 53, 95, 101–102, 164; learning process in, 105; needs assessment, 99–101; and organizational philosophy, 94–96; and organizational planning, 96–97; and pretesting, 103; staff feedback in, 105; staff involvement in technological choices, 102–103; and staff motivation and skills, 97, 101–102; systemwide support in, 99–105; and training, 97–98, 103–105; and vendor support, 103. *See also* Information technology

Teleconsults, 5

Telemedicine, 5

Telephonic triage, 9

Therapeutic Learning Program (TLP), 42–43, 45–47; design elements, 50–51; outcome studies, 52–53; problems-in-living approach, 50–52

Third-party administrator (TPA), 175, 176

Transaction processing systems, 12

Treatment progress measurement, 23

Triage, and decision support systems, 19–20

Utilization review firm, 175, 176, 177

Valley Mental Health, Salt Lake City, Utah, 127, 128, 131, 133, 134, 135, 136, 137, 138, 139, 142, 143, 146–147

Virtual communities, 250–251

Virtual group practices, 121–122

Wagman, M., 42

Weed, L., 30

Weil, M. W., 87

Weizenbaum, J., 40–41

Westin, A., 196

Workgroup for Electronic Data Interchange (WEDI), 201

World Health Organization (WHO), 256, 266

Wright, J., 432